Hiro Yoshida, Ashlesha Jain, Ajita Ichalkaranje, Lakhmi C. Jain,
Nikhil Ichalkaranje (Eds.)

Advanced Computational Intelligence Paradigms in Healthcare – 1

Studies in Computational Intelligence, Volume 48

Editor-in-chief
Prof. Janusz Kacprzyk
Systems Research Institute
Polish Academy of Sciences
ul. Newelska 6
01-447 Warsaw
Poland
E-mail: kacprzyk@ibspan.waw.pl

Further volumes of this series
can be found on our homepage:
springer.com

Vol. 30. Yukio Ohsawa, Shusaku Tsumoto (Eds.)
Chance Discoveries in Real World Decision Making, 2006
ISBN 978-3-540-34352-3

Vol. 31. Ajith Abraham, Crina Grosan, Vitorino Ramos (Eds.)
Stigmergic Optimization, 2006
ISBN 978-3-540-34689-0

Vol. 32. Akira Hirose
Complex-Valued Neural Networks, 2006
ISBN 978-3-540-33456-9

Vol. 33. Martin Pelikan, Kumara Sastry, Erick Cantú-Paz (Eds.)
Scalable Optimization via Probabilistic Modeling, 2006
ISBN 978-3-540-34953-2

Vol. 34. Ajith Abraham, Crina Grosan, Vitorino Ramos (Eds.)
Swarm Intelligence in Data Mining, 2006
ISBN 978-3-540-34955-6

Vol. 35. Ke Chen, Lipo Wang (Eds.)
Trends in Neural Computation, 2007
ISBN 978-3-540-36121-3

Vol. 36. Ildar Batyrshin, Janusz Kacprzyk, Leonid Sheremetor, Lotfi A. Zadeh (Eds.)
Preception-based Data Mining and Decision Making in Economics and Finance, 2006
ISBN 978-3-540-36244-9

Vol. 37. Jie Lu, Da Ruan, Guangquan Zhang (Eds.)
E-Service Intelligence, 2007
ISBN 978-3-540-37015-4

Vol. 38. Art Lew, Holger Mauch
Dynamic Programming, 2007
ISBN 978-3-540-37013-0

Vol. 39. Gregory Levitin (Ed.)
Computational Intelligence in Reliability Engineering, 2007
ISBN 978-3-540-37367-4

Vol. 40. Gregory Levitin (Ed.)
Computational Intelligence in Reliability Engineering, 2007
ISBN 978-3-540-37371-1

Vol. 41. Mukesh Khare, S.M. Shiva Nagendra (Eds.)
Artificial Neural Networks in Vehicular Pollution Modelling, 2007
ISBN 978-3-540-37417-6

Vol. 42. Bernd J. Krämer, Wolfgang A. Halang (Eds.)
Contributions to Ubiquitous Computing, 2007
ISBN 978-3-540-44909-6

Vol. 43. Fabrice Guillet, Howard J. Hamilton (Eds.)
Quality Measures in Data Mining, 2007
ISBN 978-3-540-44911-9

Vol. 44. Nadia Nedjah, Luiza de Macedo Mourelle, Mario Neto Borges, Nival Nunes de Almeida (Eds.)
Intelligent Educational Machines, 2007
ISBN 978-3-540-44920-1

Vol. 45. Vladimir G. Ivancevic, Tijana T. Ivancevic
Neuro-Fuzzy Associative Machinery for Comprehensive Brain and Cognition Modelling, 2007
ISBN 978-3-540-47463-0

Vol. 46. Valentina Zharkova, Lakhmi C. Jain (Eds.)
Artificial Intelligence in Recognition and Classification of Astrophysical and Medical Images, 2007
ISBN 978-3-540-47511-8

Vol. 47. S. Sumathi, S. Esakkirajan
Fundamentals of Relational Database Management Systems, 2007
ISBN 978-3-540-48397-7

Vol. 48. Hiro Yoshida, Ashlesha Jain, Ajita Ichalkaranje, Lakhmi C. Jain, Nikhil Ichalkaranje (Eds.)
Advanced Computational Intelligence Paradigms in Healthcare – 1, 2007
ISBN 978-3-540-47523-1

Hiro Yoshida
Ashlesha Jain
Ajita Ichalkaranje
Lakhmi C. Jain
Nikhil Ichalkaranje (Eds.)

Advanced Computational Intelligence Paradigms in Healthcare – 1

With 148 Figures and 15 Tables

Springer

Prof. Hiro Yoshida
Massachusetts General Hospital
Department of Radiology
Harvard University
Blossom Court 75
02114 Boston
USA

Dr. Ashlesha Jain
The Queen Elizabeth Hospital
Woodville Road
5011 Woodville
Australia

Ajita Ichalkaranje
Independant Living Centre
Blacks Road 11
5095 Adelaide
Australia

Prof. Lakhmi C. Jain
Knowledge-Based Intelligent
Engineering Systems Centre
School of Electrical
and Information Engineering
University of South Australia
Mawson Lakes Campus
South Australia, SA 5095
Australia
E-mail: Lakhmi.jain@unisa.edu.au

Dr. Nikhil Ichalkaranje
Senior Technology Advisor
Department of Communications,
IT and the Arts
Canberra, ACT 2601
Australia

ISSN print edition: 1860-949X
ISSN electronic edition: 1860-9503

ISBN 978-3-642-08001-2 e-ISBN 978-3-540-47527-9

Springer is a part of Springer Science+Business Media
springer.com

Softcover reprint of the hardcover 1st edition 2007

Cover design: deblik, Berlin

Preface

There is an ever increasing thrust to automate a range of activities in every discipline including healthcare, engineering, science, business and management. Computational intelligence paradigms have offered some advantages in automating and creating the human-like capability in healthcare sector. The primary goal of this book is to present some of the most recent research results of the applications of computational intelligence in healthcare. This book consists of ten chapters.

Chapter 1 by Sordo et al. present an Order Set Schema developed by the Clinical Knowledge Management and Decision Support Group at Partners HealthCare and the Decision Systems Group at Harvard Medical School. It provides a brief introduction to key issues involved in its implementation. The Order Set Schema is the result of a broader enterprise-wide knowledge management effort to identify and leverage current clinical knowledge across Partners institutions. The chapter includes a brief introduction to knowledge representation and management including ontologies. It includes description of the clinical content identified and presents a summary of accomplishments.

Chapter 2 by Sordo et al. is on a state-based model for management of type II diabetes. This model encompasses strategies for prevention, early diagnosis, and treatment of type II diabetes and associated complications. This effort is part of an on-going, enterprise-wide strategy to improve the quality, safety and efficiency of provided care, by maximizing the use of new clinical information technology in key issues such as complex clinical workflows, usability, controlled terminology, knowledge management and clinical decision support carried out by Partners HealthCare System. The proposed model is a disease state management system for the continuum of diabetes care that synergistically integrates patient care and education protocols at all levels of disease management, and supports the integration of evidence-based personalized care. This approach could be easily adapted to managing other chronic conditions e.g. hypertension, asthma, and coronary artery disease.

Chapter 3 by Schmidt is on case-based reasoning in medicine especially an obituary on Lothar Gierl. The research work undertaken by Gierl on

Base-Based Reasoning in Medicine (CBR-M) is discussed. A good review of the research work undertaken in the area of CBR-M is also presented. A number of case studies are included in the chapter.

Chapter 4 by Montani et al. is on assessing the quality of care in artificial intelligence environment for end stage renal failure patients. End Stage Renal Disease (ESRD) is a severe chronic condition that corresponds to the final stage of kidney failure. Hemodialysis (HD) is the widely used treatment for ESRD. This paper reports the progress made in the development of an auditing system for assessing the performance of HD centres. The authors have demonstrated that their approach is suitable for knowledge discovery and critical patterns similarity assessment on real patients' data.

Chapter 5 by Cerrito is on mining the electronic medical record to examine physician decisions. When there is a lack of accountability, there is variability in practice. Physicians typically are not held accountable for their costs in a hospital environment, nor are their patient outcomes compared to those of other physicians, with the exception of mortality rates. Therefore, there is little information available on how to examine variability in practice. With the availability of the electronic medical record, it is now possible to investigate how the variability in physician decision making impacts patient outcomes and hospital costs. This chapter examines the medical record in a hospital emergency department. Medications, charges, length of stay, and patient disposition will be analyzed using data mining techniques, including text analysis. Data were collected on approximately 14,000 patients over a six month period from a hospital emergency department. The electronic medical record (EMR) was used for all orders and charges while the patient was in the emergency department. However, medications were recorded on a separate pharmacy database that was merged into the EMR. The objective was to find ways to decrease costs while improving the quality of patient care. Payment to the hospital from Medicare, Medicaid, and private insurers is based upon an assignment of Level 1 to Level 6 care, with Level 6 generating the highest payment. Level is assignment based upon a series of points. Each item of care generates a specific number of points. However, the point-system is self-generated by the hospital, and the points assigned a particular item can vary from one hospital to another. Emergency Department care is expensive, and the longer a patient remains in the ED, the higher the cost of that care. Therefore, variability in the length of stay and reasons for that variability are also of concern.

Three fields in the data are of concern as well: charges, medications, and diagnosis. Each of the three fields has thousands of potential levels. In addition, physicians are free to insert their own information in non-standardized language. While it is possible to analyze each different diagnosis separately, the number of different diagnoses is so large that there are very few patients to be considered. Text analysis was used to reduce the number of levels, using the fact that similar words and phrases indicate similar medical issues. Then association rules were used to examine differences in physician orders for similar medical diagnoses. Once the categorical levels are reduced to manageable levels, kernel density estimation is used to investigate the relationship of levels to outcomes, in addition to predictive modelling. Once completed, the analysis showed that some physicians routinely treat patients with similar diagnoses at a higher cost compared to other physicians. Some nursing costs are routinely added as patient charges by some RNs compared to others within the same hospital setting.

This chapter demonstrates each of the techniques in the context of analyzing the EMR from the hospital emergency department. It will show that it is possible to make physicians and hospitals more accountable for their actual treatment of patients, and for the costs incurred.

Chapter 6 by Hill is on capturing and specifying multi-agent systems for the management of community healthcare. The deployment of multi-agent systems remains immature and many agent healthcare applications are developed ad hoc, with little reference to design methodologies or compliance with rigorous design requirements. It is therefore necessary to be able to model and specify, at an acceptable level of abstraction, the required characteristics of an agent-based solution to the management of community healthcare. The required characteristics should reflect the real-world view, and it follows that such specifications should also mirror the requirements of the target domain environment.

As each element of community healthcare is often delivered by independent agencies, the number of autonomous command and control systems is often considerably large, leaving the overall managers of the care (the UK Local Authority) to protect the individual bodies from disclosing sensitive and irrelevant information. Although information technology is established in community care management, it is clear that in many instances the vast quantities of disparate heterogeneous information repositories can lead to the undermining of effective system operations. Thus, using collaborative intelligent agents that overcome the difficulties of integrating disparate hardware and software platforms, queries can be mediated to the most appropriate information source. Accordingly, agent technologies have the potential to build effective co-ordinated healthcare management systems. Groups of agents such as private care providers, routine care services, nursing and medical staff, local authority manager, private care manager, and health trust agents, need to undertake considerable autonomy in order to manage the horde of messages exchanged within the community.

Contractual agreements with community healthcare agencies create a complex economic environment that must be described in a robust way if agent managed services are to be accepted commercially. Typically auction models are utilised by agent applications as they are widely understood, established, and cheap to implement, but they are too simple to capture the nuances of community care payment transactions. The author considers the 'Event Accounting' model in relation to the myriad of payment transactions within the community care environment, and proposes a robust transaction based framework for the deployment of agent-managed community care systems, to address the gulf between abstract concept and low-level, undisciplined agent system implementation.

Chapter 7 by Cortés et al. is on assistive wheelchair navigation. The world elderly population is currently increasing in a steady way, and, hence, the costs of health care are also increasing dramatically. Consequently, significant effort is being focused on technology to help individuals to remain independent in their preferred environment. Specifically, a key issue in assistance to achieve autonomy is mobility, as mobility impairment has proven to cause a downward trend in quality of life.

Mobility can be provided by different devices, ranging from walkers to traditional wheelchairs. There are several important issues to design a control system for such devices, namely the user interface, the sensory-motor hardware, and the control algorithms required to produce an output. Regarding interfaces, most works focus on user modelling. Naturally, the interface must be easy to use and accepted by the user and diverse types of interaction suited to users with different capabilities, needs and preferences. This personalization is usually achieved through activity, cognitive and affective profiles. A fundamental feature of adaptation that must be considered is the degree of autonomy that the interface provides, to check who is ultimately in control. Even though very different approaches exist as joysticks, touch screens and voice interfaces are the most common choices. The sensory motor hardware is mostly subjected to safety and health regulations and, hence, the usual choice is to employ commercial homologated wheelchairs equipped with *safe* sensors. Even though sonar has been widely used for autonomous navigation, wheelchair assisted navigation requires more precision and may rely on laser sensors instead. If localization is required, GPS may be used outdoors, whereas active beacons are feasible indoors. In most cases, wheel encoders with different precisions are used as well. The wheelchair control algorithms range from reactive to deliberative control. Reactive control maps input patterns to outputs in a straight way and it is mostly used in the field to implement emergency responses, removing control from the user only when immediate danger is detected. Deliberative control follows the sense-plan-act (SPA) paradigm and it is used to take more complex decisions like *how to reach a goal* given a location and a model of the working environment. In this case, the wheelchair is mostly controlled by the system and the user only provides high level guidelines. Hybrid solutions where control is given sometimes to the system and sometimes to the user are also feasible, but require some ranking on the user's performance or the situation at hand.

Whereas user interfaces are highly dependent on the user condition and sensory-motor hardware mostly depends on the system environment, the same control algorithms can be applied to a wide range of problems. Hence, much research has been done to this respect. It must be noted, though, that most work in the area has focused either on emergency mechanisms, curvature integration to remove shaky motion or autonomous control whenever the user can not drive the wheelchair himself/herself.

This chapter reviews current approaches to assisted wheelchair navigation control. Its main contribution is real experimental evaluation of the performance of different users presenting different pathologies depending on *how much* control they exert over their wheelchair. Results are correlated with users' pathologies to extract conclusions about the benefits of assistive navigation and how existing approaches could be improved through adaptation. It is expected that adaptive shared control would avoid loss of residual capabilities and also provide a better sense of self control to the user.

Chapter 8 by Kaiser and Miksch is on modelling treatment processes using information extraction. Clinical Practice Guidelines (CPGs) are important means to improve the quality of care by supporting medical staff. Modeling CPGs in a computer interpretable form is a prerequisite for various computer applications to support their application. However, transforming guidelines in a formal guideline representation is a difficult task. Existing methods and tools demand detailed medical knowledge, knowledge about the formal representations, and a manual modelling. In this chapter the authors have introduced methods and tools for formalizing CPGs and have proposed a methodology to reduce the human effort needed in the translation from original textual guidelines to formalized processable knowledge bases. The idea of this methodology is to use Information Extraction methods to help in the semi-automation of guideline content formalization of treatment processes. Thereby, the human modeller will be supported by both automating parts of the modelling process and making the modelling process traceable and comprehensible. The methodology, called LASSIE, represents a novel method applying a stepwise procedure. The general idea is to use this method to formalize guidelines in any guideline representation language by applying both general steps (i.e., language independent) and language-specific steps. In order to evaluate both the methodology and the Information Extraction system, a framework was implemented and applied to several guidelines from the medical subject of otolaryngology.

Chapter 9 by Brahnam et al. is on neonatal pain detection using face classification techniques. Detecting pain in neonates is a difficult problem for health care professionals yet it is very crucial since pain is a major indicator of medical conditions and untreated pain in infants results in central nervous system changes that slow development and impede child-parent bonding. This chapter presents the Infant COPE (Classification of Pain Expressions) project and the groups' research work using face classification to detect pain in a neonate's facial displays.

Aside from discussing the neonatal pain detection problem, this chapter provides a tutorial on state-of-the-art face classification techniques that is suitable for those unfamiliar with the subject. The chapter also notes other medical problems that could benefit from the application of face recognition technology.

Chapter 10 by Simo and Cavazza is on medical education interfaces through virtual patients. Virtual Patients have been used widely in simulation and medical education related to the fusion of AI Theory and Applications with knowledge in the medical field.

The authors have successfully built a system where virtual humans (virtual patients) are used for training applications in the field of cardiac emergencies. Different versions of the system integrate AI techniques for simulating medical conditions (cardiac shock states) with a realistic visual simulation of the patient in a 3D environment representing an ER room. It uses qualitative simulation of the cardio-vascular system to generate clinical syndromes and simulate the consequences of the trainee's therapeutic interventions. The use of knowledge-based simulation provides a strong basis to integrate the behavioural aspects with the graphical appearance of the patient in the virtual ER. This also supports the creation of an emotional atmosphere increasing the realism of this training.

We are grateful to the authors and the reviewers for their vision and wonderful contribution. We are indebted to Berend Jan van der Zwaag and Nandini Loganathan for their excellent help in the preparation of the camera ready copy.

Editors

Contents

Partners Healthcare Order Set Schema: An Information Model for Management of Clinical Content
Margarita Sordo, Tonya Hongsermeier, Vipul Kashyap, and Robert A. Greenes 1
1 Introduction 1
2 Knowledge Representation and Management at Partners Healthcare 2
2.1 Knowledge Management 4
2.2 Knowledge Representation 4
3 Clinical Content 6
4 Information Model and the UML 7
4.1 Information Model 7
4.2 UML 8
4.3 UML Diagrams and XML Schemas 9
5 HL7 V3 Reference Information Model 10
6 Order Set Schema (OS Schema) 13
6.1 Header Category 15
6.2 AuditData Category 15
6.3 IndicationCriteria Category 16
6.4 ClinicalSettingData Category 18
6.5 IntentionActionInteraction Category 19
6.6 TargetSpecifics Category 20
6.7 PatientData Category 20
6.8 KnowledgeRules Category 21
6.9 NotesInstructions Category 22
6.10 OrderGroup Category 22
7 Conclusions 23
References 23

A State-Based Model for Management of Type II Diabetes
Margarita Sordo, Tonya Hongsermeier, Vipul Kashyap, and Robert A. Greenes 27
1 Introduction 27
2 Diabetes Mellitus 28
3 Diabetes Management 29
3.1 Initial Diagnosis 29
3.2 Regular and Targeted Screening for Low-Risk and High-Risk Populations 30
3.3 Preventive Care 30
3.3.1 Blood Pressure Management 30
3.3.2 Lipid Management 31
3.3.3 Antiplatelet Agents 31
3.3.4 Smoking Cessation 31
3.3.5 Coronary Heart Disease 32
3.3.6 Immunization 32
3.4 Long-Term Management 33
3.5 Management and Follow-up 33
3.5.1 Diet 33
3.5.2 Physical Activity 34
3.5.3 Self Blood Glucose Monitoring 34
3.5.4 Hyperglycemia 34
3.5.5 Blood Pressure Management 34
3.5.6 Lipids Management 35
3.6 Surveillance 35
3.6.1 Nephropathy 35
3.6.2 Eye Exam 35
3.6.3 Foot Care 36
3.6.4 Antiplatelet Agents – Aspirin 36
3.6.5 Blood Pressure Management 36
3.6.6 Immunization 36
3.7 Intercurrent Illnesses 36
4 UML 2 State Machine Diagrams 37
4.1 State Diagrams 37
4.2 UML Statecharts 38
5 State Model for Management of Type II Diabetes 40
5.1 State Model – First-Level and Second-Level States 40
5.1.1 Diabetes Preventive Care 42
5.1.2 Diabetes Long-Term Management 43
5.2 Preventive Care Substates 44
5.2.1 BP State 44
5.2.2 Lipid Management 45
5.2.3 Antiplatelet Agents – Aspirin 48
5.2.4 Smoking 49

5.2.5 Coronary Heart Disease (CHD) 50
5.2.6 Immunization 51
5.3 Management Substates 51
5.3.1 Self Blood Glucose Monitoring 51
5.3.2 Diet 51
5.3.3 Physical Activity 51
5.3.4 Hyperglycemia 52
5.3.5 BP Management 55
5.3.6 Lipid Management 55
5.4 Surveillance Substates 55
5.4.1 Nephropathy (UP) 55
5.4.2 Eye Exam 55
5.4.3 Foot care 56
5.4.4 Antiplatelets – Aspirin 57
5.4.5 BP management 57
5.4.6 Immunization 57
5.5 Intercurrent Illnesses Substates 57
6 Summary 58
References 58

Case-Based Reasoning in Medicine Especially an Obituary on Lothar Gierl
Rainer Schmidt 63
1 Introduction 63
2 Obituary on Lothar Gierl 64
2.1 Diagnosis of Dysmorphic Syndromes 64
2.2 The ICONS Project 66
2.2.1 Antibiotic Therapy Advice 66
2.2.2 Time Course Prognoses of the Kidney Function 69
2.3 Influenza Forecast 73
2.3.1 Prognostic Model for Influenza 74
2.4 General Model for Time Course Prognosis 75
3 Case-Based Reasoning in Medicine 77
3.1 Three CBR in Medicine Researchers 78
3.2 Further Medical CBR Applications 79
3.2.1 Diagnostic Systems 79
3.2.2 Therapeutic and Other Support Systems 81
3.3 Medical Image Interpretation 81
4 Conclusion 82
References 82

Assessing the Quality of Care for End Stage Renal Failure Patients by Means of Artificial Intelligence Methodologies
Stefania Montani, Luigi Portinale, Riccardo Bellazzi, Cristiana Larizza, and Roberto Bellazzi 89
1 Introduction 89
2 Hemodialysis Treatment for ESRD 91
3 Data Mining for ESRD 93
4 Case-Based Retrieval for ESRD 98
5 Results 104
5.1 Testing the Data Mining Facility 104
5.2 Testing the Case-Based Retrieval System 105
6 Conclusions 109
References 111

Mining the Electronic Medical Record to Examine Physician Decisions
Patricia B. Cerrito 113
1 Introduction 113
2 Method 114
2.1 Market Basket Analysis 115
2.2 Text Analysis 115
2.3 Data Collection 116
3 Results 116
3.1 Examination of Cost Factors 118
3.2 Examination of Treatment Combinations 120
3.3 Examination of Antibiotic Use 122
4 Discussion 125
References 125

Capturing and Specifying Multiagent Systems for the Management of Community Healthcare
Richard Hill 127
1 Introduction 127
2 Developing an Agent-Based Approach 128
2.1 Event Accounting 129
2.2 Modelling Systems 130
2.3 Designing Community Care Systems 130
2.4 Representing Transactions 132
2.5 Verifying the Care Model 133
2.6 Logic and Inferencing 134
2.7 A Transaction Architecture 138
3 Agent Interoperability 139
3.1 Syntactic Interoperability 140
3.2 Semantic Interoperability 140
3.3 Communicating Intentions 142

4 Building the Model with TrAM 144
4.1 Capturing Care Scenarios and Early Requirements 144
4.1.1 Maintaining the Individual Care Plan (ICP) 144
4.1.2 Improving Quality of Life 145
4.1.3 Providing Daily Care 145
4.1.4 Emergency Support 147
4.1.5 Quality Assurance 147
4.2 Identify Agents 148
4.3 Allocate Tasks to Agents 149
4.4 Identify Collaborations 150
4.5 Apply Transaction Model 151
4.5.1 Model Concepts 152
4.5.2 Inference Model with Queries and Validate 155
5 Conclusions 159
References 161

Assistive Wheelchair Navigation: A Cognitive View
U. Cortés, C. Urdiales, R. Annicchiarico, C. Barrué, A.B. Martinez, and C. Caltagirone 165
1 Introduction 165
2 Age-Related Disability: A Clinical View 167
2.1 Disability Evaluation 167
2.2 Autonomy and Disability 168
3 Autonomous Assistive Devices 169
3.1 Sensory Hardware and User Interfaces 170
3.2 System Architectures and Shared Control 172
4 Agent-Based Personalized Assistance 176
4.1 Agents in Medicine 177
4.2 Autonomy and Agents 177
4.3 Shared Autonomy 179
5 Case Study 180
6 Conclusions 182
References 183

Modeling Treatment Processes Using Information Extraction
Katharina Kaiser and Silvia Miksch 189
1 Introduction 189
2 Modeling Computer-Interpretable Clinical Practice Guidelines 190
2.1 Markup-Based Tools 191
2.1.1 Stepper 191
2.1.2 GEM Cutter 192
2.1.3 Document Exploration and Linking Tool/Addons (DELT/A) 193
2.1.4 Uruz/Degel – Digital Electronic Guideline Library 194

2.2 Graphical Tools 195
2.2.1 AsbruView 195
2.2.2 Protégé 196
2.2.3 Arezzo 196
2.2.4 Tallis 197
2.3 Multistep Methodologies 198
2.3.1 SAGE – The Standards-Based Shareable Active Guideline Environment 199
2.3.2 MHB – A Many-Headed Bridge between Guideline Formats 200
3 LASSIE: Semiautomatic Modeling Using Information Extraction 201
3.1 Our Approach 202
3.2 The Methodology 203
3.2.1 Developing Extraction Rules 204
3.2.2 Gaining Process Information 206
3.2.3 Modeling Plans in *Asbru* 213
3.3 Results 219
4 Conclusion 220
References 221

Introduction to Neonatal Facial Pain Detection Using Common and Advanced Face Classification Techniques
Sheryl Brahnam, Loris Nanni, and Randall Sexton 225
1 Introduction 225
2 Holistic Face Classification 228
2.1 Discrete Cosine Transform 231
2.2 Sequential Forward Selection and Sequential Forward Floating Selection 232
2.3 Principal Component Analysis 232
2.3.1 PCA Classification 233
2.3.2 PCA Data Compression 235
2.3.3 Outline of PCA Face Classification 235
2.4 Linear Discriminant Analysis 235
2.5 Support Vector Machines 236
2.5.1 Outline of SVM 236
2.6 Neural Network Simultaneous Optimization Algorithm 237
2.6.1 Outline of NNSOA 238
2.7 Face Recognition Software Tools 239
3 Infant COPE Database and Study Design 240
3.1 Subjects 240
3.2 Apparatus 241
3.3 Procedure 241
3.4 Expression Categories 241

4 Method ... 243
4.1 Classification Classes ... 243
4.2 Evaluation Protocols ... 243
4.3 Outline of Experimental Procedures ... 244
5 Experiments ... 244
5.1 Experimental Results Using Protocol A ... 245
5.2 Experimental Results Using Protocol B ... 247
5.3 Current Work ... 248
6 The Future ... 249
References ... 249

Medical Education Interfaces Through Virtual Patients Based on Qualitative Simulation
Altion Simo and Marc Cavazza ... 255
1 Introduction ... 255
2 Relation to Previous Work and Motivation ... 257
3 System Overview and Architecture ... 259
4 Qualitative Simulation of the Cardiovascular System ... 263
4.1 Qualitative Processes in the Circulatory System Physiology ... 266
5 Graphics and Animations: The Interface ... 273
5.1 Mapping Simulation Parameters into Animations ... 273
5.2 Emotional Aspects of the Interface ... 276
5.3 Visualization Requirements for the Virtual Patient ... 277
6 Integrated Example ... 278
6.1 Initial Conditions and Simulation ... 278
6.2 Choice of Therapeutics and Further Simulation ... 279
7 Toward full Virtual Patients: Development and Integration Strategy ... 282
8 Conclusions and Discussions ... 284
References ... 288

List of Contributors

R. Annicchiarico
Fondazione IRCCS Santa Lucia
Rome, Italy

C. Barrué
Technical University of Catalonia
Barcelona, Spain

Riccardo Bellazzi
Dipartimento di Informatica
e Sistemistica
Università di Pavia
Italy

Roberto Bellazzi
Unità Operativa di
Nefrologia e Dialisi
S.O Vigevano, A.O. Pavia
Italy
ric@aim.unipv.it

Sheryl Brahnam
Computer Information Systems
Missouri State University
901 S. National
Springfield, MO 65804
USA
sbrahnam@missouristate.edu

C. Caltagirone
Fondazione IRCCS Santa Lucia
Rome, Italy

Marc Cavazza
School of Computing
and Mathematics
University of Teesside
Teesside, Middlesbrough TS1 3BA
UK
m.o.cavazza@tees.ac.uk

Patricia B. Cerrito
University of Louisville
Department of Mathematics
Louisville, KY 40292
USA

U. Cortés
Technical University of Catalonia
Barcelona, Spain

Robert A. Greenes
Decision Systems Group
Brigham & Women's Hospital
Harvard Medical School
Boston, MA, USA
greenes@harvard.edu
http://www.dsg.harvard.edu

Richard Hill
Sheffield Hallam University
Sheffield S1 1WB, UK
r.hill@shu.ac.uk

Tonya Hongsermeier
Clinical Knowledge Management Group
Partners Healthcare Systems, Inc
Wellesley, MA, USA
thongsermeier@partners.org

Katharina Kaiser
Vienna University of Technology
Institute of Software Technology & Interactive Systems
Vienna, Austria
kaiser@ifs.tuwien.ac.at
http://www.ifs.tuwien.ac.at

Vipul Kashyap
Clinical Knowledge Management Group
Partners Healthcare Systems, Inc
Wellesley, MA, USA
vkashyap1@partners.org

Cristiana Larizza
Dipartimento di Informatica e Sistemistica
Università di Pavia
Italy

A.B. Martinez
Technical University of Catalonia
Barcelona, Spain

Silvia Miksch
Danube University Krems
Department of Information & Knowledge Engineering
Krems, Austria
silvia@ifs.tuwien.ac.at
http://www.donau-uni.ac.at

Stefania Montani
Dipartimento di Informatica
Università del Piemonte Orientale
Italy
Corso Borsalino 54
15100 Alessandria, Italy
stefania@mfn.unipmn.it

Loris Nanni
DEIS, IEIIT – CNR
Università di Bologna
Viale Risorgimento 2
40136 Bologna, Italy
lnanni@deis.unibo.it

Luigi Portinale
Dipartimento di Informatica
Università del Piemonte Orientale
Italy
Corso Borsalino 54
15100 Alessandria, Italy
portinal@mfn.unipmn.it

Rainer Schmidt
Institute for Medical Informatics and Biometry
University of Rostock
Rembrandtstr. 16/17
D-18055 Rostock, Germany
rainer.schmidt@uni-rostock.de

Randall Sexton
Computer Information Systems
Missouri State University
901 S. National
Springfield, MO 65804
USA
rss000f@missouristate.edu

Altion Simo
National Institute of Advanced Science and Technology
Digital Human Research Center
2-41-6, Aomi, Koto-ku, Tokyo
135-0064
Japan
altion.simo@aist.go.jp

Margarita Sordo
Decision Systems Group
Brigham & Women's Hospital
Harvard Medical School
Boston, MA, USA
msordo@dsg.harvard.edu
http://www.dsg.harvard.edu

C. Urdiales
Department of Electronic
Technology ISIS group
University of Malaga
Spain

Partners Healthcare Order Set Schema: An Information Model for Management of Clinical Content

Margarita Sordo, Tonya Hongsermeier, Vipul Kashyap, and Robert A. Greenes

Summary. Developed by the Clinical Knowledge Management and Decision Support Group at Partners HealthCare and the Decision Systems Group at Harvard Medical School, the XML-based Order Set Schema presented in this chapter is the result of a broader enterprise-wide knowledge management effort to enhance quality, safety, and efficiency of provided care at Partners HealthCare while maximizing the use of new clinical information technology. We are in the process of deploying the Order Set Schema at two Partners-based, Harvard-affiliated academic medical centers the Brigham & Women's Hospital (BWH) and Massachusetts General Hospital (MGH), Boston, MA, so that existing content in the Computerized Physician Order Entry (CPOE) systems at these two institutions can be successfully extracted and mapped into the proposed schema. In this way, "hardwired" knowledge could be mapped into taxonomies of relevant terms, definitions and associations, resulting in formalized conceptual models and ontologies with explicit, consistent, user-meaningful relationships among concepts to support collaboration, and content management that will promote systematic (a) conversion of reference content into a form that approaches specifications for decision support content; (b) development and reuse of clinical content while ensuring consistency in the information; and (c) support an open and distributed review process among leadership, content matter experts, and end-users. Further, incorporating metadata into our unified content strategy will improve workflow by enabling timely review and updating of content, knowledge life-cycle management, and knowledge encoding; reduce costs and; aid authors to identify relevant elements for reuse while reducing redundant and spurious content. Ultimately, we view our knowledge management infrastructure as a key element for knowledge discovery.

1 Introduction

Real-time decision support can be incorporated in Computerized Physician Order Entry Systems (CPOE) to avoid medication errors, dosage errors, and adverse drug interactions, known patient allergies, and to calculate dosages based on patient-specific characteristics, and best practice recommendations for care [1,2]. CPOE, of course, deals with other kinds of orders, procedures,

M. Sordo et al.: *Partners Healthcare Order Set Schema: An Information Model for Management of Clinical Content*, Studies in Computational Intelligence (SCI) **48**, 1–25 (2007)
www.springerlink.com

and scheduling requests besides medication orders, and decision support can be useful for these as well. Order Sets (OSs), an important part of CPOE systems, are defined as collections of orderables aimed to improve the organization and quality of the ordering process. Order Sets are structured units of work that provide mnemonic value, convenience and efficiency, and clinical decision support during the ordering process. Sharing OSs can facilitate best practices.

As part of the five ongoing Signature Initiatives to enhance quality, safety, and efficiency of provided care, Partners HealthCare has been focusing efforts on maximizing the use of new clinical information technology. As a result, the Clinical Informatics Research and Development (CIRD) group at Partners HealthCare is leading the development of clinical systems strategies, conducting applied informatics research and development and addressing key issues in Partners enterprise clinical systems, especially those involving complex clinical workflows, usability, controlled terminology, knowledge management, and clinical decision support [3]. This work has been done in collaboration with the Decision Systems Group, a biomedical informatics research and development laboratory at Brigham and Women's Hospital (BWH) (one of the Partners-based, Harvard-affiliated academic medical centers).

The objective of this chapter is to present an OS Schema developed by the Clinical Knowledge Management and Decision Support Group at Partners HealthCare and the Decision Systems Group, and to provide a brief introduction to key issues involved in its implementation. The OS Schema is the result of a broader enterprise-wide knowledge management effort to identify and leverage current clinical knowledge across Partners institutions. This chapter has been divided into five main topics: (a) a brief introduction to knowledge representation and management, including ontologies; (b) a description of the clinical content identified in OSs, (c) an introduction to the main elements of UML, XML Schema, and Health Level Seven (HL7) as the standards we aimed to incorporate in our approach; (d) a complete description of the OS Schema developed; and, finally, (e) a summary of accomplishments.

2 Knowledge Representation and Management at Partners Healthcare

Partners Healthcare is a heterogeneous integrated healthcare system that offers patients a continuum of coordinated high-quality, safe, and efficient health care. The clinical information systems that support care across the enterprise are equally heterogeneous; hence, clinical decision support content is of varying composition and structure across Partners [4]. Several clinical information systems have been developed internally by Partners and are currently in place across Partners' hospitals. Such systems consist of a wide variety of clinical applications including a results manager to help clinic physicians review and act upon test results [5], critical event detection and alerting [2,6], and CPOE [7] to mention a few.

The CIRD group is responsible for leading the development of clinical systems strategy for Partners Healthcare, conducting applied informatics research and development, and addressing key design issues in Partners enterprise clinical systems, especially those involving complex clinical workflows, usability, controlled vocabulary and terminology, knowledge management, and decision support [3].

As part of an ongoing effort to fulfill Partners' strategic goal of becoming an effective learning organization, the CIRD knowledge management group and the DSG have carried out a series of projects to evaluate the current state of knowledge management practices across Partners entities and identify key requirements for tools and infrastructure that support collaboration and content management. This includes support for guideline definition and consensus development among leadership and subject matter experts, conversion of reference content into a form that approaches specifications for decision support content (rules, OSs, drug information, and the like), documentation of content provenance and history, tracking of responsible parties, workflow tools to enable timely review and updating of content, knowledge life-cycle management, and knowledge encoding.

Previous research initially focused on a knowledge inventory (KI) to assess ways in which various applications at the BWH utilized knowledge [8], given the long history of innovation in decision support at the hospital, that have been carried out. Although many of these are widely cited, they were to a large extent developed for the purpose of evaluation rather than long-term maintenance, and were often embedded in applications or made use of rudimentary editing tools, making maintenance and update difficult [9,10]. Based on the KI study, we carried out a more detailed analysis of the formal representation of rules to evaluate the feasibility of designing a single representation approach for encoding knowledge in the form of *if... then* statements [11], and the development of a knowledge management infrastructure for authoring, eliciting, versioning, publishing, and sharing expert knowledge [12].

The OS Schema is part of a current project that focuses on the development of a common approach for supporting the definition and management of grouped knowledge elements (KEGs) across Partners Healthcare [13]. The representation of this common approach is a UML-based schema based on the analysis of reference content of two CPOE systems currently in use at two Partners hospitals: BICS Order Entry at BWH (BICS OE), and Massachusetts General Hospital Order Entry System (MGH OE).

We envision that as a result of this effort, such a schema will foster consistency in knowledge and information extracted from current OSs and enhance usability – all in alignment with a unified content strategy with a standard infrastructure and techniques for knowledge representation and management aimed at the creation of component based, service oriented, and knowledge driven conceptual frameworks.

2.1 Knowledge Management

Knowledge Management is defined as a systematic process, by which an organization identifies, creates, acquires, shares, and leverages knowledge. In today's world, knowledge is information in context to produce an actionable understanding. Henceforth, in order for organizations to remain competitive and maximize their assets, they require clear, common objectives that can translate into actions; they need to know how to create knowledge – and manage it.

A typical organization has multiple content creators who design, create, approve, manage, and distribute information across the organization as different products, each created to serve a purpose and address particular needs of different people. From its creation, and before content reaches its target destination, it goes through a series of transformations, revisions, approvals, etc. This can lead to inconsistencies, duplication of efforts, disparities, etc. Hence, it is important to unify information to preserve consistency, and enhance its usability. This can be achieved by having a *unified content strategy* that aligns with the organizational goals.

2.2 Knowledge Representation

Knowledge Representation is a multidisciplinary subject that combines theories and techniques from Logic, Ontologies, and Computation [14]. Logic rules provide a formal structure to reason about the veracity and compatibility of statements. For example, if we measure the current body temperature of a patient, and the thermometer indicates 100.2°F, we can apply the rule in (1) to determine whether the patient has a fever or not. Sowa [15] provides an excellent introduction to logical, philosophical and computational aspects of Knowledge Representation.

$$\text{If patient's temperature} > 98.6^{\circ}\text{F then, the patient has fever.} \quad (1)$$

Ontologies are conceptualizations of a specific domain. Without these underlying conceptualizations, it is not possible to develop data models or schemas to represent such knowledge domains. Representation of knowledge is carried out in terms of objects and the relationships between objects within a domain or application. A vocabulary provides the terms necessary to describe objects, their attributes and behavior, and the relationships between objects. An interesting approach for creation and maintenance of structured clinical documentation is presented in [16]. Without ontologies, it is not possible to represent knowledge coherently. A well-defined ontology will support:

- Coherent and cohesive reasoning
- Sharing of knowledge
- Reusability

Thus, the first step in developing an effective knowledge representation and vocabulary is to perform an ontological analysis of the domain at hand, in terms of:

- Objects that exist in a domain
- Objects that have attributes with values
- Objects have relationships with other objects in the domain
- A characterization or enumeration of the potential states of an object. These states may be modeled as values of one or more attributes
- The value of attributes of objects can change over time
- Events can occur at different times
- Events can trigger other events
- Events can trigger transitions in states
- Objects can belong to one or more classes
- Classes can have generalization and specialization relationships with each other
- Classes can have constraints specified on the values of various attributes
- Axioms that enable complex definition of a class in terms of other classes and constraints on various attributes can also be represented in an ontology

The resulting ontology must capture the intrinsic structure of a domain in terms of concepts and their relationships. For example, let us imagine that in a simplistic clinical domain there are four classes of people: doctors, patients, males, and females. A common way to organize such information would be first to define a human class, with both doctors and patients as types-of human. Similarly, both males and females are also types-of human (Fig. 1).

The first problem that arises with the ontology representation in Fig. 1 is that doctors can also be patients, and patients can be patients at times, but not all the time. This indicates that doctor and patient are not types of humans, but actually are *roles* that humans can play. Further, male and female are values that *gender* as an attribute of humans can take. A more appropriate ontological representation for our example is depicted in Fig. 2, with two classes: human and role. Gender is an attribute of the human class. The role class can take one of two possible values: doctor or patient. There is

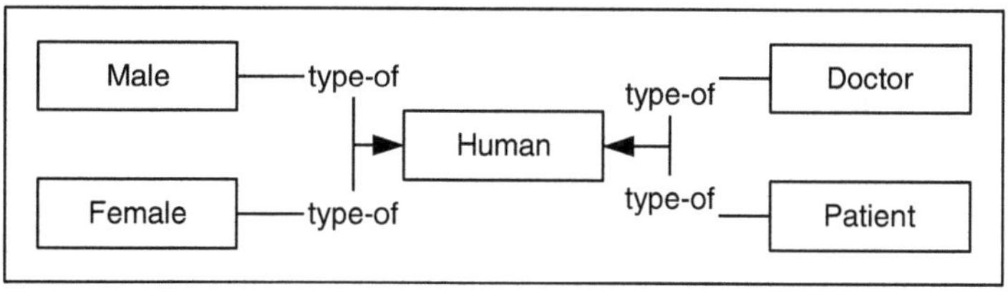

Fig. 1. An ontology representation depicting the class human and the *Doctor, Patient, Male,* and *Female* classes as *types-of* the class *Human*

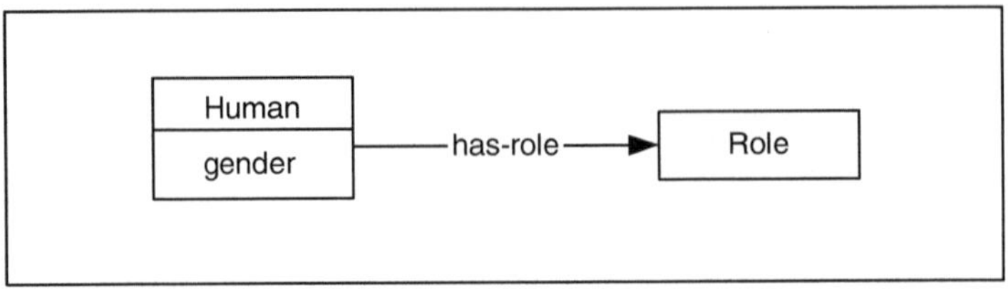

Fig. 2. An ontology representation depicting two classes: (1) *Human*, with the attribute gender, and (2) *Role*, the relationship *has-role* indicates the roles a human can play: doctor or patient

also the *has-role* relationship which connects Human with Role. This conceptualization is similar to that used by the HL7 Reference Information Model (RIM). A section is dedicated to the description of the HL7 RIM core classes used to represent a clinical domain.

A sound knowledge representation is vital if we want to preserve consistency and foster reusability and shareability. One of the advantages of ontologies is that the notation used to represent knowledge is not committed to a particular platform, or implementation. The ontology simply represents knowledge in a logical manner, regardless of the means we choose to implement such knowledge.

Computation supports the development of knowledge-based applications. However, ontologies remain independent from whatever means we choose to implement them. For example, the ontology representation in Fig. 2 could be implemented as a relational or object-oriented database. Similarly, we could choose one programming language over another. None of these choices will affect our representation.

3 Clinical Content

As noted previously, the analysis presented herein focuses on the reference content of two CPOE systems currently in use, at two hospitals: BICS OE and MGH OE. CPOE systems have been designed to support clinical processes, by automating the ordering processes, and providing the clinician with relevant, valuable information at the point of decision making. CPOEs provide real-time decision support for medication errors, dosage error, and adverse drug interactions, known patient allergies, calculate dosages based on the patient, and standardized care [1, 2]. The Institute of Medicine report on medical errors has also drawn attention to CPOE systems as a means of reducing errors [17]. Several authors have indicated that the use of OSs derived from best-practice standards reduce errors and improve physicians' acceptance of CPOE systems [18, 19]. Also, OSs help organize the ordering process into structured units of work serving as important elements of clinical decision support, time management, and sharing of clinical knowledge.

Partners Healthcare System OSs are organized by clinical discipline as the main criterion, with secondary indexing keys. Our OS Schema is a composite of orders involving multiple items including header, audit data, indication criteria, clinical setting, intention–action–interaction, target specifics, patient data, knowledge rules, notes and instructions, and order specifics.

Our catalog of orders consists of 24 types including admission, monitoring, nursing, medications, tubes and drains, lines and IVs, Imaging and Rx–Dx, laboratory tests, allergy, consults, diet, wound care, patient activity, discharge procedures, blood products, respiratory, patient preparation, immunization, health maintenance, follow-up, consequent orders, corollary orders, transfer, and others. The OS Schema proposed herein will be described in detail in a subsequent section.

4 Information Model and the UML

4.1 Information Model

An information model, or conceptual schema, defines the structure of information in a given domain. It represents relationships between domain objects without indicating how those relationships would be structured. An information model typically contains entities, relationships and associations between entities, and constraints on the relationships. A key feature of information models is the semantic description of the fact types, or associations. An information model is not simply a structure for containing data, but also an expression of the semantics behind the data.

Information modeling fosters appropriate design, implementation, planning and extensibility, stages along the development process. It facilitates visualization and communication of design concepts, provides a basis for assessment of compatibility with standards and foreign systems, and encourages the clarification of definitions of terms.

The net result is a better understanding of the structural themes in clinical information, possible candidate solutions to system requirements, and the possibility of incorporating additional features or refining existing features as needed.

The information modeling method used in this project was Unified Modeling Language (UML) [20]. Additional information for standards-based information modeling can be found in [21–23].

The conceptual schema designed for OSs has several important capabilities. This schema is intended to provide part of the foundation needed for business intelligence, data mining, and clinical research applications. When coupled with the appropriate mapping mechanisms, the OS Schema will serve as a repository into which current clinical information from disparate sources could be mapped, hence providing a standard representation for clinical data. Further, given that the OS Schema is expressed in terms of elementary object types, this facilitates subsequent additions to the schema.

4.2 UML

The Unified Modeling Language (UML) is a visual language for constructing and documenting the artifacts of software-intensive systems. UML is used particularly in software and business modeling. UML is also often used for information modeling and logical data modeling, where classes are used to represent entities. The UML uses graphical notations to express the design of software projects. It is a valuable tool to help project teams communicate, explore potential designs, and validate the architectural design of the software [20,23].

UML class diagrams are used to describe objects and their relationships. A class diagram is represented by a rectangle, divided into three sections: the name of a class, its attributes, and operations. The name of an attribute is followed by a colon and a valid type, as depicted in Fig. 3, where the attribute name of the class Patient is defined as:

Name: Char.

Operations are normally used to retrieve, manipulate, and compute attribute values. For example, the *age* operation in the Patient class (Fig. 3) takes the current date and the patient's DOB as input parameters and returns the age of the patient in number of years. The notation for operations is as follows:

Operation (parameter list): Return Type

The parameter list contains the input parameter passed to the operation using the following notation:

[Parameter: Type, . . . , parameter: Type]

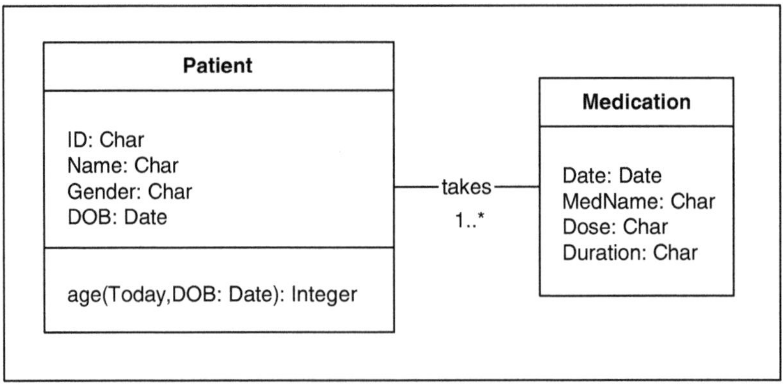

Fig. 3. UML diagram representing two classes (*Patient* and *Medication*) with their attributes, and one relationship

Input parameters are optional. However, for clarity it is best to include them whenever possible. Relationships between classes are represented by binary associations. For example, in Fig. 3, the line segment connecting the classes Patient and Medication indicates a relationship. The multiplicity or cardinality of an association may be indicated numerically, e.g., as 1..* in Fig. 3. The cardinality of an association is denoted by $Minimum \dots Maximum$, where *Minimum* indicates the minimum number of instances of an entity type that may be associated with each instance of any other entity type, and *Maximum* is the maximum number of instances of an entity type that may be associated with each instance of any other entity type.

This section is meant as an introduction to the UML classes. A more detailed description, including N-ary associations, aggregations, subtyping and statechart diagrams with additional sources can be found in [24].

4.3 UML Diagrams and XML Schemas

XML is a markup language that focuses on the organization of information. It allows the creation of structured documents that can be visually rendered with the appropriate tools. The W3C XML Schema Definition Language is an XML language for describing and structuring the content of XML documents [25]. Similar to a DTD, an XML Schema helps defining the building blocks of an XML document. An XML Schema defines:

- The elements that can appear in a document
- The attributes that can appear in a document
- Data types for elements and attributes
- Default and fixed values for elements and attributes
- Which elements can be child elements
- The order of child elements
- The number of child elements

Besides providing a structured representation, XML Schemas use the XML <*tag*> syntax, allow the definition of data types, and support extensibility. Hence, with XML Schemas, it is possible to describe permissible content, validate the correctness of data, map data to/from databases and other structured sources, define restrictions and data formats, and convert data between different data types. Further, XML Schemas support reusability, use of data types derived from standard types, and references to multiple schemas from the same document.

In a continuum of models, ranging from informal, unstructured depictions of the world, to precise modeling, a UML model provides a formal, yet simplified graphic representation of the real world, while an XML schema provides the most precise representation. The rationale behind each modeling technique shifts from the readability and simplicity of a UML model to a precise, formal, structured representation of an XML schema.

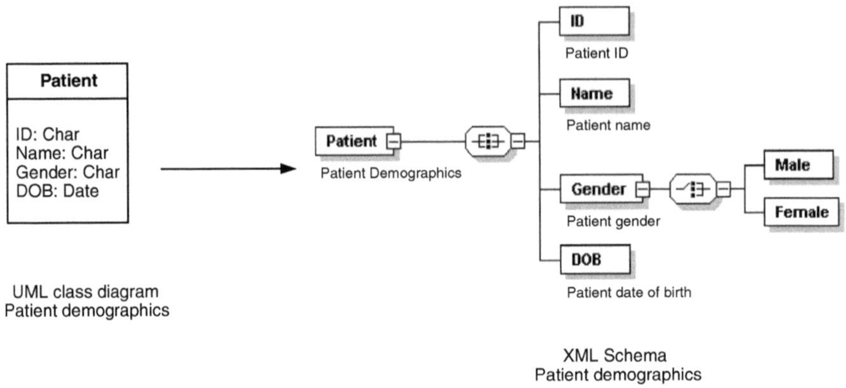

Fig. 4. An UML class diagram and its equivalent XML Schema

When developing an XML schema for a specific UML diagram, the structure of each element in the diagram must be detailed. For example, the UML class diagram for Patient demographics depicted in the left hand side of Fig. 4 consists of a patient ID, name, gender, and date of birth (DOB). Each attribute in the UML class diagram is mapped into an element in the schema by specifying its name and type. The right-hand side of Fig. 4 is a visual rendering in the form of a tree of the XML schema that corresponds to the UML class Patient demographics. The actual XML schema appears in Fig. 5.

It is possible to automate the transformation process of a UML class diagram into an XML schema. Automated derivation relies on a mapping transformation where every UML concept (class, attribute, association, etc.) that is represented in the UML metamodel, becomes an XML element. A stylesheet simply transforms `UML:Class` from XMI into an `xs:element` in the XML Schema. An excellent instruction to designing XML schemas using UML can be found in [26, 27].

5 HL7 V3 Reference Information Model

The Health Level Seven, Inc (HL7) is a standards development organization that produces standards for the exchange, integration, and management of clinical and administrative data in health care with an emphasis on interoperability of information systems [28]. The HL7 V3 standard is an object-oriented development methodology based on a RIM [29]. HL7 V3 also includes a number of other more specific information models as well as data types, vocabulary domains, and a messaging model.

The HL7 V3 RIM is a static information model on which all other HL7 V3 information models are based. It also provides the basis for the information content of all HL7 V3 protocol standards. The RIM is expressed as

```
<?xml version="1.0"?>
<xs:schema xmlns:xs="http://www.w3.org/2001/XMLSchema" elementForm
Default="qualified" attributeFormDefault="unqualified">
  <xs:element name="Patient">
    <xs:annotation>
      <xs:documentation>Patient Demographics</xs:documentation>
    </xs:annotation>
    <xs:complexType>
      <xs:all>
        <xs:element name="ID">
          <xs:annotation>
            <xs:documentation>Patient ID</xs:documentation>
          </xs:annotation>
          <xs:complexType />
        </xs:element>
        <xs:element name="Name">
          <xs:annotation>
            <xs:documentation>Patient name</xs:documentation>
          </xs:annotation>
        </xs:element>
        <xs:element name="Gender">
          <xs:annotation>
            <xs:documentation>Patient gender</xs:documentation>
          </xs:annotation>
          <xs:complexType>
            <xs:choice>
              <xs:element name="Male" />
              <xs:element name="Female" />
            </xs:choice>
          </xs:complexType>
        </xs:element>
        <xs:element name="DOB">
          <xs:annotation>
            <xs:documentation>Patient date of birth</xs:documentation>
          </xs:annotation>
        </xs:element>
      </xs:all>
    </xs:complexType>
  </xs:element>
</xs:schema>
```

Fig. 5. Instance document for the patient demographics XML schema depicted in Fig. 4

a UML class diagram. The core of the RIM is a metamodel that specifies the kinds of associations that may exist between the various classes in the other information models of HL7 V3. The HL7 RIM also includes the inheritance relationships for subclasses that are derived from the core classes. The structure of the RIM core classes is depicted Fig. 6.

The HL7 RIM specifies that an *Entity* may play a *Role* that has a *Participation* in an *Act*. For example, a person entity may play a patient role that participates as the subject of a medication administration act. An *Entity* may also "scope" a *Role* being played by a given *Entity* in the sense of defining, guaranteeing, or acknowledging that the *Role* is played by the given *Entity*. A relationship between two acts (e.g., one act is a component of another act) is represented by an *ActRelationship*. A relationship between two roles (e.g., one role has direct authority over another role) is represented by a *RoleLink*.

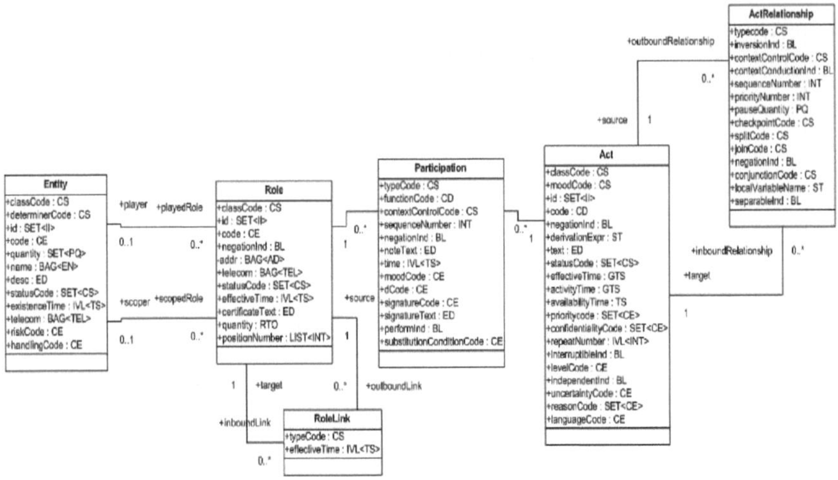

Fig. 6. HL7 V3 Reference Information Model core classes

The *Entity* class is used to represent a physical thing or an organization. For example, an *Entity* may be a living subject, a place, an organization, a material, a device, or a container. The *Role* class represents the competency or suitability of an *Entity* to play a given role while participating in appropriate acts. For example, a *Role* may be a patient, an employee, or equipment certified to perform specific functions. The *Participation* class represents the way that a *Role* participates in an *Act*, for example a performer, a subject, a witness, or a referrer. The *Act* class represents an intentional action. For example, an *Act* may be an observation, a procedure, a substance administration, or a patient encounter. An A*ct* represented by this class may be in the process of occurring, have already occurred, or be intended or requested to occur. It may also simply be an act that could occur.

One of the strategies fostered by HL7 is to develop coherent, extensible standards that permit structured, encoded health care information of the type required to support patient care, to be exchanged between computer applications while preserving meaning. The RIM is an essential part of the HL7 V3 development methodology, as it provides an explicit representation of the semantic and lexical connections that exist between the information carried in the fields of HL7 messages. The HL7 Structured Documents Technical Committee (authors of the CDA – Clinical Document Architecture) and the Templates SIG of the Modeling and Methodology Technical Committee in HL7 are addressing the creation of standards for clinical documents [14] and templates [30]. Without such standards, unstructured content is loosely communicated across an organization. In this framework, OSs can be seen as instances of structured documents containing tagged concepts and relationships between concepts.

6 Order Set Schema (OS Schema)

Order Sets are predefined groups of orders for specific clinical settings, diagnoses or treatments. They provide decision support to help clinicians improve the outcome of treatments by prompting clinical alerts about current patient's condition; diagnosis support by highlighting key symptoms and finding; medication ordering by suggesting appropriate medications and dosages based on the medical condition of a patient; cost reduction by suggesting effective alternative treatments, and medications. Such decision support can be incorporated into computerized systems in a variety of ways:

- Representation and interpretation of data
- Modeling patient information
- Representation of medical concepts
- Abstraction and interpretation of data
- Modeling processes
- Representation of actions
- Organization of plans
- Modeling decisions
- Representation of goals and intentions

In alignment with the proposed enterprise-wide unified content strategy to support consistency, interoperability, and reusability of components that can easily be integrated into applications, the initial step of our modeling process was the definition of an OS (as described above), and the elements involved. It is particularly important to have a clear definition of what is to be modeled, because an information model is about the semantics behind the data. A clear semantic definition promotes semantic interoperability between applications and information systems. Generally speaking, a definition used with a model is considered reasonably clear if the structure of the model and the way the model is used are robust with respect to variation within the range of uncertainty in the definition. The benefits derived from a clear definition also apply to the semantics of the relationships and associations in the model.

The next step in the modeling process was the analysis and categorization of reference content of the two CPOE systems, BICS OE and MGH OE, currently in use at the two main academic medical centers of Partners. In this step we identified and defined all the logically independent components (metadata categories) involved in the OSs of these two CPOE systems. The result was a list of categorized metadata representing the internal structure of the analyzed OSs, as depicted in Fig. 7. The following are the definitions of the identified metadata categories:

- *Header* – contains general information about the OS as a whole, including OS name, unique identifier, version, description of the purpose of the OS, and intended user.
- *Audit Data* – includes information that supports the editorial process from creation of content to version management and ownership.

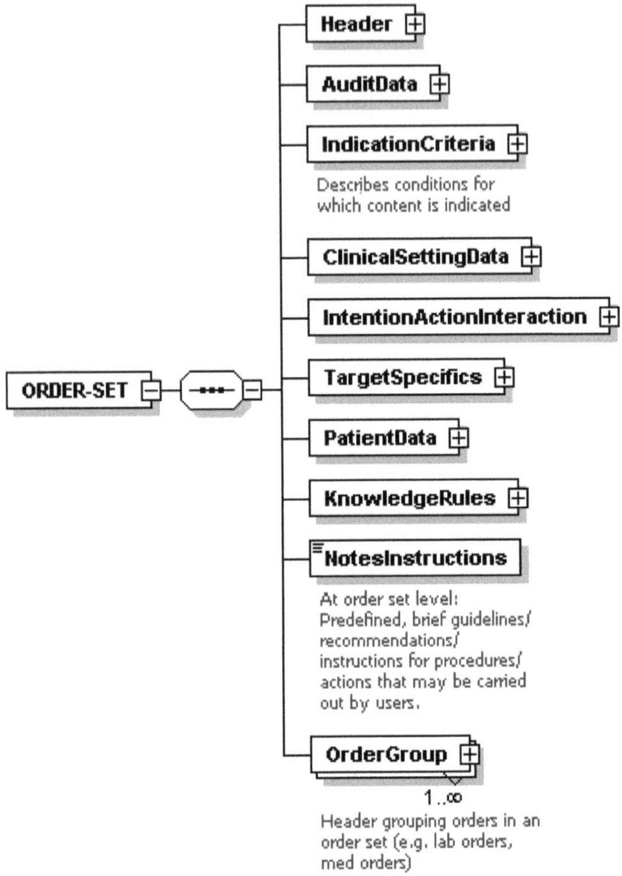

Fig. 7. Overall structure of the XML OS Schema. The *plus sign* indicates that the element has multiple attributes and can be expanded

- *Indication Criteria* – describes clinical conditions to which the clinical knowledge applies.
- *Clinical Setting* – includes venues, and clinical disciplines to which the content applies.
- *Intention-Action-Interaction* – indicates the type of encounter to which the current content applies, the reasons and goals for the OS, and the processes involved. This category includes an ontology of intentions which will be described below.
- *Target Specifics* – indicates the suitability of the OS for specific target groups in terms of age, gender, and acuity of symptoms.
- *Patient Data* – contains patient-specific data, such as past clinical history (e.g., medications, laboratory test results, allergies, previous diagnoses, family history), and current diagnosis.

- *Knowledge Rules* – provides real-time decision support for medication errors, dosage error, and adverse drug interactions, known patient allergies, calculate dosages based on the patient, and standardized care. It also provides links to alternative, complementary supporting knowledge.
- *Notes and Instructions* – contains predefined, brief guidelines, recommendations, and instructions for procedures and actions that may be carried out by users.
- *Order Group* – header grouping similar orders in an OS.

The Schema in Fig. 7 captures the metadata categories of the OS information model. Each category consists of group or cluster of related content elements. As content is grouped and categorized, a taxonomy automatically starts to appear, and terms in the taxonomy become metadata that can be used as an index to retrieve content. Element metadata identifies content at the element level (finer granularity), based on the elements defined in the information model. Element metadata helps authors manage content through the authoring process, further fostering reusability, retrieval, and tracking issues. Following is a more detailed description of the elements in each category.

6.1 Header Category

The Header metadata category in Fig. 8 is formed by the following elements:

- *OrderSetID* – a unique identifier for the OS.
- *Name* – a descriptive or general heading.
- *Version* – latest version of the OS.
- *IsCurrent* – *(Y/N)* indicates whether this is the current version of the OS or not. For audit purposes all versions – reflecting changes – are kept in a repository.
- *Description* – contains a more detailed, extended description of the OS.
- *IntendedUser* – Role/actor for which order related content would be of interest. Content is applicable for this audience (from a content template builder perspective or knowledge management). The actual role specific permission resides in the application – and content is not permission level dependent.

6.2 AuditData Category

The AuditData category in Fig. 9 holds the content required to analyze how clinical content is, created, used, reused, modified, and delivered to various audiences. The AuditData category is formed by the following elements:

- *IsPersonal* – Boolean attribute used to distinguish personal OSs from departmental ones.
- *ContentOwner* – This is a complex object with attributes including name and contact information of person(s) responsible for content. The expanded elements are depicted in Fig. 10.

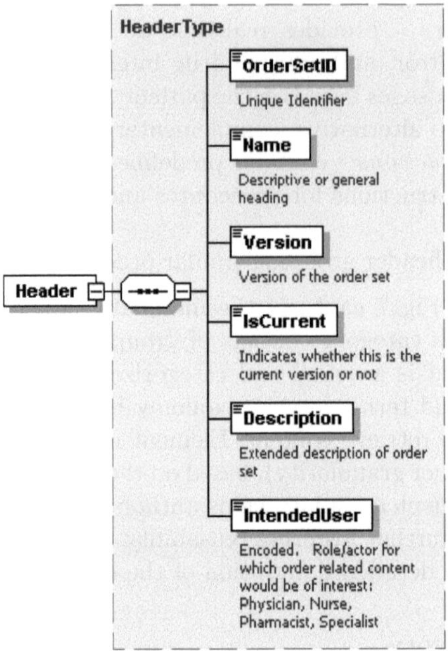

Fig. 8. Diagram showing the Schema for the *Header* metadata

- *CreationDate* – Date of creation of content.
- *EffectiveDate* – Effective date of OS.
- *ExpirationDate* (optional) – Expiration date of OS.
- *ScheduledRevisionDate* – Scheduled upcoming date for reviews, changes, deletions, and updates of content. It is always prefilled with a future date. If overdue, it should be flagged.
- *TrackingChanges* (optional) – Keeps track of the history of changes, including date of changes, revisions, deletions, and updates of content. *RevisionDate* is the actual date the content was reviewed. It documents changes, reasons for changing the content in the OS, name of the person(s) responsible for the changes, and name of the person(s) who authorized the changes. Also, it indicates whether the OS was moved from another discipline or category, or if the OS replaces (optional) another OS. The expanded diagram is depicted in Fig. 11.
- *ComparableContent* (optional) – Identifies content on the same topic by means of unique OS identifier(s).

6.3 IndicationCriteria Category

The IndicationCriteria category in Fig. 12 describes the conditions for which content is indicated, e.g., what makes a patient a candidate for a procedure or action.

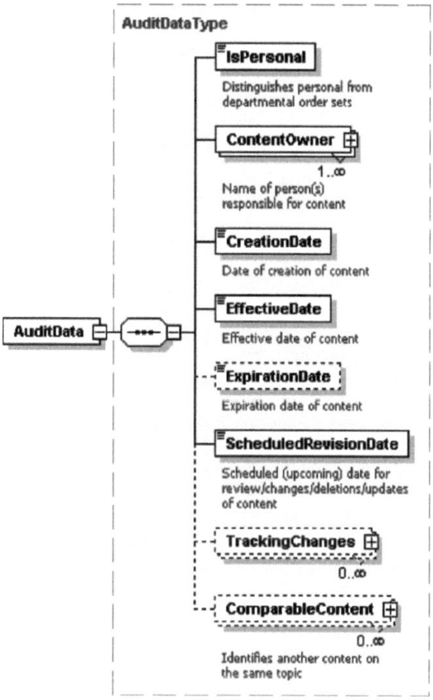

Fig. 9. Diagram for the *AuditData* category and its elements. *Dotted lines* indicate the element is optional, *solid lines* indicate the element is required. The *plus sign* indicates that the element has multiple attributes and can be expanded

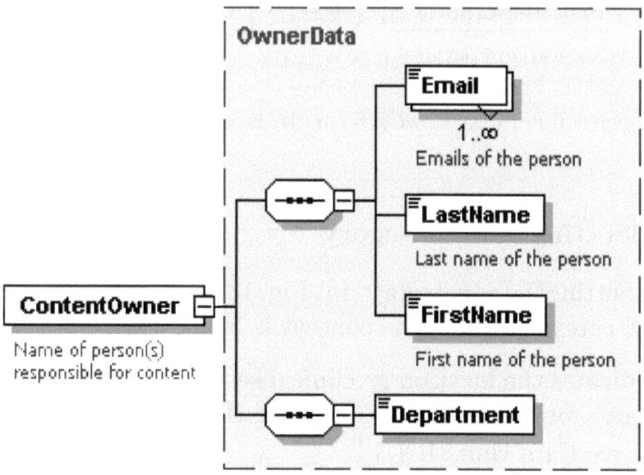

Fig. 10. *ContentOwner* diagram

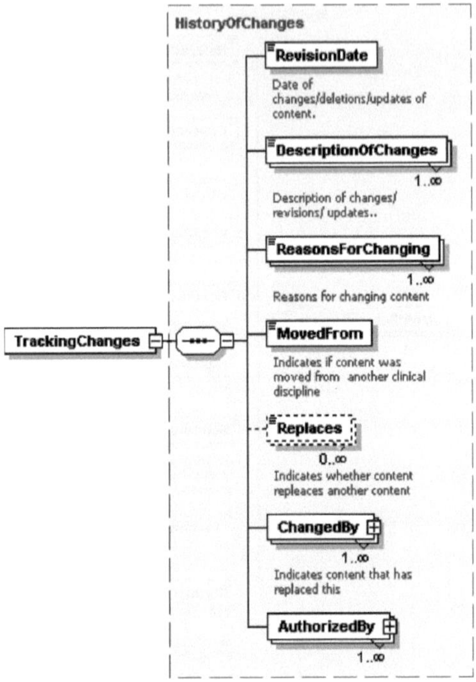

Fig. 11. Diagram for *TrackingChanges* category and its elements. *Dotted lines* indicate the element is optional, *solid lines* indicate the element is required. The *plus sign* indicates that the element has multiple attributes and can be expanded

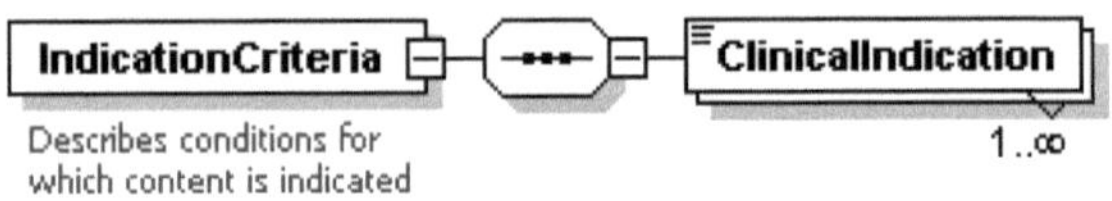

Fig. 12. Diagram for *IndicationCriteria*. It is a collection of applicable clinical indications

6.4 ClinicalSettingData Category

The ClinicalSettingData category in Fig. 13 indicates the venue, clinical discipline and category where the content is being used:

(a) *Venue* indicates the location or clinical setting where the content is being used as one – or more – of the following (list is not exhaustive):
  - Intensive Care Unit (ICU)
  - Ambulatory/Outpatient
  - Acute
  - Emergency
  - Perioperative
  - Pediatrics

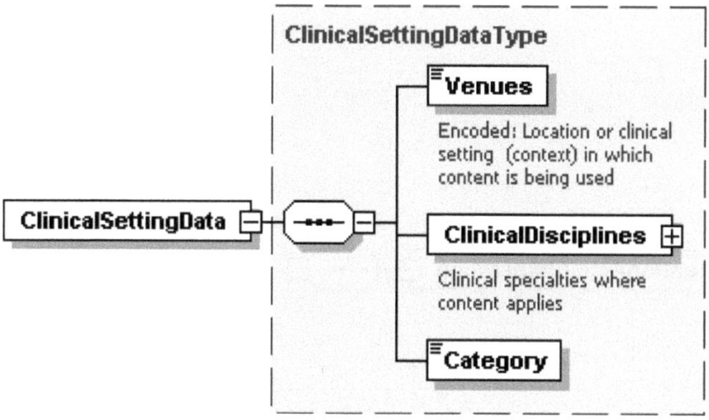

Fig. 13. Diagram for *ClinicalSettingData*. The *plus sign* indicates that the element has multiple attributes and can be expanded

(b) *ClinicalDisciplines* represents the clinical specialty where the content of the OS applies as one or more of the following (list is not exhaustive):
   - Anesthesiology/Perioperative medicine
   - Behavioral medicine
   - Burn management
   - Cardiology
   - Oncology surgery
   - Orthopedic
   - Otolaryngology – Head and neck surgery
   - Pediatric surgery
   - Urology/Renal
   - Urology/Renal surgery
   - Vascular surgery

6.5 IntentionActionInteraction Category

The IntentionActionInteraction category in Fig. 14 indicates the type of encounter, processes, intentions, and goals regarding the use of an OS during a patient–physician encounter.

(a) *Type of encounter* indicates the type of interaction between the physician and a patient as one or more of the following:
   - Initial consult
   - Follow-up
   - Review of symptoms
   - Disease management
   - Pre- or Post-procedure
   - Procedure

(b) *Process* refers to a series of actions or operations conducting to an end:
   - Pre-, Post-procedure
   - Admission

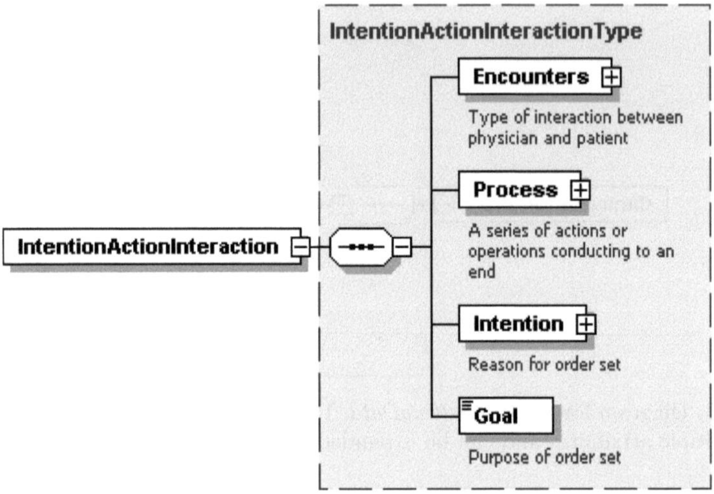

Fig. 14. Diagram for *IntentionActionInteraction* category and its elements. The *plus sign* indicates that the element has multiple attributes and can be expanded

  - Transfer
  - Discharge

(c) *Intention* is the reason for the OS, e.g., an intention can be for gathering knowledge about a patient during a physician–patient encounter, or as the execution of an action to, e.g., admit a patient, address the condition of a patient by preventing, or treating a disease.
(d) *Goal* defines the purpose of the OS.

6.6 TargetSpecifics Category

TargetSpecifics category in Fig. 15 contains information about identified groups of patients the clinical content applies to in terms of age groups, gender, and acuity (e.g., acute, chronic, and emergency).

6.7 PatientData Category

The PatientData category in Fig. 16 contains past and current patient information.

- *PatientPastData* contains the patient and family histories in the form of collections of observations – consistent with the HL7 RIM classes. Family history triggers alerts and decision support recommendations that are diagnosis specific, e.g., a high risk for colon cancer could trigger a colonoscopy. PatientPastData also contains information about

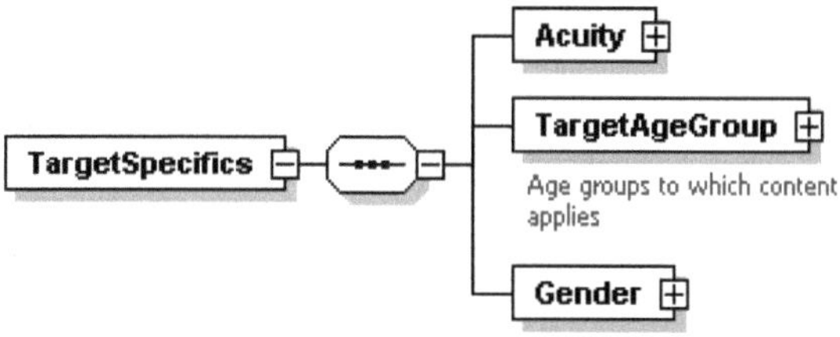

Fig. 15. Diagram for *TargetSpecifics* category and its elements. The *plus sign* indicates that the element has multiple attributes and can be expanded

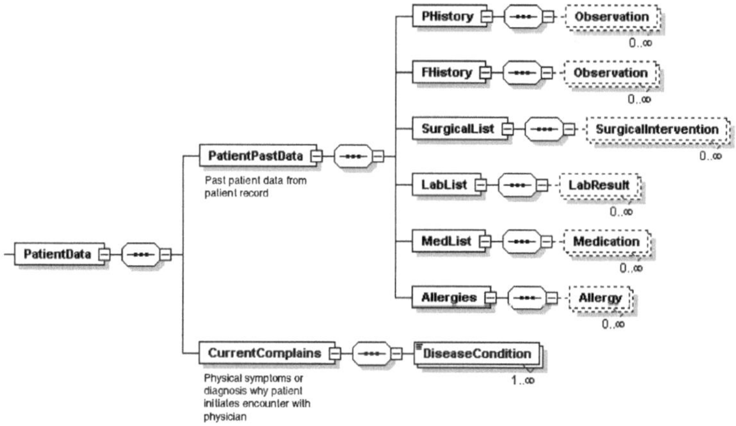

Fig. 16. Diagram for *PatientData* category and its elements. It is divided in two main subcategories: Past and Current patient information

surgical interventions, laboratory test results, medications, and known allergies. Given the importance of allergies, they are explicitly displayed independently of Patient's history.
- *CurrentComplains* contains information about physical symptom(s) or diagnosis, e.g., why patient initiates encounter with physician.

6.8 KnowledgeRules Category

The KnowledgeRules category in Fig. 17 contains associated knowledge in the form of links to additional, supporting knowledge, e.g., articles, clinical guidelines, and identifiers to rules in a central repository. The associated rules provide context- and patient-specific decision support in the form actions, and recommendations about e.g., medication options, medication suggestions, medication dosages, discharge protocols, consequent rules, and corollary orders.

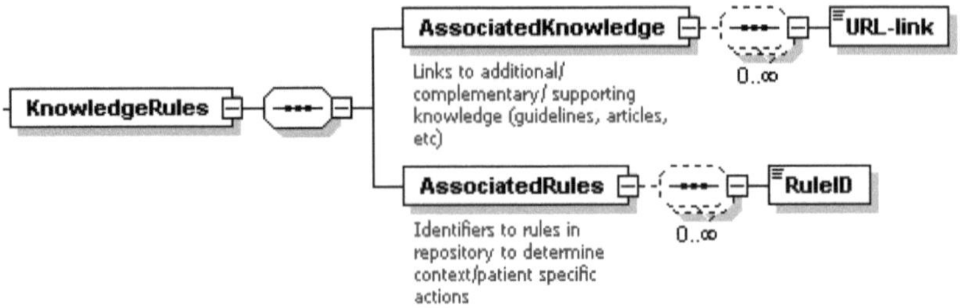

Fig. 17. Diagram for *KnowledgeRules* category. This category consists of *Associated Knowledge* – a collection of links to additional, supporting knowledge, and *Associated Rules* – identifiers to a repository of decision support rules

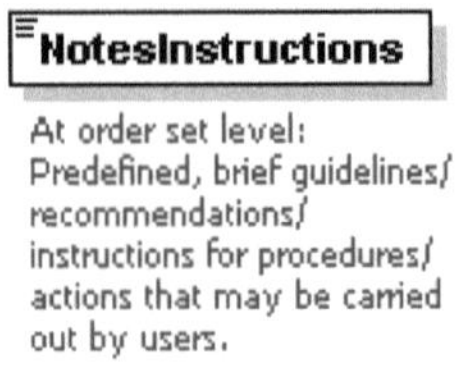

Fig. 18. Diagram for *NotesInstructions* category. This category consists of predefined, brief guidelines, recommendations and instructions for procedures and actions. They are not patient specific

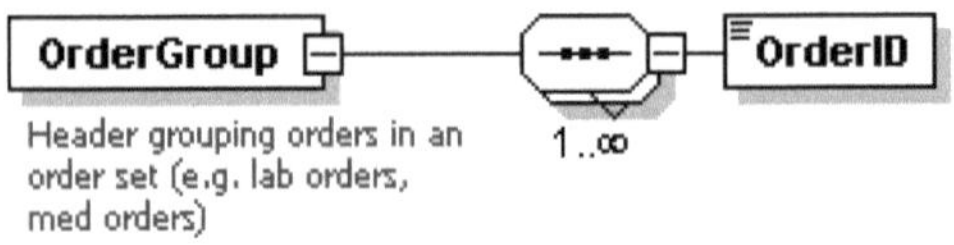

Fig. 19. Diagram for *OrderGroup* category. This category consists of a series of links – denoted by the *OrderID* unique identifier – to orders

6.9 NotesInstructions Category

The NotesInstructions category in Fig. 18 contains predefined, brief guidelines, recommendations and instructions for procedures and actions that could be carried out by users. As opposed to the KnowledgeRules category, these notes and instructions are not patient specific, but rather, they are specific to the OS itself, e.g., "call attending if ...".

6.10 OrderGroup Category

OrderGroup category in Fig. 19 groups orders in an OS by type. Orders are referred to by OrderID – a unique identifier for each order. An order type can be any of following (list not exhaustive): Admission, Monitoring, Nursing, Medications Tubes–Drains, Lines-IVs, Image Rx–Dx, Laboratory Results, Allergy, Consults, Diet, Wound Care, Patient Activity, Discharge List,

Procedures, Blood Products Respiratory, Patient Preparation, Immunization, Health Maintenance, Follow-up, Consequent, Corollary, Transfer, Other.

7 Conclusions

The proposed OS Schema presented in this chapter is part of the infrastructure to expand and support content development at Partners HealthCare System. Our first step is to deploy the OS Schema so that existing content in the OSs in both BWH and MGH CPOE systems can be successfully extracted and mapped into the proposed schema. In this way, "hardwired" knowledge could be mapped into taxonomies of relevant terms, definitions and associations, resulting in formalized conceptual models and ontologies with explicit, consistent, user-meaningful relationships among concepts.

We envision that the proposed schema, as part of an enterprise-wide knowledge management infrastructure to support collaboration and content management, will promote systematic (a) conversion of reference content into a form that approaches specifications for decision support content; (b) development and reuse of clinical content while ensuring consistency in the information; and (c) support an open and distributed review process among leadership, content matter experts and end-users. Further, incorporating metadata into our unified content strategy will improve workflow by enabling timely review and updating of content, knowledge life-cycle management, and knowledge encoding; reduce costs and; aid authors to identify relevant elements for reuse while reducing redundant and spurious content. Ultimately, we view our knowledge management infrastructure as a key element for knowledge discovery.

Acknowledgments

This project was supported by a grant from the Partners HealthCare Information Systems Research Council. We would like to thank Judith Colecchi, Martha Muffie Martin and Cathyann Harris for their valuable input.

References

1. Bates DW, Teich JM, Lee J, Seger DL, Kuperman GJ, Ma'Luf N, et al. The impact of computerized physician order entry on medication error prevention. J Am Med Inform Assoc 1999;6:313–321
2. Horsky J, Kuperman GJ, Patel V. Comprehensive analysis of a medication dosing error related to CPOE. J Am Med Inform Assoc 2005;12(4)
3. Clinical Informatics Research and Development (CIRD). Partners Healthcare. http://www.partners.org/cird/AboutUs.asp

4. Partners Healthcare System. http://www.partners.org
5. Poon EG, Wang SJ, Gandhi TK, Bates DW, Kuperman GJ. Design and implementation of a comprehensive outpatient Results Manager. J Biomed Inform 2003;36(1–2):80–91
6. Jha AK, Kuperman GJ, Teich JM, Leape L, Shea B, Rittenberg E, Burdick E, Seger DL, Vliet MV, Bates DW. Identifying adverse drug events. Development of a computer-based monitor and comparison with chart review and stimulated voluntary report. J Am Med Inform Assoc 1998;5(3):305–314
7. Kaushal R, Bates DW. Computerized Physician Order Entry (CPOE) with Clinical Decision Support Systems (CDSSs) in Making health care safer: A critical analysis of patient safety practices. Evidence Report/Technology Assessment: Number 43. AHRQ Publication No. 01-E058, July 2001. Agency for Healthcare Research and Quality, Rockville, MD. http://www.ahrq.gov/clinic/ptsafety/
8. Boxwala AA, Kuperman GJ, Denekamp Y, Scott-Wright A, Middleton BL, Greenes RA. Survey and evaluation of electronic knowledge use for clinical decision support at Brigham and Women's Hospital 2003, Technical Report DSGTR 2002-007, http://www.dsg.harvard.edu/gello/KnowledgeInventoryReport.doc
9. Kuperman GJ, Cooley T, Tremblay J, Teich JM, Churchill WW. Decision support for medication use in an inpatient physician order entry application and a pharmacy application. Medinfo 1998;9:467–471
10. Kuperman GJ, Teich JM, Gandhi TK, Bates DW. Patient safety and computerized medication ordering at Brigham and Women's Hospital. Jt Comm J Qual Improv 2001;27:509–521
11. Greenes RA, Sordo M, Zaccagnini D, Meyer M, Kuperman GJ. Design of a standards-based external rules engine for decision support in a variety of application contexts: Report of a feasibility study at Partners HealthCare system. Proceedings of medical informatics association (Medinfo), September, 2004
12. Hongsermeier T, Kashyap V, Sordo M. Case study: Knowledge management infrastructure: Evolution at Partners Healthcare system in medical decision support. In computer-based approaches to improving healthcare quality and safety. Elsevier, November, 2006
13. Sordo M, Palchuk M. Grouped knowledge elements. In computer-based approaches to improving healthcare quality and safety. Elsevier, November, 2006
14. Alschuler L. HL7's CDA, clinical document architecture: An overview, May 2002. Available from www.hl7.org as Document ID# 620
15. Sowa JF. Knowledge representation: Logical, philosophical, and computational foundations, Brooks Cole, Pacific Grove, CA, 2000. Actual publication date, 16 August 1999
16. Kashyap V, Morales A, Hongsermeier T, Li Q. Definitions management: A semantics-based approach for structured clinical documentation. Proceedings of the 4th International Semantic Web Conference (ISWC 2005), November, 2005
17. Kohn L, Corrigan J, Donaldson M. To err is human: Building a safer health system. Washington, DC: Committee on quality of health care in America, Institute of Medicine, National Academy, 1999
18. Bates DW, Shu K, Narasimhan D, Horsky J. Comparing time spent writing orders on paper and physician computer order entry. Proc AMIA Symp 2000:965
19. Lee F, Teich JM, Spurr CD, Bates DW. Implementation of physician order entry: User satisfaction and self-reported usage patterns. J Am Med Inform Assoc 1996;3:42–55

20. Object management group – UML. http://www.uml.org/
21. Cattell RGG, Barry DK, Berler M, Eastman J, Jordan D, Russell C, Schadow O, Stanienda T, Velez F. The object data standard: ODMG 3.0. Morgan Kaufmann, 2000
22. Tkach D, Puttick R. Object technology in application development. Redwood City, CA: Benjamin/Cummings, 1994
23. Warmer J, Kleppe A. The object constraint language. Precise modeling with UML. Reading, MA: Addison Wesley, 1999
24. Gooch, T. Unified Modeling Language (UML) Tutorial. http://atlas.kennesaw.edu/~dbraun/csis4650/A&D/UML_tutorial/what_is_uml.htm
25. W3C XML Schema. http://www.w3.org/XML/Schema
26. Malik A. Designing XML schemas using UML. http://www-128.ibm.com/developerworks/library/x-umlschem/
27. Marchal B. Working XML: UML, XMI, and code generation, Part 1. Design XML vocabularies with UML tools. http://www-128.ibm.com/developerworks/xml/ library/x-wxxm23/
28. Health Level Seven. HL7. http://hl7.org
29. HL7 Reference Information Model (RIM). http://www.hl7.org/Library/data-model/RIM/modelpage_mem.htm
30. Kernberg M. Template and archetype architecture draft for San Antonio. January 2004. Available from www.hl7.org as Document ID#1209

A State-Based Model for Management of Type II Diabetes

Margarita Sordo, Tonya Hongsermeier, Vipul Kashyap, and Robert A. Greenes

Summary. The Decision Systems Group at the Brigham & Women's Hospital, Boston, USA and the Clinical Knowledge Management Group at Partners HealthCare Systems, Inc. have developed a computational model that encompasses strategies for prevention, early diagnosis, and treatment of type II diabetes and associated complications. This effort is part of an on-going, enterprise-wide strategy to improve the quality, safety, and efficiency of provided care, by maximizing the use of new clinical information technology in key issues such as complex clinical workflows, usability, controlled terminology, knowledge management, and clinical decision support carried out by Partners HealthCare System. The proposed model is a disease state management system for the continuum of diabetes care that synergistically integrates patient care and education protocols at all levels of disease management, and supports the integration of evidence-based personalized care. Our approach could be easily adapted to managing other chronic conditions e.g., hypertension, asthma, and coronary artery disease.

1 Introduction

Diabetes mellitus is the leading cause of morbidity and mortality in the United States. From 1980 to 2004, the number of Americans with diabetes more than doubled (from 5.8 million to 14.7 million), with older adults (aged 65 years or older) accounting for almost 40% of the population with diabetes [1]. An estimated 16 million Americans suffer from type II diabetes, and about 800,000 new cases are diagnosed each year [2, 3].

Although a lifelong disease, patients who suffer from diabetes can have a reasonably normal lifestyle if they comply with the appropriate medical and educational guidelines aimed to maintain healthy blood glucose levels and reduce the likelihood and progression of adverse macrovascular complications, e.g., coronary artery disease (CAD), stroke, and peripheral vascular

M. Sordo et al.: *A State-Based Model for Management of Type II Diabetes*, Studies in Computational Intelligence (SCI) **48**, 27–61 (2007)
www.springerlink.com

disease, and microvascular complications, e.g., retinopathy, nephropathy, and neuropathy.

Diabetes and its concomitant complications require comprehensive models for prevention, detection, and treatment at all levels of care. Guidelines have been developed that provide effective management strategies for diabetes care [4–6].

The Decision Systems Group at the Brigham & Women's Hospital, Boston, USA and the Clinical Knowledge Management Group at Partners HealthCare Systems, Inc have developed a computational model that encompasses strategies for prevention, early diagnosis, and treatment of diabetes and associated complications. The proposed model is a disease state management system for the continuum of diabetes care. The computational representation is consistent with Unified Modeling Language (UML) 2 state machine diagrams.

The current effort is part of the Partners Healthcare System enterprise-wide strategy to improve the quality, safety, and efficiency of provided care, by maximizing the use of new clinical information technology in key issues such as complex clinical workflows, usability, controlled terminology, knowledge management, and clinical decision support [7].

This chapter is divided in six sections. We start with a brief introduction to diabetes in general, and type II diabetes specifically. This is followed by a description of the main elements involved in diabetes management including regular screening, initial diagnosis, preventive care, management of diabetes complications, and intercurrent illnesses, surveillance, and follow-up. We introduce the UML 2 state machine diagrams as means of representing the state model. Next, we devote a section to our state model for management of type II diabetes, and finally, we summarize and our accomplishments.

2 Diabetes Mellitus

Diabetes mellitus is a metabolic syndrome characterized by chronic hyperglycemia due to insulin deficiency, insulin resistance or both. Diabetes is a chronic illness that requires long-term continuing medical care and patient self-management education in order to reduce the risk of acute complications. Diabetic patients can have a reasonably normal lifestyle if they comply with the appropriate medical and educational guidelines aimed to maintain healthy blood glucose levels and reduce the likelihood and progression of adverse macrovascular complications, e.g., CAD, stroke, and peripheral vascular disease; and microvascular complications, e.g., retinopathy, nephropathy, and neuropathy.

Noninsulin-dependent diabetes mellitus or type II diabetes is relatively common in all populations, with higher prevalence rates in people of African,

Caribbean, Native American, Latino, and South Asian ancestry. Type II diabetes and its concomitant complications require comprehensive models for prevention, detection, and treatment at all levels of care. Guidelines have been developed that provide effective management strategies for diabetes care [4–6].

Given the multidisciplinary nature of the work presented in this chapter, we devote the following section exclusively to the issues related to the management of type II diabetes, from initial diagnosis, regular, and targeted screening of low- and high-risk populations, to preventive care, and long-term management of diabetes, including management and follow-up, surveillance, and management of intercurrent illnesses.

3 Diabetes Management

Motivated by the need of standards of care intended to provide clinicians and patients with the key components of diabetes care, the American Diabetes Association has published a series of recommendations focused on diagnostic and therapeutic actions believed to favorably affect the outcomes of patients with diabetes. Their recommendations include the criteria for diagnosis of type II diabetes in nonpregnant adults; regular and targeted screening of asymptomatic adults, particularly those individuals at high risk; criteria for a complete initial evaluation of newly diagnosed patients and; customized long-term management. Long-term management includes a variety of strategies and techniques aimed at providing adequate glycaemic and lipid control; prevention of complications; support for lifestyle changes, e.g., physical activity, diet, smoking cessation; routine follow-up, and immunization [8].

3.1 Initial Diagnosis

Polyuria, thirst, and weight loss is the classic triad of symptoms of diabetes. Initial diagnosis is usually confirmed by measurement of plasma glucose by one of the following tests:

- A single plasma glucose $\geq 11.1\,\mathrm{mmol\,l^{-1}}$
- Fasting plasma glucose (FPG) $> 7.0\,\mathrm{mmol\,l^{-1}}$
- 2-h plasma glucose (PG) $> 11.1\,\mathrm{mmol\,l^{-1}}$ during an oral glucose tolerance test (OGTT)

As part of the initial diagnosis, a complete medical evaluation should be performed to overrule any possible complications, and a complete management plan should be formulated.

3.2 Regular and Targeted Screening for Low-Risk and High-Risk Populations

Regular screening for asymptomatic adults should be performed as follows:

1. **Low Risk** – Regular screening every 3 years for low risk, asymptomatic adults older than 45 years of age and with no prior diagnosis of diabetes.
2. **High Risk** – Targeted screening for younger, overweight patients, and patients older than 45 years of age with any of the following high risk factors:
   (a) Physically inactive
   (b) Member of a high-risk ethnic population, e.g., African American, Native American, Latino, Asian American, Pacific Islander
   (c) Hypertensive (BP $> 140/90$ mmHg)
   (d) HDL cholesterol level ≥ 0.90 mmol l^{-1} and/or triglyceride level ≥ 2.82 mmol l^{-1}
   (e) Family history of diabetes
   (f) Polycystic ovary syndrome (women)
   (g) Delivered a baby weighing $>$ 9lb or have been diagnosed with gestational diabetes mellitus (women)
   (h) History of impaired glucose tolerance (IGT) or impaired fasting glucose (IFG)
   (i) Any other clinical conditions associated with insulin resistance
   (j) History of vascular disease

3.3 Preventive Care

Preventive care aims to improve delivery of appropriate clinical preventive services by helping patients to maintain and/or develop healthy lifestyle habits and eliminate high-risk behaviors. In the context of managing type II diabetes, there are several health factors that require close observation, e.g., blood pressure, lipid management, antiplatelet agents, smoking cessation, coronary heart disease (CHD) and immunization. These factors are explained in more detail in the following sections.

3.3.1 Blood Pressure Management

High blood pressure is a common comorbidity in patients with diabetes, and a strict control is necessary to prevent adverse outcomes [5]. Several studies have demonstrated that an improved control of blood pressure greatly reduces the risk for both macrovascular complications e.g., CAD [9–11], and microvascular complications [12,13]. The American Diabetes Association recommended values are < 130 mmHg for systolic and < 80 mmHg for diastolic blood pressure [8].

3.3.2 Lipid Management

Lipid management focuses at reducing LDL cholesterol, elevating HDL cholesterol, and reducing triglycerides. The recommended values for non-pregnant adults are: LDL < 2.6 mmol l^{-1}, HDL > 1.1 mmol l^{-1}, and triglycerides < 1.7 mmol l^{-1} [8]. The benefits of healthy lipid levels are manifold, particularly on reducing the risk of cardiovascular events in patients with a high risk of CAD. Initial treatment focuses on dietary and lifestyle changes, e.g., physical activity, smoking cessation, and weight loss, aimed at reducing lipid levels. However, such interventions may be complemented with pharmacological treatment if lifestyle and diet changes alone do not produce an adequate response. Evidence suggests that lipid-lowering medication leads to 22–24% reduction of major cardiovascular complications, statins being the medication of choice, in patient with diabetes [4].

3.3.3 Antiplatelet Agents

Unless contraindicated, aspirin is the most commonly prescribed medication to prevent adverse cardiovascular events. When contraindicated, other antiplatelet agents are available for patients with high cardiovascular risks. Most common contraindications include allergic reactions to aspirin, bleeding, anticoagulant therapies, gastrointestinal bleeding, and clinically active hepatic disease.

Studies have demonstrated the benefits of aspirin as primary and secondary therapy to prevent cardiovascular events in both diabetic and nondiabetic patients, particularly on those at high risk [12–15]. The American Diabetes Association recommends a dose of 75–162 mg/day of aspirin as primary prevention therapy for patients with type II diabetes with increased cardiovascular risk, including patients over 40 years of age with additional risk factors e.g., hypertension, family history of CDV, smoking history [8].

3.3.4 Smoking Cessation

There is a high incidence of smoking-related deaths in the US in the general population, with even higher rates in diabetic patients. Several epidemiological studies have linked smoking with insulin resistance, an early and potentially modifiable metabolic defect in the pathogenesis of type II diabetes [16, 17]. They have also shown a correlation between tobacco consumption and the incidence of diabetes [18, 19], and cardiovascular complications [10, 20].

The routine assessment of tobacco use and smoking cessation counseling is of vital importance in the preventive care and long-term management of type II diabetes.

3.3.5 Coronary Heart Disease

Early identification and treatment of CAD in patients with diabetes is important for optimal prevention of cardiovascular events. Asymptomatic patients should be screened at least annually to determine the presence of any CAD symptoms. CHD risk factors include dyslipidemia, hypertension, smoking, family history of premature coronary disease, and presence of micro- or macroalbuminuria [8, 21].

Recommendations issued by the American Diabetes Association include the following [22]:

1. Evaluate patients based on the risk criteria outlined above
2. Refer patients with symptoms to cardiologist for further evaluation
3. Metformin is contraindicated in patients with treated congestive heart failure.
4. ACE inhibitors should be considered to reduce the risk of cardiovascular events in patients matching the following criteria:
   (a) Age older than 55 years
   (b) With or without hypertension
   (c) Presence of any of the following cardiovascular risk factors:
      - History of cardiovascular disease
      - Dyslipidemia
      - Microalbuminuria
      - Smoking
5. β-blockers should be considered in patients with prior myocardial infarction or in patients undergoing major surgery

3.3.6 Immunization

Although limited, epidemiological studies have demonstrated that patients with diabetes are at higher risk for complications, hospitalization, and death from influenza and pneumococcal disease, and may benefit from vaccination [23]. Immunization of diabetic patients has the potential of reducing hospital admissions during influenza epidemics and the morbidity and mortality related to these diseases. The Centers for Disease Control and Prevention recommend that all persons over 65 years of age, as well as all diabetic patients regardless of their age receive annual influenza and pneumococcal vaccinations [24]. Similarly, the American Diabetes Association recommends that [22]:

1. All diabetic patients 6 months of age and older should receive an influenza vaccine every year.
2. Adult patients with diabetes should receive at least one lifetime pneumococcal vaccination

3. One-time pneumococcal revaccination is recommended for
   (a) Patients older than 64 years of age, if they were immunized when they were < 65 years old, and the vaccine was administered more than five years ago
   (b) If patient suffers from
   - Nephrotic syndrome
   - Chronic renal failure
   - Immunocompromised

3.4 Long-Term Management

Type II diabetes is not an isolated disease, but rather, a complex metabolic abnormality often involving hypertension, obesity, dyslipidemia, renal function, and a spectrum of cardiovascular diseases. Appropriate management of diabetes requires multiple strategies aimed to improve the patient's glycaemic control, and minimize the risk of complications, based on individual preferences, comorbidities, and the overall prognosis. The key element for a successful outcome, however, is cooperation from the patient. Adequate information about the risks of diabetes and potential benefits of good self-management should be discussed with the patient. Basic guidelines for long-term management include diet and exercise therapies; blood glucose, blood pressure, and lipids management as described in Sect. 3.5.

Diabetes is a risk factor for micro- and macrovascular complications. Characteristic of diabetes, microvascular complications affect small blood vessels throughout the body, with particular danger in three sites: retina (diabetic retinopathy), renal glomerulus (diabetic kidney), and nerve sheaths (diabetic neuropathy). Macrovascular complications affect diabetics and nondiabetics alike. However, there is an excess risk to diabetics compared with the general population. For example, diabetics are twice as likely to suffer a stroke, myocardial infarction is 3–5 times more likely to occur to diabetics, and amputation of a foot due to gangrene is 50 times more likely. Diabetes-related risks for cardiovascular complications are additive to other risk factors, e.g., smoking, overweight, or Hyperlipidemia. We will further address these issues as part of surveillance strategies for the long-term management of diabetes.

Infections, trauma, myocardial infarction, surgery, and other common illnesses produce increased insulin resistance and worsen glycaemic control in diabetics. Hence, diabetic patients with intercurrent illnesses may require more frequent monitoring of blood glucose.

3.5 Management and Follow-up

3.5.1 Diet

Diet for diabetic patients is no different from a health diet for the regular population. Caloric intake should be tailored to the needs of the patient. Patients on insulin or oral agents should eat the same amount of food at the same time every day. Patients on insulin may require small snacks between meals and before bedtime to help maintain stable, healthy blood glucose levels and buffer the effect of injected insulin. Care should be taken in the consumption of alcohol and simple sugars. Alcohol intake may cause hypoglycemia, while refined sugars may cause rapid swings in blood glucose levels.

3.5.2 Physical Activity

Regular exercise helps weight control, improves blood glucose levels, and reduces the risk of cardiovascular diseases. An activity program adapted to the patient specific needs is recommended.

3.5.3 Self Blood Glucose Monitoring

Day-to-day glucose measurement provides an excellent assessment for glucose control, and the importance of regular measurements should be emphasized to the patient. If properly instructed, patients should be able to provide reasonably accurate results – and essential strategy for maintaining healthy blood glucose levels. Results should be evaluated regularly by health care providers.

3.5.4 Hyperglycemia

Glycaemic control is best assessed by reviewing both the patient's day-to-day self blood glucose monitoring results and the HA1C values. HA1C test represent the average blood sugar level for the previous 2–3 months [25]. The frequency for performing the HA1C test should be determined by the clinician based on the clinical status of a patient, and treatment options. The American Diabetes Association recommends that HA1C test should be performed at least twice a year in patients with stable glycaemic controls and quarterly in patients who do not meet their glycaemic goals [22].

3.5.5 Blood Pressure Management

As described above, hypertension is common comorbidity of diabetes. High blood pressure increases the risk of cardiovascular disease and microvascular complications. Maintaining a systolic blood pressure < 130 mmHg and diastolic pressure < 80 mmHg in diabetic persons is of great benefit [26,27]. Blood pressure should be measured at every visit. Drug therapy e.g., ACE inhibitors, ARBs, β-blockers, diuretics, and calcium channel blockers, in addition to behavioral and lifestyle changes is advised.

3.5.6 Lipids Management

As described in the corresponding section, patients with type II diabetes are particularly susceptible to lipid abnormalities. Lipid management strategies should be aimed at reducing LDL cholesterol, raising HDL cholesterol, and lowering triglycerides. Healthy lipid levels have shown to reduce the risk of cardiovascular complications and mortality. Lifestyle changes including nutritional changes, physical activity, smoking cessation, and weight loss should be considered as initial strategies to achieve lipid levels. Drug therapy including statins, fibrates, and niacin is indicated when lifestyle changes alone are ineffective.

Patients with healthy lipid levels should be tested once a year, while patients who do not meet the lipid goal levels should be monitored more often.

3.6 Surveillance

3.6.1 Nephropathy

Diabetic nephropathy is the kidney disease that occurs as a result of diabetes and is also a sign of worsening blood vessels throughout the body. It is a leading cause of end-stage renal disease in Europe and the USA. Albumin, a large blood protein, is an early marker for development of nephropathy in patients with type II diabetes. As nephropathy starts to develop, there is a progressive leak of large protein molecules from the kidneys into the urine.

It has been observed that patients who progress from microalbuminuria (albumin/creatinine ratio 3–299 $\mu g\ mg^{-1}$) to macroalbuminuria (albumin/creatinine ratio $\geq 300\ \mu g\ mg^{-1}$) are likely to progress to end-stage renal failure [28]. Healthy blood glucose levels have shown to delay the onset of microalbuminuria and the progression of microalbuminuria into macroalbuminuria in patients with type II diabetes [22]. Strategies for slowing the progression of diabetic nephropathy include managing hypertension [29], optimizing glycaemic control [14], and using angiotensin-converting enzyme (ACE) inhibitors or angiotensin receptor blockers (ARBs) [2, 30–32].

Continued surveillance is required to assess response to treatment and evolution of the disease. Recommendations by the American Diabetes Association include performing an annual test in all type II diabetes patients [22].

3.6.2 Eye Exam

Diabetes damages the blood vessels in the retina by increasing the thickness of the basement membrane and the permeability of the retinal capillaries. Normal blood glucose levels have shown to prevent and/or delay the onset of diabetic retinopathy [29]. Other contributing factors in the development of retinopathy in type II diabetics include high blood pressure, and nephropathy.

Patients with type II diabetes should have an initial comprehensive eye exam immediately after being diagnosed with diabetes, with regular, once-a-year examinations, unless retinopathy is progressing, in which case more frequent exams should be performed.

3.6.3 Foot Care

Diabetes can damage peripheral nervous tissue with the consequent loss of protective sensation. Increased risk factors include having diabetes for more than 10 years, being male, having poor glucose control, and having cardiovascular, renal or retinal complications. Patients should be advised to recognize early symptoms including loss of vibration sense, pain sensation, and temperature sensation in the feet.

The American Diabetes Association recommends a multidisciplinary approach to management of foot ulcers and high-risk feet, particularly those with a history of ulcers or amputations. High risk patients should be referred to specialists for preventive care and life-long surveillance. Initial screening should include a history for claudication and assessment of pedal pulses. An annual exam should be performed on diabetic patients to identify risk factors predictive of foot ulcers and amputations [22].

3.6.4 Antiplatelet Agents – Aspirin

Antiplatelet agents are part of disease prevention in diabetic patients at risk of developing cardiovascular complications and also part of the surveillance and long-term management of diabetes. The guideline for antiplatelet treatment is the same during preventive care and surveillance. For a description see corresponding antiplatelet agents in Sect. 3.3.

3.6.5 Blood Pressure Management

See Sect. 3.3.1, and Management and follow-up sections above.

3.6.6 Immunization

See Sect. 3.3.6.

3.7 Intercurrent Illnesses

Intercurrent illnesses may cause increased insulin resistance and worsen glycaemic control in diabetics. Early, newly developed symptoms should be promptly investigated and, if appropriate immediate care must be provided to prevent future complications. Any new treatments and the health condition of the patient should be closely followed.

This section presented an overview of relevant issues involved in the management of type II diabetes. Section 4 introduces the basic concepts and definitions for the UML 2 State Machine Diagrams.

4 UML 2 State Machine Diagrams

4.1 State Diagrams

State diagrams are a graphical representation of finite state machines. A finite state machine (FSM) or finite automaton models the behavior of a system in terms of states, transitions, and actions. An FSM is a tuple of the form:

$$\mathrm{FSM} = (S, \Sigma, S_0, \delta, \alpha) \qquad (1)$$

where S is a [finite] set of all possible states, S_0 is the initial state where $S_0 \in S, \Sigma$ is an alphabet with all possible symbols, $\delta = \Sigma x\, S \rightarrow S$ is a transition function that indicates a state change. The condition(s) for such a change to take place is defined by rule(s), and α is the set actions or behaviors to describe what is to be performed at a given state. An action can be one of the following:

- entry action – executed when entering a state
- exit action – executed when exiting a state
- input action – executed based on the current state and input conditions
- transition action – executed while a transition from a state to another is taking place

Figure 1 illustrates an FSM for turning on/off a lamp. It consists of two states: lamp on and lamp off; two transitions: lamp on → lamp off, and lamp off → lamp on. Transitions are triggered when the condition becomes true. The lamp is turned on/off as a result of an entry action to the corresponding state.

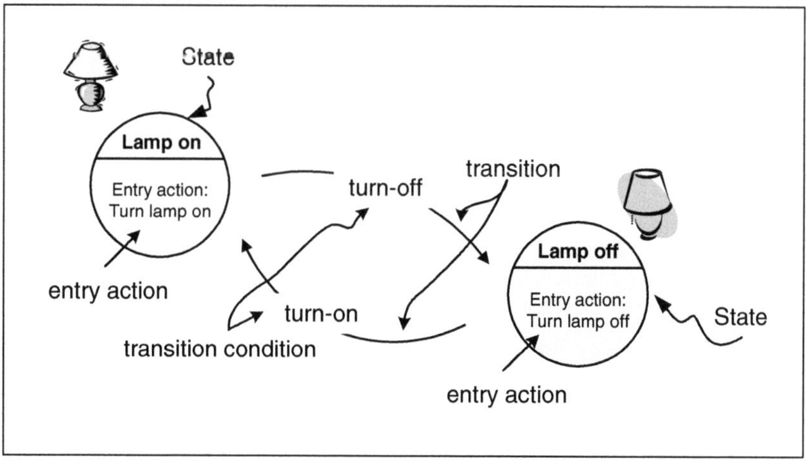

Fig. 1. Finite State Machine consisting of states, transitions and actions. The example shows a Finite State Machine for turning on/off a lamp. It consists of two states: Lamp On and Lamp Off; two transitions to change states, and two entry actions: "turn lamp on", and "turn lamp off"

4.2 UML Statecharts

The UML is a standard object modeling language that defines the notation and semantics often used for information and logical data modeling. In the context of the UML, classes are used to represent entities, exhibiting some sort of state behavior [33]. This behavior can be captured by state machines, or the UML equivalent, statecharts.

UML statecharts are used to model transitions from state to state as a result of a triggering event – represented by the transition condition. Like FSM, statecharts consist of three main elements: states, actions, and transitions.

A state is a condition during the life of an object. An object will remain in a state as long as it satisfies the given condition(s), performs some action or awaits the occurrence of an event. The graphic representation of a state is depicted in Fig. 2. The rounded rectangle with a name is most basic representation of a state (e.g., S1 in Fig. 2). A state, like S0 contains a name, and two substates with transitions. It also has a list of internal actions that are to be performed as in response to events. S0 has two actions: an entry and exit actions.

States can be refined as disjoint *or-states*, or as concurrent *and-states*. Unless otherwise indicated, states are considered *or-states*, meaning that an object can only be in one state at a given time. *And-states* however represent independent aspects of the same object, each modeled by a substate.

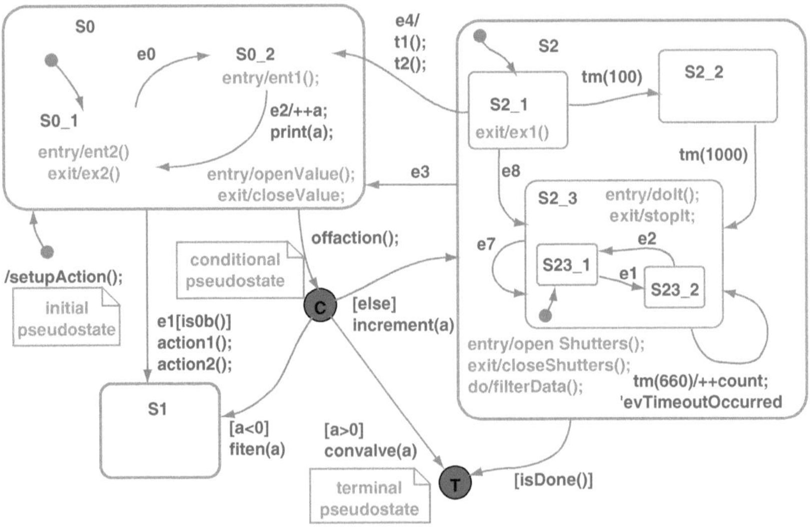

Fig. 2. Notation of a UML statechart (from [34]) consists of three main states (S0, S1, and S2) and several substates. Transitions depicted as arrows connecting states. Actions are indicated by name, and occur while entering, during or exiting a state, or during a transition

Pseudostates are notational devices used to indicate that an object may not be in such a state but must transit to an actual state. Normally, pseudostates are used to indicate the initial entry state of a state machine; dynamic choice points are used to decide the next state from various candidate states, based on the defined *guards*; history states to keep tract of the transitions of the state machine; termination pseudostates to close the state just existed; and final states to represent the completion of activity in a closing state. For example, in Fig. 2, there is an initial pseudostate at the bottom left-hand side of the diagram, a dynamic choice point indicated by the shaded circle with a C, and a termination point T.

Transitions are the means by which objects can change states if the conditions for the transition are satisfied. Transitions are the response of a state machine to events. For example, in Fig. 2, state S0_1 has a transition to S0_2. This transition will take place if and only if the event e0 occurs. Transitions affecting a superstate (e.g., S0) will apply at all levels inside that superstate. In other words, transitions affecting S0 will affect S0_1 and S0_2. In other words, transitions affecting a superstate are *inherited* by all its substates.

Transitions represent the response of a state machine to events. Events that are not explicitly defined and associated to a state are ignored. For example, only three events affect S0_1: e0, causing a transition to S0_2; e1, from the superstate S0, causing a transition to S1; and e5, also from superstate S0, causing a transition to the conditional pseudostate C.

Transitions can also be triggered by timeout events. For example, in Fig. 2, state S2 has a timer tm(660) event, which will trigger upon reaching the time limit, unless another event causes a transition.

In UML, there are four types of events:

- Signal event due to an external asynchronous process
- Call event caused by the execution of an operation/action within the object
- Change event caused by the change on the value of an attribute
- Time event due to the passage of time

The notation for events is as follows:

event-name (argument-list)-[guard()]/action-list,^ event-list

The *argument list* is enclosed within parenthesis, as in the case of the time event tm(660).

Guards are Boolean conditions written in terms of parameters of the triggering event, and are used as transition conditions. A transition takes place only if an event triggering that transition occurs, and the condition(s) specified by the guards is/are true. Guards can also be used in dynamic choice pseudostates to determine, based on which of the guards is true, the transition that will take place (see the dynamic choice pseudostate C in Fig. 2). Note that only one guard should evaluate to true.

Actions invoke operations that are executed if and when the transition fires. They are considered atomic and may not be interruptible. An action must be executed entirely before any other actions are considered. Actions are separated from the event guard by a "/." The action list may contain zero or more actions.

Actions can be associated with states, and when explicitly defined, they are executed in a predefined order: exit actions from source state are executed first, followed by transition actions, and finally entering actions at the target state.

This section presented an overview of finite state machines and UML 2 statecharts as means of graphically representing the behavior of objects in terms of states, transitions and actions. Section 5 describes the state model for management of type II diabetes we implemented using the aforementioned UML statecharts.

5 State Model for Management of Type II Diabetes

The proposed state model is a chronic disease state management system for the continuum of diabetes care. Developed by the Decision Systems Group at the Brigham & Women's Hospital, Boston, USA and the Clinical Knowledge Management Group at Partners HealthCare Systems, Inc., the state model aims to provide integrated care across the entire spectrum of the disease and its complications, and the prevention of comorbidities.

The clinical expertise reflected in the state model has been developed by Partners HealthCare Systems, Inc. and is consistent with national [1,8,22,24] and international [14, 29, 35] standards of care. The rest of this section is devoted to the description of the state model, starting with a high-level view of the system, followed by a description of each state and substates. The graphic representation and semantic interpretation of the model is consistent with that of the UML 2.0 statechart described in Sect. 4.2.

5.1 State Model – First-Level and Second-Level States

In this section we describe the state model at two levels of granularity. The first level consists of two main states: diabetes preventive care and diabetes long-term management (top and bottom of Fig. 3, respectively). Each main state consists of three substates (second level).

The diabetes preventive care state (top half of Fig. 3) focuses on providing regular screening for early detection of symptoms and complications; initial diagnosis of type II diabetes; and preventive services to help patients develop and maintain healthy lifestyle habits, and minimize the risk for complications.

The diabetes long-term management (bottom half of Fig. 3) focuses on the long-term management of diabetes, regular monitoring (surveillance) for early detection and management of diabetes-related complication, as well as regular monitoring for diagnosis, treatment, and follow-up of intercurrent illnesses.

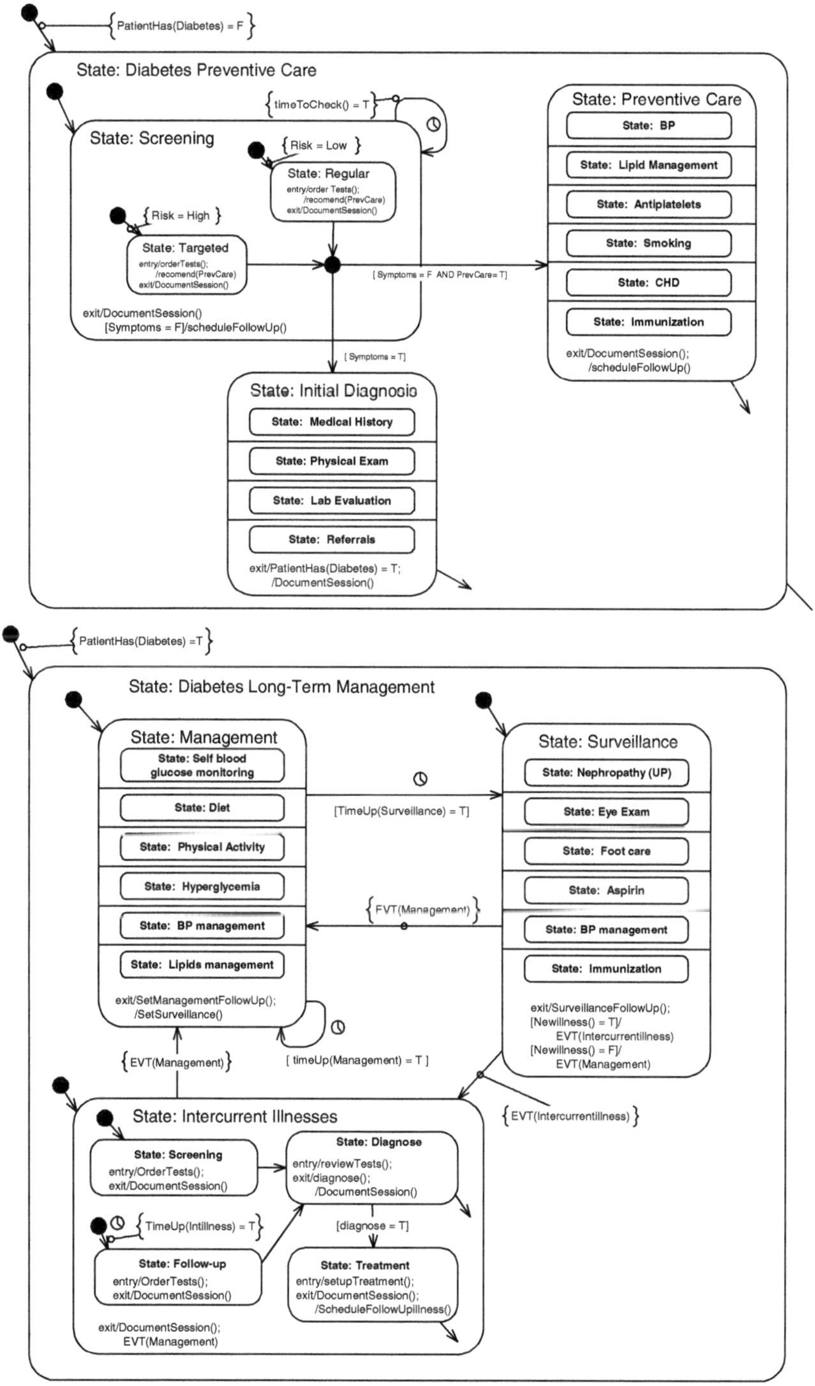

Fig. 3. High-level view of the state model for management of type II diabetes. There are two main states: diabetes preventive care and diabetes long-term management

Note that both main states have a guard used as a transition condition to enter each state. The guard {PatientHas(Diabetes) = F} allows a patient to enter the diabetes preventive care state – she/he has not been diagnosed with diabetes. However, the moment a patient is diagnosed with diabetes, the Boolean value of this guard will automatically change to {PatientHas(Diabetes) = T} as an exit action of the initial diagnosis state. This will trigger the transition of the patient to the diabetes long-term management state. This is explained in more detail in the following paragraphs.

5.1.1 Diabetes Preventive Care

The diabetes preventive care state consists of three substates: screening, preventive care, and initial diagnosis.

Screening

The screening state contains two substates: Regular, aimed at low-risk patients – as indicated by the guard {Risk = Low}; and Targeted {Risk = High}, aimed at high-risk patients. The risk level is determined by the criteria described in the Sect. 2 dedicated to diabetes mellitus. Inside both states similar actions are performed.

Upon entering the regular – and the targeted – state, a series of tests are ordered, as indicated by the entry event entry/orderTests(). If applicable preventive care is recommended/recommend(PrevCare). The session is documented on exiting the state.

Both states converge at a dynamic choice pseudostate. If a patient has no symptoms and preventive care of some sort is recommended (transition with guard [Symptoms = F AND PrevCare = T]), the patient will leave the current state and will enter the preventive care state. However, if the patient presents any symptoms consistent with diabetes ([Symptoms = T]), she/he will enter the initial diagnosis state, where she/he will be diagnosed and will move into long-term management. Note that when exiting the screening state two actions are carried out: the session is documented, and if the patient has no symptoms, a follow-up is scheduled. This action is indicated by [Symptoms = F]/scheduleFollowUp(). scheduleFollowUp() sets up a timer that eventually will trigger the event TimeToCheck(), recalling the patient for another screening procedure.

Preventive Care

The preventive care state consists of six concurrent substates: BP for blood pressure management, lipid management, antiplatets, smoking, CHD, and immunization. These states will be described in detail in the following sections.

There are two actions that are executed while leaving the preventive care state: exit/DocumentSession(), and /scheduleFollowUp(), the latter sets up a timer for a future screening session.

Initial Diagnosis

The Initial Diagnosis state consists of four concurrent substates aimed at reviewing the medical history of the patient, performing a physical exam, laboratory evaluation, and scheduling the appropriate referrals. Upon exiting the state the session is documented and the guard PatientHas(Diabetes) is set to T. This guard will trigger the transition event from the diabetes preventive care state to the diabetes long-term management state.

5.1.2 Diabetes Long-Term Management

The diabetes long-term management state consists of three substates: management, surveillance, and intercurrent illnesses. A patient will enter, and remain in this state when the guard PatientHas(Diabetes) becomes true.

Management

The management state consists of six concurrent substates: self blood glucose monitoring, diet, physical activity, hyperglycemia, blood pressure management, and lipid management. These states will be described in detail in the following sections. The management state has two exit actions, both setting up timers for upcoming management and surveillance visits: exit/SetManagementFollowUp(), and /SetSurveillance().

Surveillance

The surveillance state consists of six concurrent substates: nephropathy, eye exam, foot care, antiplatelets – aspirin, BP management, and immunization. These states are described in detail in the upcoming sections. exit/SurveillanceFollowUp() sets up a timer for a future surveillance visit. This action is executed upon exiting the Surveillance state. There are also two guards that, if true, will trigger two different transition events: [NewIllness() = T]/EVT (IntercurrentIllness) triggers a transition event to the intercurrent illnesses state if there is a new illness that needs to be treated. Note that the transition to the Intercurrent Illnesses state is guarded by {EVT(IntercurrentIllness)}, which has to be true so the transition can take place. Similarly, [NewIllness() = F]/EVT(Management) triggers a transition event back to the management state, since there are no new illnesses detected. The transition from Surveillance back to management is guarded by {EVT(Management)}.

Intercurrent Illnesses

The Intercurrent Illnesses state consists of four substates: screening, diagnose, treatment, and follow-up. They are described below. Upon exiting this state, two actions take place: exit/DocumentSession(), and EVT(Management). The latter triggers a transition event from this state back to the management state. The transition is guarded by {EVT(Management)} which has to be true for the transition to take place.

5.2 Preventive Care Substates

5.2.1 BP State

The BP state in Fig. 4 monitors and manages hypertension. This state is part of the preventive care, diabetes/management, and diabetes/surveillance substates. The criteria for monitoring and managing high blood pressure are the same in all three states. We will describe the BP state in detail in this section and will refer the reader back here where appropriate.

The BP overdue state is triggered if a patient's blood pressure has not been checked. Upon entering the state, the patient's blood pressure is measured by the action entry/takeBP() and the reading is recorded exit/record(BP). Abnormal BP values systolic $>$ 130 or diastolic $>$ 80, will trigger a transition to the BP $>$ Goal state, guarded by {Systolic BP $>$ 130 or diastolic BP $>$ 80}.

Upon entering the BP $>$ Goal state, several actions take place, all aimed at regulating the patient's blood pressure. These actions include lifestyle modifications, laboratory tests to evaluate specific markers, drug therapies, and referrals to specialists for further treatment. The session is documented on exiting the state.

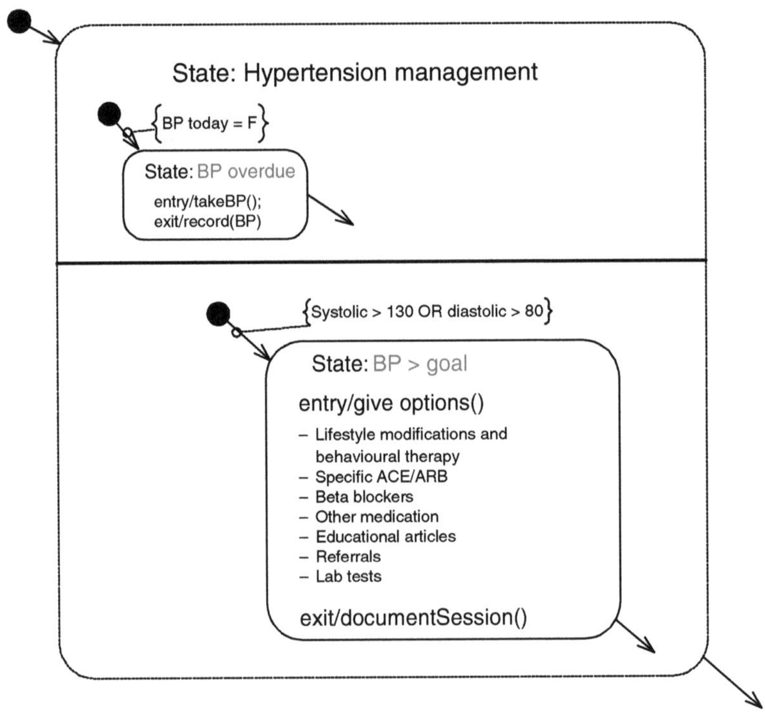

Fig. 4. Blood Pressure (BP) State. It consists of two substates aimed at monitoring and managing a patient's blood pressure

5.2.2 Lipid Management

- Patients with type II diabetes are particularly susceptible to lipid abnormalities. The lipid management state in Fig. 5 consists of a series of strategies for monitoring lipid levels, reducing LDL cholesterol, raising HDL cholesterol and lowering triglycerides:
  - *Lipids Monitoring.* A patient enters the lipids monitoring state in Fig. 6 if she/he has CAD, as denoted by the guard {PatientHas(CAD) = T}. This state consists of four concurrent states. The top two states check for overdue lipid exams. The lipids' 1 year follow up state schedules a follow-up visit, while lipids panel overdue presents a series of lipid test options. Note that all these substates have PatientHas(CAD) = T as part of their guards. This is redundant, since as described in the UML 2.0 statechart section, all substates inherit the guards of a superstate. However, this condition was included in the guards for the sake of clarity.
  - *LDL > Goal.* LDL > Goal state in Fig. 7 is formed by seven concurrent substates aimed at managing medication and referral strategies to help lowering LDL levels. These states contain the appropriate criteria for prescribing and/or adjusting the dose of a medication. Due to space limitations, from the seven concurrent states, only the Patient not on Statins state is depicted in Fig. 8. A patient will enter this state if she/he has CAD AND the LDL value > 100 AND the patient is not on statins, AND statins are not contraindicated, OR if the patient's LDL value > 100 AND the patient is not on statins, AND statins are not contraindicated, as illustrated by the state guard. Upon entering the state, a series of prescription options are presented. When exiting the state, the session is documented.

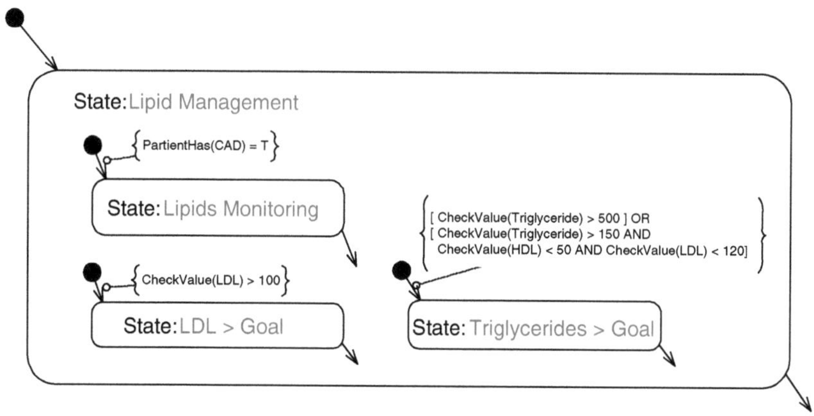

Fig. 5. Lipids management state consisting of three substates for monitoring lipids, and managing LDL cholesterol and triglycerides levels

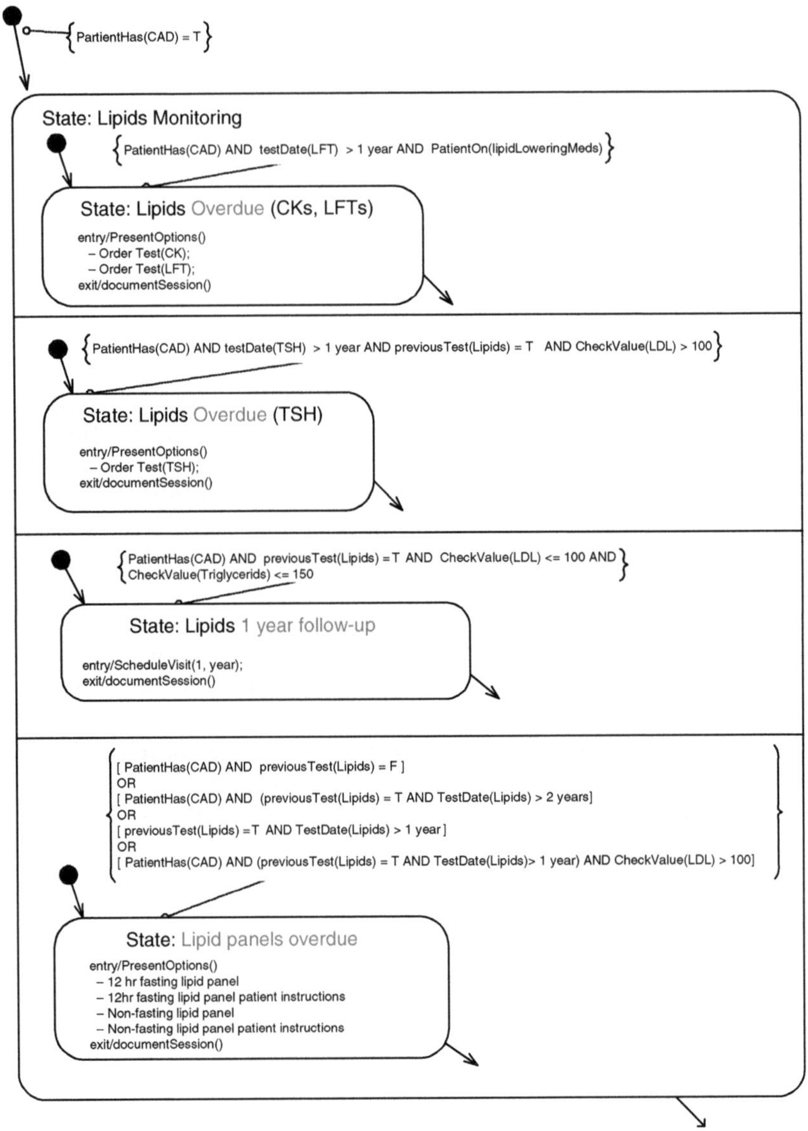

Fig. 6. Lipids monitoring state. This is a substate of the lipids management state depicted in Fig. 5. It consists of four concurrent states aimed at performing overdue lipids and lipid panel exams, and scheduling follow-up visits

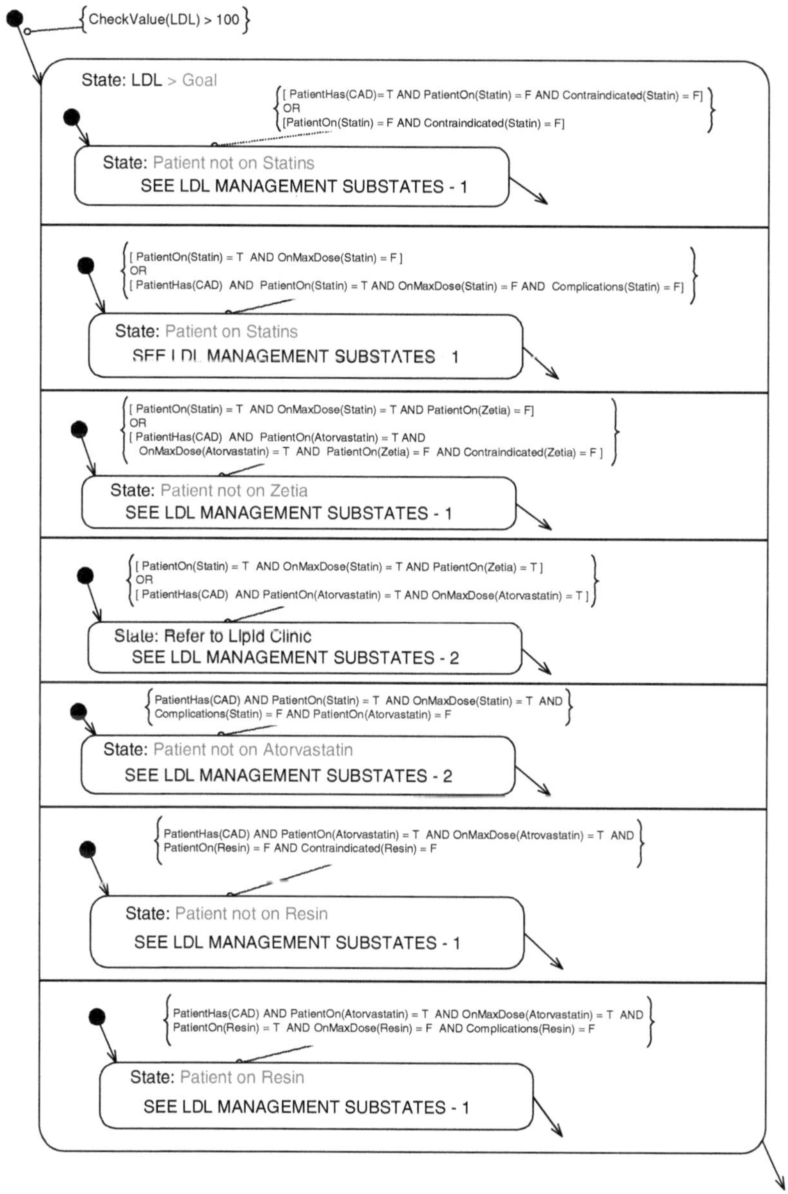

Fig. 7. LDL > Goal state. This state is formed by seven concurrent substates; all aimed at managing medication and referral strategies to help lowering LDL levels

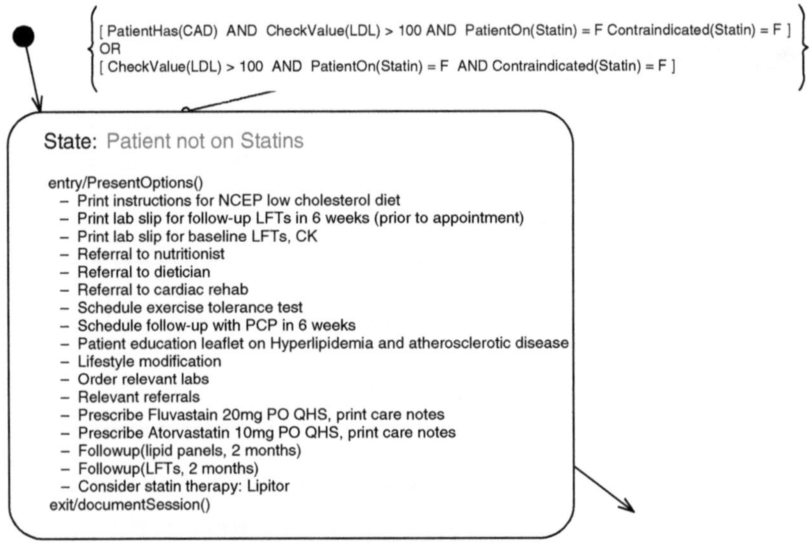

Fig. 8. Patient not on Statins substate is a concurrent state in LDL > Goal state. Upon entering the state, a series of prescription options are presented. When exiting the state, the session is documented

- *Triglycerides > Goal.* Triglycerides > Goal state in Fig. 9 is formed by seven concurrent states of suitable medication therapies and lifestyle modifications intended to lowering a patient's triglycerides levels. A state guard will allow a patient to enter the state if the triglycerides value is > 500 OR if the triglycerides are > 150 and the HDL Cholesterol is < 50 AND the LDL Cholesterol is < 120. At each substate, a series of medication options, dosages, laboratory tests, and lifestyle changes are presented. Due to space limitations they are not presented.

5.2.3 Antiplatelet Agents – Aspirin

The Aspirin (antiplatelet agents) state in Fig. 10 consists of two substates. A patient is not eligible for aspirin therapy if she/he suffers from MI, VB Surgery, Stroke, TIA, PVD, Claudication, or Angina, is allergic to aspirin, suffers from bleeding, recent GI bleeding, has a clinically active hepatic disease, or is on anticoagulant therapy – as described by the aspirin contraindicated state.

On the other hand, a patient is eligible for aspirin treatment if she/he is older than 40 years, has family history of CDV, suffers from hypertension, is a smoker, has dyslipidemia or albuminuria, and she/he is not allergic to aspirin, has no bleeding, no recent GI bleeding, has no clinically active hepatic disease, and is not on anticoagulant therapy.

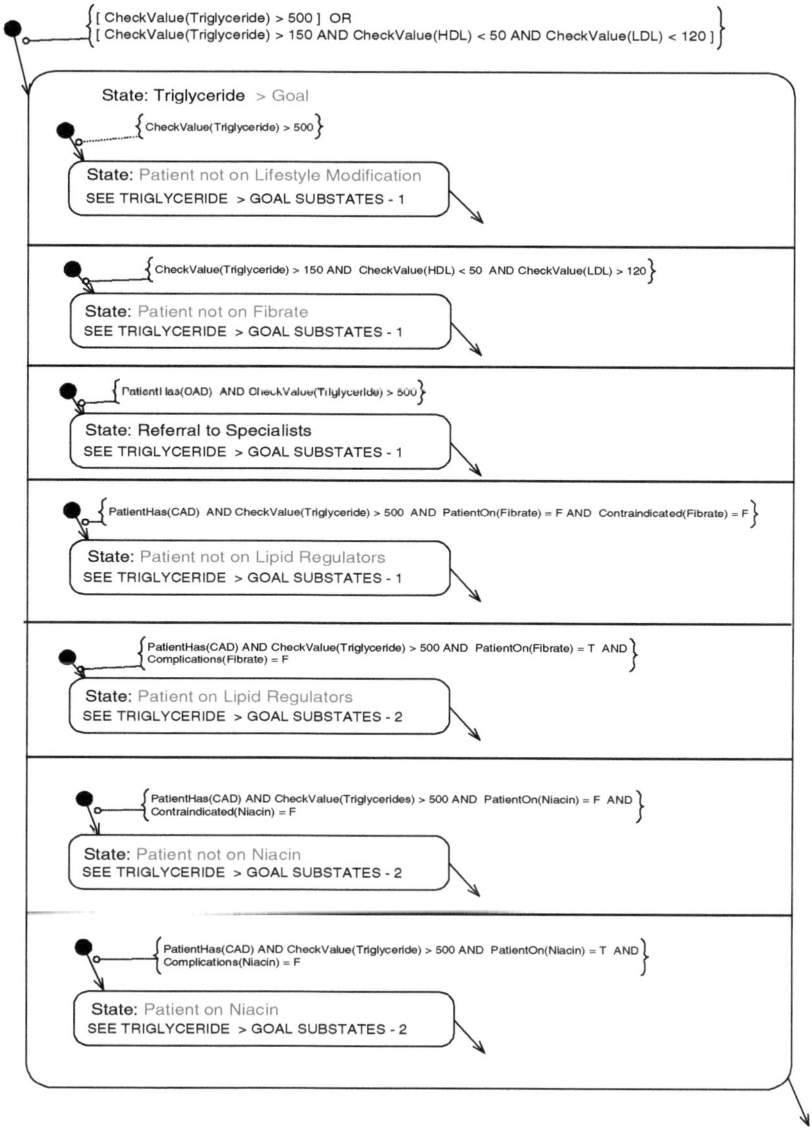

Fig. 9. Triglycerides > Goal state consists of seven concurrent states of medication therapies and lifestyle changes to lower triglycerides levels

5.2.4 Smoking

The Smoking state in Fig. 11 presents upon entering a series of options ranging from counseling and behavioral changes to medication. A patient enters the state if she/he is a smoker. The session is documented when patient exits the state.

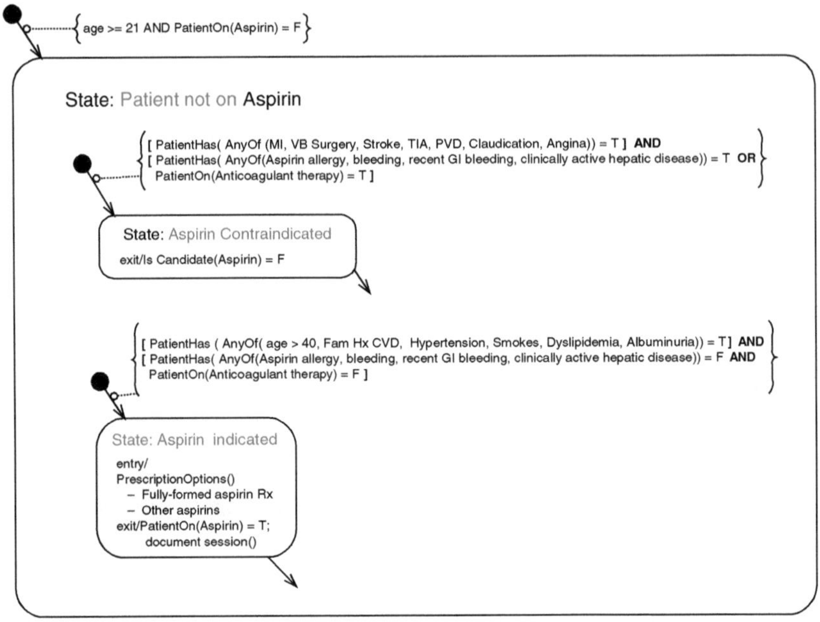

Fig. 10. Antiplatelet agents – Aspirin State. Unless contraindicated, aspirin is the antiplatelet agent to prescribe

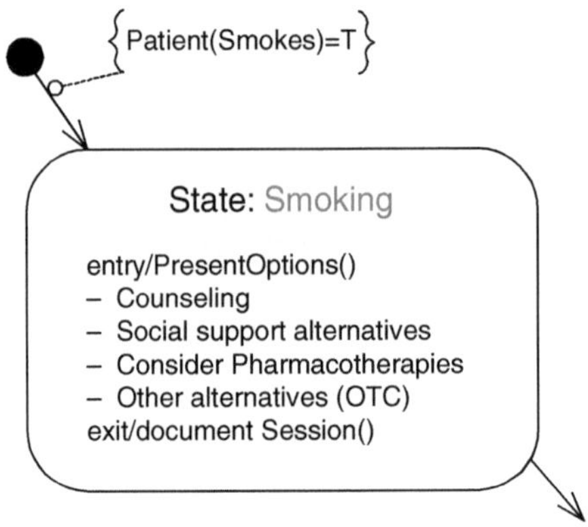

Fig. 11. Smoking state. Upon entering a series of options ranging from counseling and behavioral changes to medication are presented. The session is documented when patient exits the state

5.2.5 Coronary Heart Disease (CHD)

The CHD state in Fig. 12 evaluates information provided by the other concurrent states in the preventive care state, and if appropriate, the patient is referred to a specialist. All the necessary information about risk factors is provided by the BP, lipids management, antiplatelet agents, and smoking states.

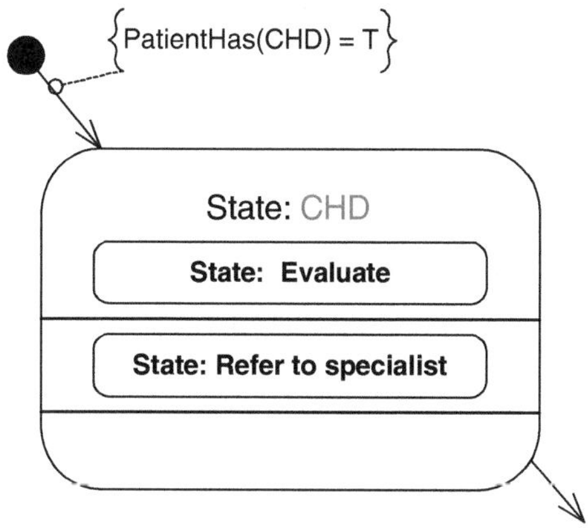

Fig. 12. The Coronary Heart Disease (CHD) State evaluates information provided by the other concurrent states in the preventive care state, and if appropriate, refers the patient to a specialist

5.2.6 Immunization

The immunization state in Fig. 13 consists of two states that check for overdue Pneumococcal and flu vaccinations. If immunization is appropriate, the patient is vaccinated and the session is documented.

5.3 Management Substates

5.3.1 Self Blood Glucose Monitoring

The Self Blood Glucose Monitoring in Fig. 14 contains two substates: monitoring overdue that becomes active if a patient misses a glucose measurement. Upon entering the state, a patient measures the glucose level. When leaving the state she/he records the glucose value. A patient enters the Glucose > Goal state if she/he has abnormal glucose levels for the time of the day – as indicated by the guard.

5.3.2 Diet

Diet is the first line of treatment for patients with type II diabetes. A Patient enters the diet state (not shown) when she/he requires diet therapy to maintain good glycaemic levels.

5.3.3 Physical Activity

Physical activity is essential in managing diabetes. A patient will enter this state (not shown) as part of a maintenance regime designed to control glycaemic levels, and weight, and to reduce the risk of cardiovascular complications.

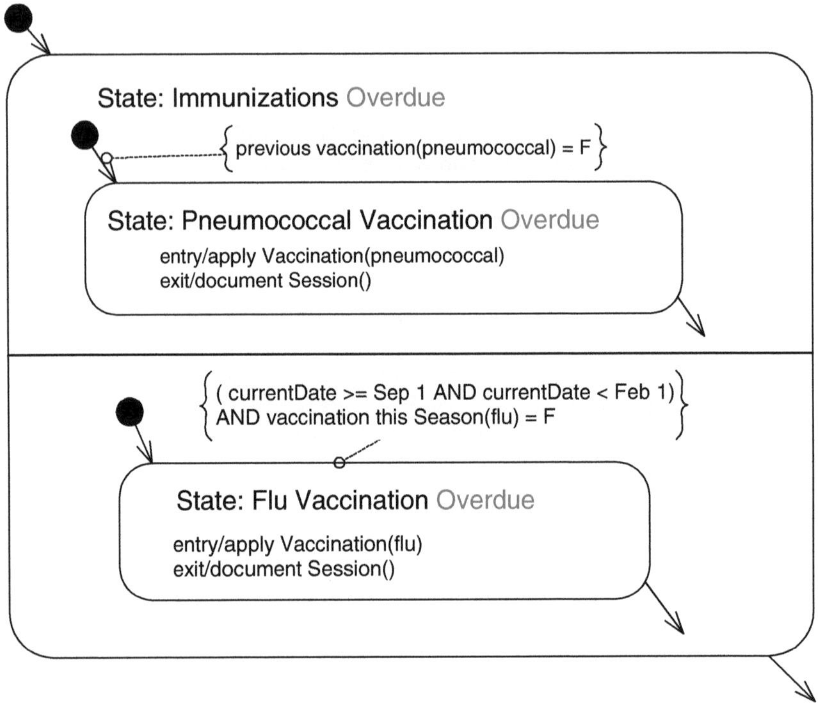

Fig. 13. Immunization State. If the patient is overdue, the appropriate vaccinations are administered and the session is documented

5.3.4 Hyperglycemia

Hyperglycemia is the hallmark of diabetes. All patients with type II diabetes need careful monitoring and management of glucose levels. The Hyperglycemia state is divided in two large substates aimed at monitoring and regular testing for HA1C (Fig. 15) and treatment with medication therapies and insulin (Fig. 16).

A patient enters the Hyperglycemia Monitoring – HA1C Overdue state if she/he has no record of previous HA1C tests (e.g., when first diagnosed with diabetes), or if the last test was normal but it was performed more than six months ago, or if the last test was performed more than 3 months ago and the HA1C result was $> 7\%$ (the recommended maximum value). Upon entering the state a HA1C test is performed, and when leaving the state, the session is documented.

A patient enters the Hyperglycemia Monitoring – Follow-up HA1C state if the last HA1C result was normal (HA1C $<= 7\%$) and the test was performed between 3 and 6 months to the date; or the test was performed less than 3 months to the date. Upon entering the state a follow up exam is scheduled and on exit, the session is documented.

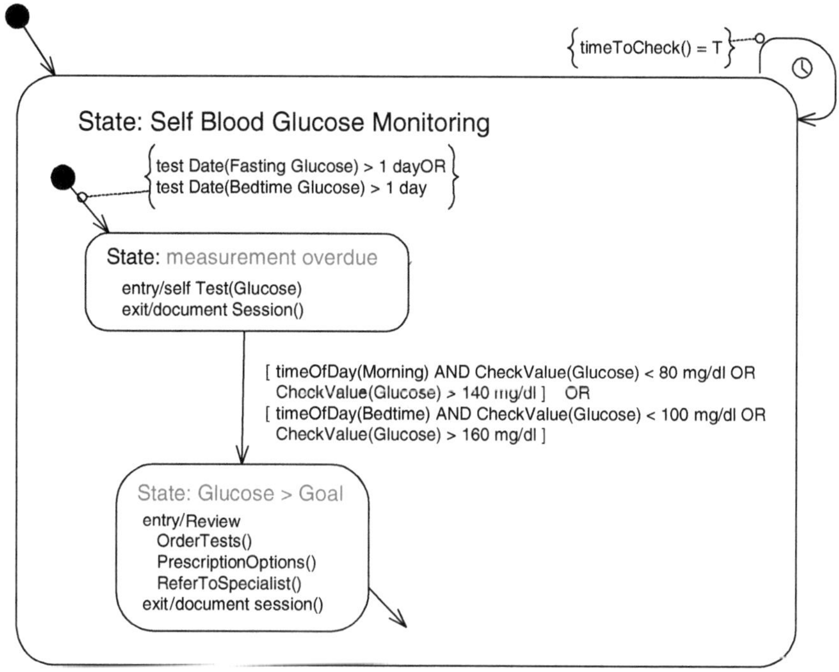

Fig. 14. Self blood glucose monitoring state. This state has a timer to regulate the frequency of testing. A patient enters the measurement overdue state if a measurement is missing. A transition event is triggered if the measured glucose value is above goal. This is determined by the time of the day the measurement was taken and the corresponding glucose values

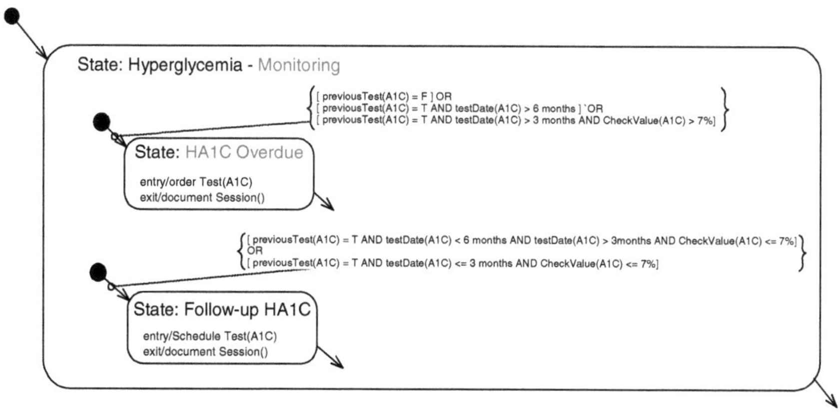

Fig. 15. Hyperglycemia monitoring state is a substate of Hyperglycemia devised to regularly measure HA1C levels in patients, and to schedule timely follow-ups

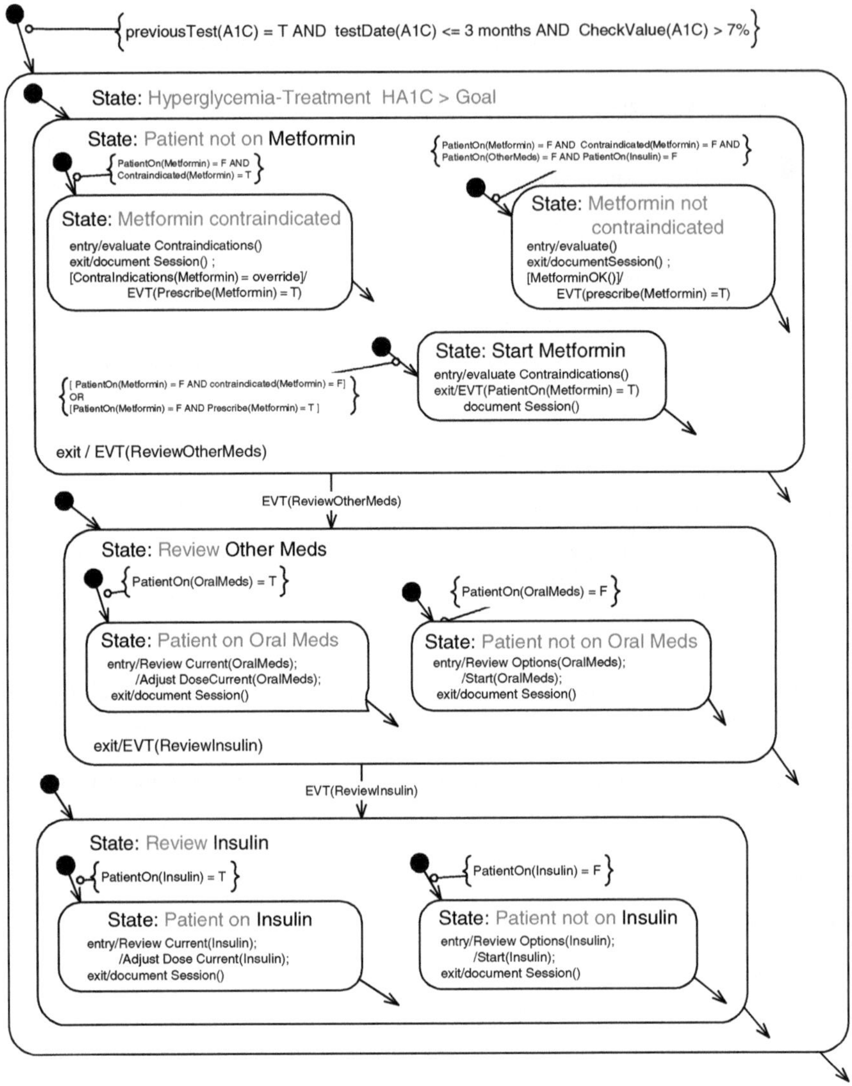

Fig. 16. Hyperglycemia Treatment – HA1C > Goal State is formed by three substates to devise the most appropriate medication and insulin treatments for a patient with abnormally high HA1C levels

A patient enters the Hyperglycemia Treatment HA1C > Goal state (Fig. 16) if the last HA1C result was abnormal and the test was performed 3 months ago or less. Unless contraindicated, a patient starts treatment with Metformin by entering the Patient not on Metformin state. Upon exiting the session is documented and a transition event EVT(ReviewOtherMeds) is triggered, and the patient moves into the Review Other Meds state where current oral medication doses are re-evaluated (Patient on Oral Meds), or additional oral medications are considered (Patient not on Oral Meds). Upon exiting, the EVT(ReviewInsulin) is triggered. If appropriate, the patient starts an insulin regime, or if she/he is currently taking insulin, the dosage is revised.

5.3.5 BP Management

See Sect. 3.3.1.

5.3.6 Lipid Management

See Sect. 3.3.2.

5.4 Surveillance Substates

5.4.1 Nephropathy (UP)

The Nephropathy (Urine Protein) state consists of two substates aimed at monitoring and regular testing for Urine Protein (top state in Fig. 17) and treatment with medication therapies for patients with abnormal ratio values of Ualb/Crea (bottom state in Fig. 17). A patient enters the Urine Protein Overdue state if she/he suffers from diabetic retinopathy, micro-albumia, end-renal disease, CRF, renal insufficiency, or acute renal failure or the patient is under dialysis, hemodialysis, or peritoneal dialysis; or if the patient has no record of previous Ualb/Cre tests or if the latest test that was performed is more than one-year old. Upon entering the state, a Ualb/Cre laboratory exam is ordered. Prior to leaving the state, the session is documented.

A Patient enters the Ualb/Cre Ratio > Goal state if she/he has Ualb/Crea Ratio > 30. If a patient is currently on ACE inhibitors or Angiotensin II Receptor Blocker (ARB) (Patient on Renal Meds), the prescription options are revised and medications are re-evaluated, dosages are adjusted. Also, other medications are considered and appropriate tests are ordered. If necessary, the patient is referred to a specialist and patient education is provided. If the patient is not on renal medication, treatment options include starting drug therapy with ACE or ARB medications, and considering other medications. Appropriate lab tests are ordered, patient information is provided, and she/he is referred to a specialist. Upon leaving, the session is documented.

Patients starting or currently taking renal medications are scheduled for follow-up test, and consequent orders in a timely manner. Upon leaving the state, the session is documented.

5.4.2 Eye Exam

The eye exam state in Fig. 18 checks for overdue eye examinations. If appropriate, the patient is referred to an ophthalmologist or optometrist for a comprehensive exam and the session is documented.

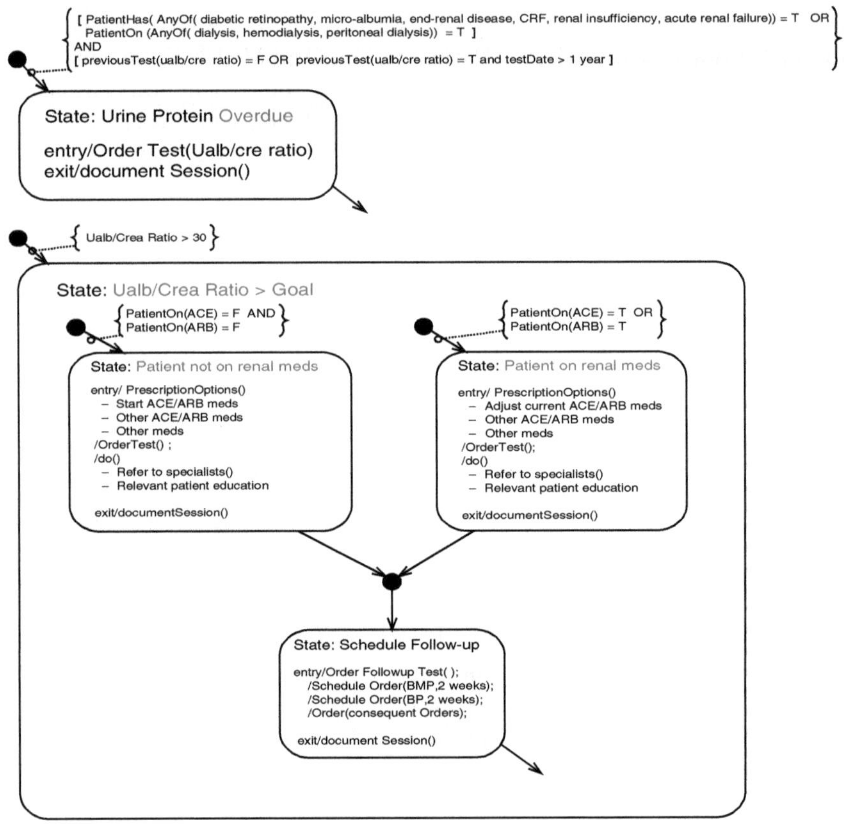

Fig. 17. Nephropathy State is formed by two substates devised to regularly measure urine protein (UP), and provide appropriate medication treatment, and regular follow-up evaluations

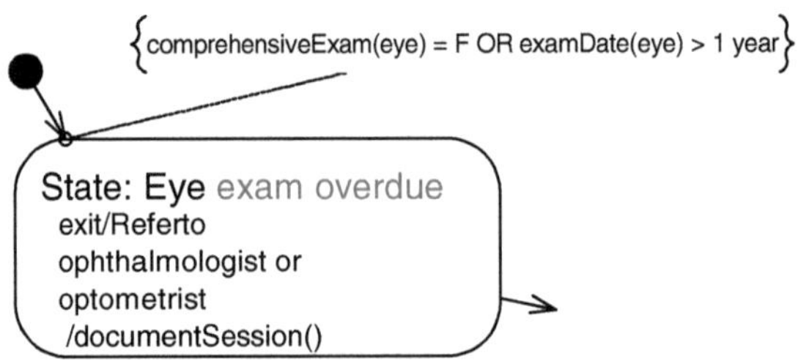

Fig. 18. Eye Exam State. A patient enters this state if an eye exam is overdue or has never been performed

5.4.3 Foot care

A patient enters the foot care state (Fig. 19) if she/he is overdue for a foot exam or has never had one. Upon entering the state a clinician is reminded

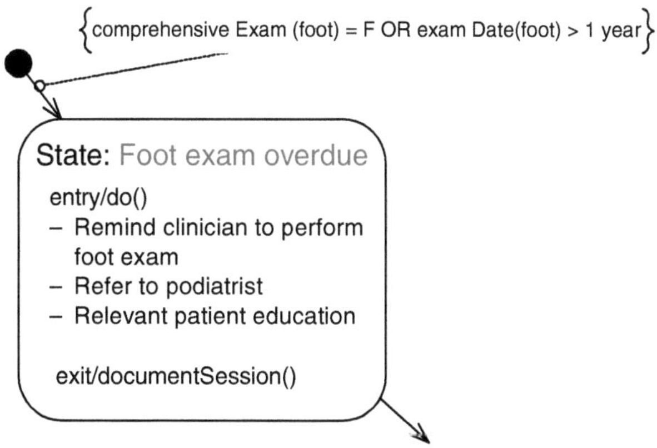

Fig. 19. Foot Exam State. A patient enters this state if a foot exam is overdue

to perform the exam, provide relevant educational information to the patient and refer her/him to a podiatrist for a comprehensive exam. Before leaving the state the session is documented.

5.4.4 Antiplatelets – Aspirin

See Sect. 3.3.3.

5.4.5 BP management

See Sect. 3.3.1.

5.4.6 Immunization

See Sect. 3.3.6.

5.5 Intercurrent Illnesses Substates

The Intercurrent Illnesses State in Fig. 20 focuses on monitoring for newly developed symptoms that may require investigation and immediate care to prevent future complications. Any new treatments and the patient's health should be closely followed.

A patient enters this state when a transition event is generated by the surveillance state. Upon entering, a series of tests are ordered and reviewed, and if appropriate, treatment is started. Follow-ups are scheduled in a timely manner to monitor patient's health. Before leaving the state and substates, each session is documented.

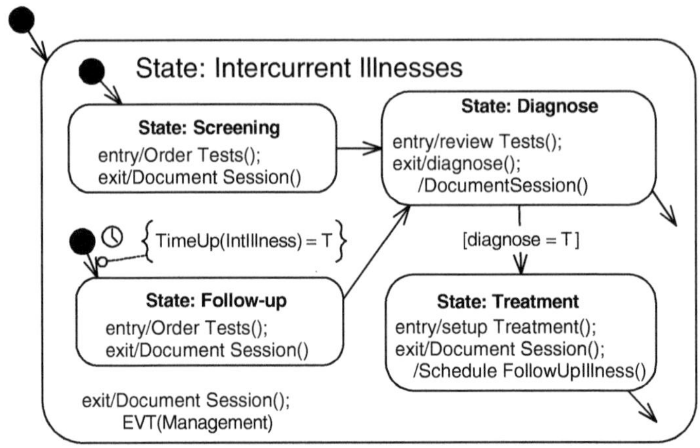

Fig. 20. Intercurrent Illnesses State consists of four states aimed a regularly screening for new symptoms, diagnosing, and treating new diseases and providing regular follow-up

6 Summary

We believe that systematic education and disease management of patients with chronic conditions like type II diabetes is an effective way of improving the quality, safety, and efficiency of provided care. Our synergistic approach integrates patient care and education protocols at all levels of disease management, and supports the integration of evidence-based personalized care. Further, we believe that our approach could be easily adapted to managing other chronic conditions e.g., hypertension, asthma, and coronary artery disease.

Our approach departs from the traditional acute, episodic illness treatment towards a more integrated system that provides a continuum of care. We envision that the implementation of the proposed state model for long-term management of type II diabetes will result in a more efficient use of health care resources, and a decrease is healthcare costs.

Acknowledgments

This project was supported by a grant from the Partners Health Care Information Systems Research Council.

References

1. National Center for Chronic Disease Prevention and Health Promotion. National Diabetes Surveillance System. http://www.cdc.gov/diabetes/statistics/prev/national/index.htm

2. Appel GB. Improved outcomes in nephrotic syndrome. Cleve Clin J Med. 2006; 73(2):161–167. Review
3. Diabetes Disparities among Racial and Ethnic Minorities. Agency for Healthcare Research and Quality Fact Sheet. Accessed at http://www.ahrq.gov/research/diabdisp.htm
4. Snow V, Aronson MD, Hornbake ER, Mottur-Pilson C, Weiss KB. Lipid control in the management of type 2 diabetes mellitus: a clinical practice guideline from the American College of Physicians. Ann Intern Med. 2004; 140(8):644–649
5. Vijan S, Hayward RA. Treatment of hypertension in type 2 diabetes mellitus: blood pressure goals, choice of agents, and setting priorities in diabetes care. Ann Intern Med. 2003; 138:593–602
6. Vijan S, Hayward RA. Pharmacologic lipid-lowering therapy in type 2 diabetes mellitus: background paper for the American College of Physicians. Ann Intern Med. 2004; 140:650–658
7. Clinical Informatics Research and Development (CIRD). Partners Healthcare. http://www.partners.org/cird/AboutUs.asp
8. American Diabetes Association. Consensus development conference on the diagnosis of coronary heart disease in people with diabetes (Consensus Statement). Dia Care. 1998; 21:1551–1559
9. Curb JD, Pressel SL, Cutler JA, Savage PJ, Applegate WB, Black H, Camel G, Davis BR, Frost PH, Gonzalez N, Guthrie G, Oberman A, Rutan GH, Stamler J. Effect of diuretic-based antihypertensive treatment on cardiovascular disease risk in older diabetic patients with isolated systolic hypertension. Systolic hypertension in the Elderly Program Cooperative Research Group. JAMA. 1996; 276(23):1886–1892. Erratum in: JAMA 1997; 277(17):1356
10. Fuller J, Stevens LK, Chaturvedi N, Holloway JF. Antihypertensive therapy for preventing cardiovascular complications in people with diabetes mellitus. Cochrane Database Syst Rev. 2000; (2):CD002188
11. Staessen JA, Thijs L, Fagard R, Celis H, Birkenhager WH, Bulpitt CJ, de Leeuw PW, Fletcher AE, Forette F, Leonetti G, McCormack P, Nachev C, O'Brien E, Rodicio JL, Rosenfeld J, Sarti C, Tuomilehto J, Webster J, Yodfat Y, Zanchetti A. Systolic hypertension in Europe (Syst-Eur) trial investigators. Effects of immediate versus delayed antihypertensive therapy on outcome in the systolic hypertension in Europe trial. J Hypertens. 2004; 22(4):847–857
12. Hayden M, Pignone, M, Phillips C, Mulrow C. Aspirin for the primary prevention of cardiovascular events: A summary of the evidence for the U.S. preventive services task force. Ann Intern Med. 2002; 136:161–172
13. Parving HH, Lehnert H, Brochner-Mortensen J, Gomis R, Andersen S, Arner P. Irbesartan in patients with type 2 diabetes and Microalbuminuria Study Group. The effect of irbesartan on the development of diabetic nephropathy in patients with type 2 diabetes. N Engl J Med. 2001; 345(12):870–878
14. UK Prospective Diabetes Study Group. Efficacy of atenolol and captopril in reducing risk of macrovascular and microvascular complications in type 2 diabetes: UKPDS 39. UK Prospective Diabetes Study Group. BMJ 1998; 317:713–720
15. US Preventive Services Task Force: Aspirin for the primary prevention of cardiovascular events: recommendation and rationale. Ann Intern Med. 2002; 136: 157–160
16. Barret-Connor E, Khaw K-T. Cigarette smoking and increased central adiposity. Ann Intern Med. 1989; 111:783–787

17. Facchini FS, Hollenbeck CB, Jeppesen J, Chen YD, Reaven GM. Insulin resistance and cigarette smoking. Lancet. 1992; 339:1128–1130
18. Kawakami N, Takatsuka N, Shimizu H, Ishibashi H. Effects of smoking on the incidence of non-insulin-dependent diabetes mellitus. Am J Epidemiol. 1997; 145:103–109
19. Rimm EB, Chan J, Stampfer MJ, Colditz GA, Willett WC. Prospective study of cigarette smoking, alcohol use, and the risk of diabetes in men. BMJ 1995; 310:555–559
20. Bazzano LA, He J, Muntner P, Vupputuri S, Whelton PK. Relationship between cigarette smoking and novel risk factors for cardiovascular disease in the United States. Ann Intern Med. 2003; 138(11):891–897
21. Leiter LA, Fitchett D. Optimal care of cardiovascular disease and type 2 diabetes patients: Shared responsibilities between the cardiologist and diabetologist. Atheroscler Suppl. 2006; 7(1):37–42
22. American Diabetes Association. Standards of medical care in diabetes. Dia Care. 2004; 27(Suppl. 1): S15–S35
23. Smith SA, Poland GA: The use of influenza and pneumococcal vaccines in people with diabetes (Technical Review). Dia Care. 2000; 23:95–108
24. Centers for Disease Control and Prevention. Advisory Committee on Immunization Practices (ACIP): Prevention and control of influenza: Recommendations of the Advisory Committee on Immunization Practices (ACIP). http://www.cdc.gov/
25. Sacks DB, Bruns DE, Goldstein DE, Maclaren NK, McDonald JM, Parrott M. Guidelines and recommendations for laboratory analysis in the diagnosis and management of diabetes mellitus. Clin Chem. 2002; 48(3):436–472
26. Chobanian AV, Bakris GL, Black HR, Cushman WC, Green LA, Izzo JL Jr, Jones DW, Materson BJ, Oparil S, Wright JT Jr, Roccella EJ; Joint National Committee on Prevention, Detection, Evaluation, and Treatment of High Blood Pressure. National Heart, Lung, and Blood Institute; National High Blood Pressure Education Program Coordinating Committee. Seventh report of the Joint National Committee on Prevention, Detection, Evaluation, and Treatment of High Blood Pressure. Hypertension. 2003; 42(6):1206–1252
27. Hansson L, Zanchetti A, Carruthers SG, Dahlof B, Elmfeldt D, Julius S, Menard J, Rahn KH, Wedel H, Westerling S. Effects of intensive blood-pressure lowering and low-dose aspirin in patients with hypertension: principal results of the Hypertension Optimal Treatment (HOT) randomised trial. HOT Study Group. Lancet. 1998; 351(9118):1755–1762
28. Gall MA, Hougaard P, Borch-Johnsen K, Parving HH. Risk factors for development of incipient and overt diabetic nephropathy in patients with non-insulin dependent diabetes mellitus: prospective, observational study. BMJ. 1997; 314(7083):783–788
29. UK Prospective Diabetes Study Group. Intensive blood-glucose control with sulphonylureas or insulin compared with conventional treatment and risk of complications in patients with type 2 diabetes (UKPDSG 33). Lancet. 1998; 352:837–853
30. Shoda J, Kanno Y, Suzuki H. A five-year comparison of the renal protective effects of angiotensin-converting enzyme inhibitors and angiotensin receptor blockers in patients with non-diabetic nephropathy. Intern Med. 2006; 45(4):193–198

31. Bakris GL, Williams M, Dworkin L, Elliott WJ, Epstein M, Toto R, et al. Preserving renal function in adults with hypertension and diabetes: a consensus approach. National Kidney Foundation Hypertension and Diabetes Executive Committees Working Group. Am J Kidney Dis. 2000; 36:646–661
32. Herman WH, Shahinfar S, Carides GW, Dasbach EJ, Gerth WC, Alexander CM, Cook JR, Keane WF, Brenner BM. Lozartan reduces the costs associated with diabetic end-stage renal disease: the RENAAL study economic evaluation. Dia Care. 2003; 26(3):683–687
33. Object Management Group - UML. http://www.uml.org/
34. Douglass BP. UML Statecharts. http://www-md.e-technik.uni-rostock.de/ma/gol/ilogix/umlsct.pdf
35. UK Prospective Diabetes Study Group. Tight blood pressure control and risk of macrovascular and microvascular complications in type 2 diabetes: UKPDS 38. UK Prospective Diabetes Study Group. BMJ. 1998; 317(7160):703–713

Case-Based Reasoning in Medicine Especially an Obituary on Lothar Gierl

Rainer Schmidt

Summary. In the early 1990s case-based reasoning (CBR) emerged. Since then it has become a successful technique in many application domains. Medicine is a much more complicated area, where usually more problems arise for all intelligent techniques. This holds for CBR too, though it seems to be very appropriate in medicine, because doctors reason with cases anyway. Nevertheless, in the last 15 years a whole string of medical CBR systems have been developed, some of them are quite successful. Overviews about these systems usually categorise them either concerning their medical purposes (e.g. diagnosis, therapy) or their computational tasks (e.g. planning, classification). We have chosen a different approach. Since 1993 yearly international CBR conferences are taking place. Here we introduce the CBR for medicine researchers and research groups that regularly presented their work in this community. In the last two decades of his life, the main research focus of Prof. Lothar Gierl was on CBR for Medicine. Thus, here we summarise his main medical CBR research projects.

1 Introduction

Case-based reasoning (CBR) means to use previous experience represented as cases to understand and solve new problems. A case-based reasoner remembers former cases similar to the current problem and attempts to modify solutions of former cases to fit for the current problem.

The fundamental ideas of CBR came up in the late 1980s (e.g. [1]). In the early 1990s CBR emerged as a method that was firstly described by Kolodner [2]. Later on Aamodt and Plaza presented a more formal characterisation of the CBR method. Figure 1 shows the CBR cycle developed by Aamodt and Plaza [3], which consists of four steps: retrieving former similar cases, adapting their solutions to the current problem, revising a proposed solution, and retaining new learned cases. However, there are two main subtasks in CBR [2,3]: The retrieval, the search for a similar case, and the adaptation, the modification of solutions of retrieved cases. Since differences between two cases are sometimes very complex, especially in medical domains, many case-based

R. Schmidt: *Case-Based Reasoning in Medicine Especially an Obituary on Lothar Gierl*, Studies in Computational Intelligence (SCI) **48**, 63–87 (2007)
www.springerlink.com

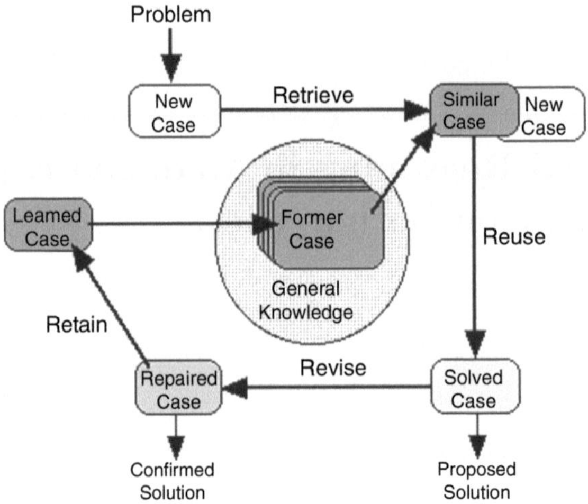

Fig. 1. The Case-based reasoning cycle developed by Aamodt

systems are so-called retrieval-only systems. They just perform the retrieval task, visualise current and similar cases, and sometimes additionally point out the important differences between them.

Though medicine has never been one of the main application domains for CBR, a whole string of medical CBR systems have already been developed, for overviews see [4–6].

2 Obituary on Lothar Gierl

In the last two decades of his life, the main research focus of Prof. Lothar Gierl, Head of the Institute for Medical Informatics and Biometry, University of Rostock, deceased in December 2004, was on CBR for Medicine. Thus here we summarise his main medical CBR research projects.

Already in the 1980s, before CBR emerged as a method, a case-oriented system for the diagnosis of dysmorphic syndromes was developed [7, 8].

In the 1990s, within the ICONS project two case-based systems were built. The first one provides antibiotic therapy advice [9]. Inspired by the second one, which deals with analyses and prognoses of kidney function courses [10], subsequently a temporal CBR method was developed [11]. This method has been applied in the recent TeCoMed project to predict approaching influenza waves [12].

2.1 Diagnosis of Dysmorphic Syndromes

When a child is born with dysmorphic features or with multiple congenital malformations or if mental retardation is observed at a later stage, finding the correct diagnosis is extremely important. Knowledge of the nature and the aetiology of the disease enable the paediatrician to predict the patient's future course. So, an initial goal for medical specialists is to diagnose a patient to a recognised syndrome. Genetic counselling and a course of treatments may then be established.

A dysmorphic syndrome describes a morphological disorder and it is characterised by a combination of various symptoms, which form a pattern of morphologic defects. An example is Down's syndrome which can be described in terms of characteristic clinical and radiographic manifestations such as mental retardation, sloping forehead, a flat nose, short broad hands, and generally dwarfed physique [7].

The main problems of diagnosing dysmorphic syndromes are as follows [7]:

- More than 200 syndromes are known
- Many cases remain undiagnosed with respect to known syndromes
- Usually many symptoms are used to describe a case (between 40 and 130)
- Every dysmorphic syndrome is characterised by nearly as many symptoms

Furthermore, knowledge about dysmorphic disorders is continuously modified, new cases are observed that cannot be diagnosed, and sometimes even new syndromes are discovered. Usually, even experts of paediatric genetics only see a small count of dysmorphic syndromes during their lifetime.

GS.52 is a prototype-based expert system that was routinely used in the children's hospital of the University of Munich for many years [7, 8]. It is a diagnostic support system for dysmorphic syndromes. In GS.52 each syndrome is represented by a prototype (prototypical case) that contains its typical features. Two-thirds of the prototypes were taken from literature or defined by medical experts. One-third of them was acquired by expert consultation sessions, in which a physician selects at first a new or an already existing syndrome and secondly typical cases for this syndrome. Subsequently, GS.52 determines the relevant features and their relative frequency (see Table 1).

The diagnostic support occurs by searching for the most adequate prototypes concerning a query case. A similarity value between each prototype and the query case is calculated and the prototypes are ranked according to these values.

Table 1. Portion of an example of a generated prototype

Heart murmur	30%	Depressed nasal bridge	23%
Diminished postnatal growth rate	77%	Anteverted nares	63%
Hypercalcaemia	30%	Prominent lips	17%
Prenatal onset	75%	Long philtrum	17%
Mild microcephaly	67%	Fullness of peri-orbital region	75%
Full cheeks	46%	Medial eyebrow flare	25%

The numbers are the relative frequency in percentages the features occurred in the cases of the prototype

GS.52 differs from typical CBR systems, because it does not consider single case but cases are clustered into prototypes that represent diagnoses and the retrieval searches among these abstract prototypes. The adaptation consists of two examinations of the probable prototypes: A plausibility check with general rules (constraints) and a check of evidences for or against specific syndromes (some syndromes are nearly a proof for or against some diagnoses).

2.2 The ICONS Project

Within the ICONS project two case-based systems were built. The first one provides antibiotic therapy advice, the second one deals with analyses and prognoses of kidney function courses.

2.2.1 Antibiotic Therapy Advice

ICONS is an antibiotics therapy adviser for intensive care patients who develop an infection as additional complication. The identification of the pathogen that causes the infection needs at least 24 h in the laboratory. In contrast to normal patients where physicians usually can wait for the results of the laboratory, intensive care patients need immediate introduction of an appropriate antibiotics therapy. Since the real pathogen is still unknown, a spectrum of probable pathogens has to be calculated. The aim of ICONS is to give rapid antibiotic therapy advice. Besides the expected pathogen spectrum, which has to be covered by the antibiotics, the current resistance situation, contraindications of the patient against some antibiotics, and the sphere of activity of the antibiotics have to be considered. CBR techniques are used to speed up the process of finding suitable antibiotics therapies (the right path in Fig. 2).

Antibiotics Selection Strategy. Since ICONS is not a diagnostic system, it does not attempt to deduce evidence for the diagnosis of symptoms, frequencies and probabilities. Instead, the following strategy is pursued (the left path in Fig. 2): Find all possible solutions and reduce them using the patient's contraindications and the complete coverage of the calculated pathogen spectrum (establish-refine strategy). First, it is distinguished between different groups of patients and affected organs to determine the calculated pathogen spectrum. A first list of antibiotics is generated by a susceptibility relation. For each group of pathogens it returns all antibiotics that usually have therapeutic effects. This list contains those antibiotics that can control at least a part of the considered pathogen spectrum. A second list of antibiotics is obtained by reducing the first one by applying criteria such as the patient's contraindications and the desired sphere of activity. Using the antibiotics of this second list, general rules are applied to generate sensible antibiotics combinations. Subsequently, the generated antibiotics combinations have to be proofed for their ability to completely cover the calculated spectrum.

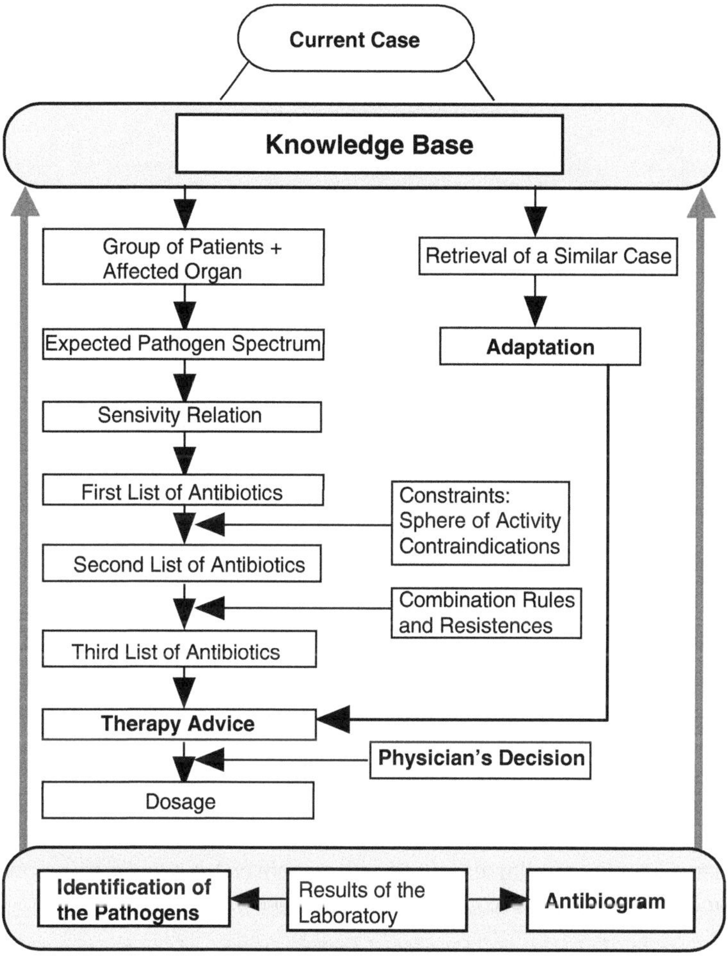

Fig. 2. ICONS process flowchart

Before the user chooses one therapy, he can investigate potential side effects of the antibiotics (Fig. 3 shows the output menu). Moreover, he may obtain information about the calculated spectrum and the daily costs of each suggested therapy. After the physician has chosen one therapy, ICONS computes the recommended dosage.

Adaptation of Similar Cases. The principal argument for CBR [2, 3] that it is often faster to solve a new problem by modifying the solution of a similar case applies to the process of finding adequate therapies. Considering the close relation concerning the group of patients and the affected organ, a similar case is retrieved from a hierarchically and generalising storage structure containing prototypes as well as single cases.

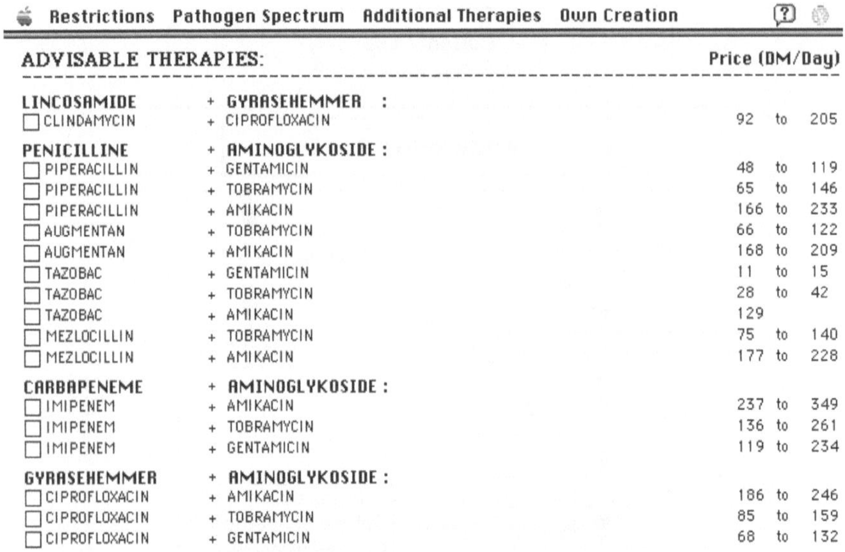

Restrictions Pathogen Spectrum Additional Therapies Own Creation

ADVISABLE THERAPIES:		Price (DM/Day)
LINCOSAMIDE	+ GYRASEHEMMER :	
CLINDAMYCIN	+ CIPROFLOXACIN	92 to 205
PENICILLINE	+ AMINOGLYKOSIDE :	
PIPERACILLIN	+ GENTAMICIN	48 to 119
PIPERACILLIN	+ TOBRAMYCIN	65 to 146
PIPERACILLIN	+ AMIKACIN	166 to 233
AUGMENTAN	+ TOBRAMYCIN	66 to 122
AUGMENTAN	+ AMIKACIN	168 to 209
TAZOBAC	+ GENTAMICIN	11 to 15
TAZOBAC	+ TOBRAMYCIN	28 to 42
TAZOBAC	+ AMIKACIN	129
MEZLOCILLIN	+ TOBRAMYCIN	75 to 140
MEZLOCILLIN	+ AMIKACIN	177 to 228
CARBAPENEME	+ AMINOGLYKOSIDE :	
IMIPENEM	+ AMIKACIN	237 to 349
IMIPENEM	+ TOBRAMYCIN	136 to 261
IMIPENEM	+ GENTAMICIN	119 to 234
GYRASEHEMMER	+ AMINOGLYKOSIDE :	
CIPROFLOXACIN	+ AMIKACIN	186 to 246
CIPROFLOXACIN	+ TOBRAMYCIN	85 to 159
CIPROFLOXACIN	+ GENTAMICIN	68 to 132

Fig. 3. ICONS therapy recommendations

As features the contraindications and as methods, a variation of the similarity measure of Tversky [13] and the Hash-Tree-Retrieval algorithm developed by Stottler, Henke, and King [14] are applied. Furthermore a criterion for adaptability is used during the retrieval, because similar cases with additional contraindications in comparison to the query patient are not adaptable. The adaptation is done by a solution transfer of the advisable therapies of a similar case and subsequently by a reduction concerning additional contraindications of the query patient.

Adaptation to Laboratory Results. Identifications of pathogens and sensitivity tests (antibiograms) made in the laboratory are used as control mechanisms. When the actual pathogen is identified, the calculated pathogen spectrum is replaced by this pathogen and the already started therapy has to be checked if it fits for the identified pathogen. The set of possible antibiotic therapies is reduced by the antibiogram to those antibiotics the pathogens are not resistant to.

The frequently changing parts of the knowledge base are updated by an interpretation of the laboratory findings. That means each theoretically determined pathogen spectrum is supplemented by an empirically justified one, due to identified pathogens. The information about resistances is updated concerning antibiogram results.

For both adaptations, those to the findings of query patients and those parts of the knowledge base, no retrieval but an evaluation and a statistical interpretation is performed.

2.2.2 Time Course Prognoses of the Kidney Function

Intensive care patients are often no longer able to maintain adequate fluid and electrolyte balances themselves due to impaired organ functions, renal failures, or medical treatments, e.g. parenteral nutrition of mechanically ventilated patients. Therefore physicians need objective criteria for the monitoring of the kidney function and to diagnose therapeutic interventions as necessary. So, at our intensive care unit in Munich a renal function monitoring system, NIMON [15], existed that provided daily renal reports. These reports consisted of 13 measured and 33 calculated parameters of those patients where renal function monitoring was applied. But the interpretation of all reported parameters was quite complex and required special knowledge of the renal physiology.

The aim was to develop a system that provides automatic interpretation of the renal state to elicit impairments of the kidney function on time. In the domain of fluid and electrolyte balance, neither prototypical courses in ICU settings are known nor exists complete knowledge about the kidney function. Especially, knowledge about the behaviour of the various parameters over time is yet incomplete. So, a method had to be designed to deal with course analyses of multiple parameters without prototypical courses and without a complete domain theory.

We developed a method that consists of three main steps, two abstractions plus CBR retrieval. The idea of abstracting many parameters into one single parameter was taken from RÉSUMÉ [16] where the course of this single parameter is analysed by means of a complete domain theory. The comparison of parameter courses with well-known course pattern is performed in many medical knowledge based systems (e.g. Haimowitz and Kohane [17]). Since no such pattern were known for the kidney function, single courses and incrementally learned prototypes are used instead of well-known course pattern to compare with. Course patterns were partly learned by structuring the case base by prototypes.

The procedure for interpretation of the kidney function can be described as follows. First, everyday the monitoring system NIMON gets 13 measured parameters from the clinical chemistry and calculates 33 meaningful kidney function parameters. Since the interpretation of all parameters is too complex, they are abstracted into meaningful kidney function states (Fig. 4 shows the definition of the state "reduced kidney function"). The states are organised in a hierarchy with five levels: normal kidney function, some impairments like tubular damage, reduced function, sharply reduced function, and kidney failure.

Based on the kidney function states, characterised by obligatory and optional conditions for selected renal parameters, we first check the obligatory conditions. For each state that satisfies the obligatory conditions we calculate a similarity value concerning the optional conditions. We use a variation of Tversky's [13] measure of dissimilarity between concepts. Only if two or more states are under consideration, ICONS presents them to the user

Reduced Kidney Function

Obligatory Condtion:	c_kreat 40–80	
Optional Conditions:		
Retention Rates:	p_kreat_se	< 2
	p_urea_se	< 150
Tubular Function:	u_osmol 320–600	
	u_p_osmol	1.1–1.8
	u_kreat 10–40	
	u_p_kreat	20–50
Urine Volume:	urine1 volume	0.7–3.0
	osmol_ex	800–3000

Fig. 4. Definition of the reduced kidney function state. Abbreviations: c, clearance; p, plasma; u, urine; kreat, kreatinin; osmol, osmolality; se, serum; ex, excretion

(sorted according to their similarity values) together with information about the satisfied and not satisfied optional conditions.

The next step is a temporal abstraction of a patient's sequence of daily kidney function states within a time period of the last seven days. Experts consider longer time periods to be irrelevant for the current situation of a patient.

First, we have fixed five assessment definitions for the transition of the kidney function state of one day to the state of the respectively next day. These assessment definitions are related to the grade of renal impairment:

- *Steady*: both states have the same severity value.
- *Increasing*: exactly one severity step in the direction towards a normal function.
- *Sharply Increasing*: at least two severity steps in the direction towards a normal function.
- *Decreasing*: exactly one severity step in the direction towards a kidney failure.
- *Sharply Decreasing*: at least two severity steps in the direction towards a kidney failure.

These assessment definitions are used to determine the state transitions from one qualitative value to another. Based on these state transitions, we generate three trend descriptions. Two trend descriptions especially consider the current state transitions.

Short-term trend:	current state transition; Abbreviation: T1
Medium-term trend:	looks recursively back from the current state transition to the one before and unites them if they are both of the same direction or one of them has a "steady" assessment; Abbreviation: T2
Long-term trend:	characterises the considered course of at most seven days; Abbreviation: T3

For the long-term trend description we additionally introduced four new assessment definitions. If none of the five former assessments fits the complete considered course, we attempt to fit one of these four definitions in the following order:

Alternating: at least two up and two down transitions and all local minima are equal.

Oscillating: at least two up and two down transitions.

Fluctuating: the distance of the highest to the lowest severity state value is greater than one.

Nearly Steady: the distance of the highest to the lowest severity state value equals one.

Only if there are several courses with the same trend descriptions, we use a minor fourth trend description T4 to find the most similar among them. We assess the considered course by adding up the state transition values inversely weighted by the distances to the current day. Together with the current kidney function state these four trend descriptions form a course depiction that abstracts the sequence of the kidney function states.

Looking back from a time point t, these four trend descriptions form a pattern of the immediate course history of the kidney function considering qualitative and quantitative assessments.

Example. The following kidney function states may be observed in this temporal sequence (Fig. 5):

- Selective tubular damage, reduced kidney function, reduced kidney function, selective tubular damage, reduced kidney function, reduced kidney function, sharply reduced kidney function

So we get these six state transitions:

- Decreasing, steady, increasing, decreasing, steady, decreasing.

With these trend descriptions:

- Current state: sharply reduced kidney function.
- T1: decreasing, reduced kidney function, one transition.
- T2: decreasing, selective tubular damage, three transitions.
- T3: fluctuating, selective tubular damage, six transitions.
- T4: 1.23.

In this example, the short-term trend description T1 assesses the current state transition as "decreasing" from a "reduced kidney function" to a "sharply reduced kidney function". Since the medium-term trend description T2 accumulates steady state transitions, T2 determines a "decrease" in the last four days from a "selective tubular damage" to a "sharply reduced kidney function". The long-term trend description T3 assesses the entire course of seven days as "fluctuating", because there is only one increasing state transition and the difference between the severity values of a "selective tubular damage" and a "sharply reduced kidney function" equals two.

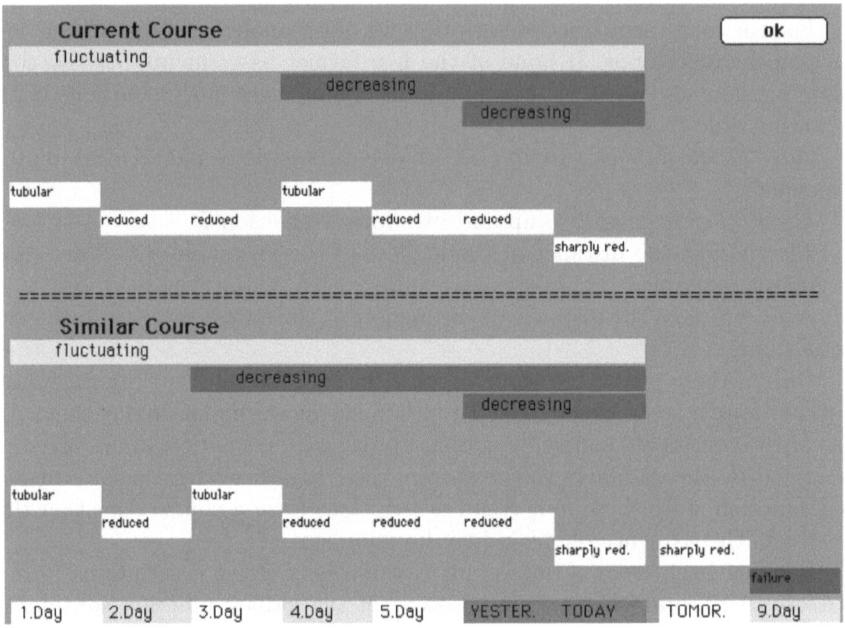

Fig. 5. Presentation of a current and a similar course

Subsequently, CBR retrieval methods [13,18,19] use the parameters of the trend descriptions to search for similar courses. The result, a current query course is depicted in comparison to similar ones to the user (Fig. 5), the course continuations of the similar courses serve as prognoses.

Since the aim was to develop an early warning system, a prognosis is needed. As there are many different possible continuations for the same previous course, it is necessary to search for similar courses and different projections. Therefore, the search space is divided into nine parts corresponding to the possible continuation directions. Each direction forms an own part of the search space. During the retrieval these parts are searched separately and each part may provide at most one similar course.

Before the main retrieval, a prototype that matches most of the trend descriptions is searched. Below this prototype the main retrieval starts. It consists of two steps for each projection part. First an activation algorithm [18] concerning qualitative features is applied.

Subsequently, the retrieved cases are checked with an adaptability criterion that looks for sufficient similarity, because even the most similar course may differ from the current one significantly.

If several courses are selected in the same projection part, in a second step a sequential similarity measure is used concerning the quantitative features. It is a variation of TSCALE [19] and goes back to Tversky [13].

As there may be too many different aspects between both patients, the adaptation of a retrieved similar course to the current query course is not done automatically. In fact, ICONS displays not just one comparison but theoretically in each of the nine projection parts a similar case can be found. In practise, in just few projection parts (usually two or three) similar kidney function courses are found.

ICONS offers only diagnostic and prognostic support, the user has to decide about the relevance of all displayed information. When presenting a comparison of a current and a similar course, ICONS supplies the user with the ability to access further information. Namely about additional renal syndromes, courses of single parameter values of the kidney function during the relevant time period, and information about how typical the retrieved former course is (a prototypical case or a single case).

2.3 Influenza Forecast

The general idea of tour TeCoMed project was to discover regional health risks in the German federal state Mecklenburg Western Pomerania by keeping spreads of infectious diseases under surveillance. A program was developed that computes early warnings against forthcoming waves or even epidemics of infectious diseases that are characterised by cyclic but irregular occurrences. The program has mainly been applied on influenza [11], later on additionally on bronchitis [20].

Since influenza results in many costs, especially in an increased number of days of unfitness for work, many of the most developed countries have started to generate influenza surveillance systems. The idea is to predict influenza waves or even epidemics as early as possible and to indicate appropriate actions like starting vaccination campaigns or advising high-risk groups to stay at home.

Though a couple of factors are influencing influenza (e.g. weather conditions, mutations of the influenza virus, and outbreaks in foreign countries) no proper knowledge about these influences is available. Consequently all surveillance systems focus on observed counts of infections. Furthermore, all influenza surveillance systems make use of former influenza seasons. Most of them have tried statistical methods, so far only with modest results. The usual idea is to compute mean values and standard courses based on weekly incidences of former seasons and to analyse deviations from a statistic normal situation. Influenza waves usually occur only once a season, but they start at different time points and have extremely different intensities. So, Farrington already pointed out that statistical methods are inappropriate for diseases (like influenza) that are characterised by irregular cyclic behaviour of temporal spreads [21].

Instead, in the TeCoMed we applied CBR again. So, former influenza seasons are considered more explicitly. Those parts of former seasons that are most similar to the current situation are searched and used to decide whether warnings are appropriate. Here, just the method is summarised. For more details and for results see [11].

2.3.1 Prognostic Model for Influenza

Influenza seasons start in early October and end in late March. They consist of 26 weeks. The choice to consider weekly incidences instead of, e.g. daily ones is common practice in influenza surveillance. Since warnings seem to be appropriate in at most up to four weeks in advance, we consider courses that consist of four weekly incidences. In some other influenza systems this period of time is used too (e.g. in [22]). So, every influenza season is split into 23 courses, each of them consists of four weekly incidences. Figure 6 shows the prognostic model.

Temporal Abstraction. Firstly, three trends are defined that characterise the changes from last week to this week, from last but one week to this week, and from last but two weeks to this week. The assessments for these trends are "enormous decrease", "sharp decrease", "decrease", "steady", "increase", "sharp increase" and "enormous increase". They are based on the percentage of alteration. Together with the four weekly incidences these assessments are used to determine similarities between a query course and all four-week courses stored in the case base.

The intention for using these two sorts of parameters is to ensure that a query course and an appropriate similar course are on the same level (similar weekly data) and that they have similar changes on time (similar assessments).

Searching for Similar Courses. Subsequently, distances between a query course and all four-week courses stored in the case base are computed. The considered attributes are the three nominal valued trend assessments and the four weekly incidences.

Sufficient Similarity. The result of computing distances is a very long list of all former four weeks courses sorted according to their distances. The next

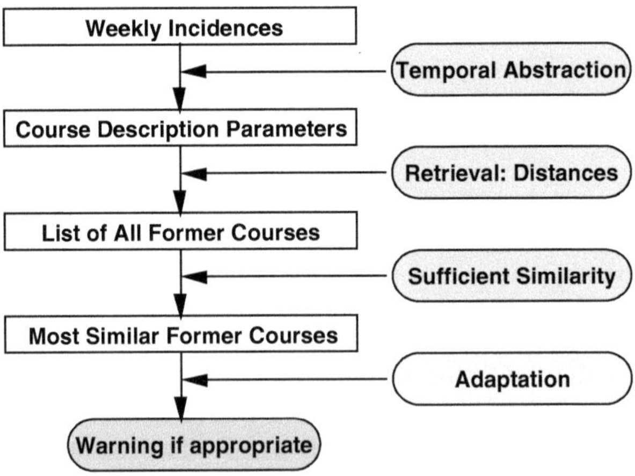

Fig. 6. The prognostic model to forecast influenza

step means to find the most similar ones. One idea might be to use a fixed number, e.g. the first two or three courses in the sorted list. Unfortunately, this has two disadvantages.

First, even the most similar former course might not be similar enough, and secondly, vice versa, e.g. the fourth, fifth, etc. course might be nearly as similar as the first one.

So, the most similar courses are found by applying sufficient similarity criteria, namely two thresholds. First, the difference concerning the three trend assessments between the query course and a most similar course has to be below a first threshold. This guarantees similar changes on time. And secondly, the difference concerning the incidences of the current weeks must be below a second threshold. This guarantees an equal current incidence level.

Adaptation. Now the list of the most similar former courses usually is very small. However, the question arises how these courses can help to decide whether early warnings are appropriate. Those time points of the former courses are marked where, in retrospect, a first warning was appropriate. This means that a solution of a four weeks course is a binary mark, either a warning was appropriate or not.

For the decision to warn, the list of the most similar courses is split in two lists. One list contains courses where a warning was appropriate; the second list gets the other ones. For both of these new lists their sums of the reciprocal distances of their courses are computed to get sums of similarities. Subsequently, the decision about the appropriateness to warn depends on the question: which of these two sums is bigger.

In Fig. 7, past influenza seasons of Mecklenburg, Western Pomerania are depicted. The squares indicate time points for first warnings which can easily be computed. Circles indicate time points for earlier warnings. Since these points are difficult to discriminate from normal situations, the computation of these earlier warnings is not so easy. For details about experimental results about these two ideas when to warn see [11]. Later the same method has also been applied on data from Scottish Health Centres (for results see [23]), where the distinction between influenza waves and normal situations was easier than for the data of Mecklenburg, Western Pomerania.

2.4 General Model for Time Course Prognosis

Based on experiences with time course prognosis of the kidney function (Sect. 2.2.2) and with influenza forecast (Sect. 2.3) a general model for time course prognosis was developed (Fig. 8). It is similar to the CBR cycle proposed by Aamodt and Plaza (see Fig. 1), which consists of retrieving former similar cases, adapting their solutions to a current problem, revising proposed solutions, and retaining new learned cases [3].

Since in both our applications the idea is to give information about a specific development and its probable continuations, a revision of proposed

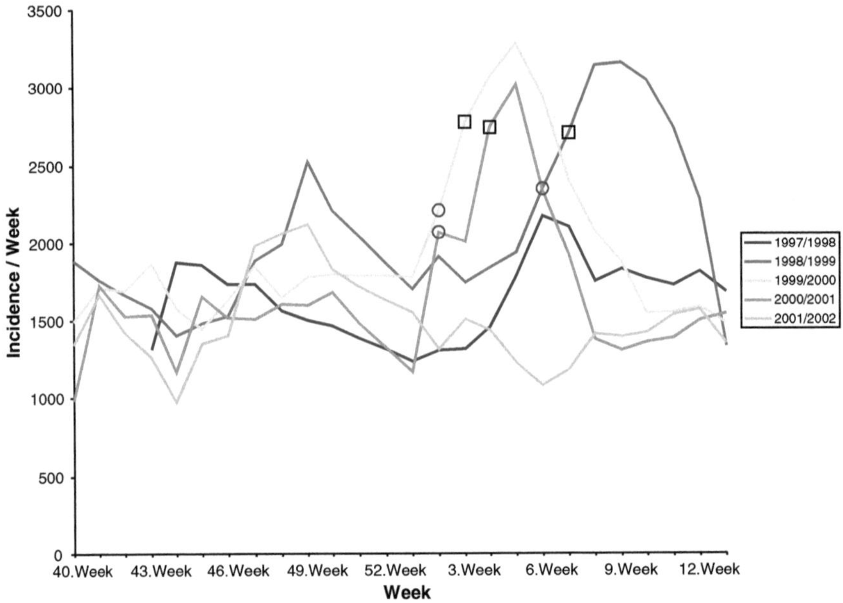

Fig. 7. Influenza seasons of Mecklenburg, Western Pomerania

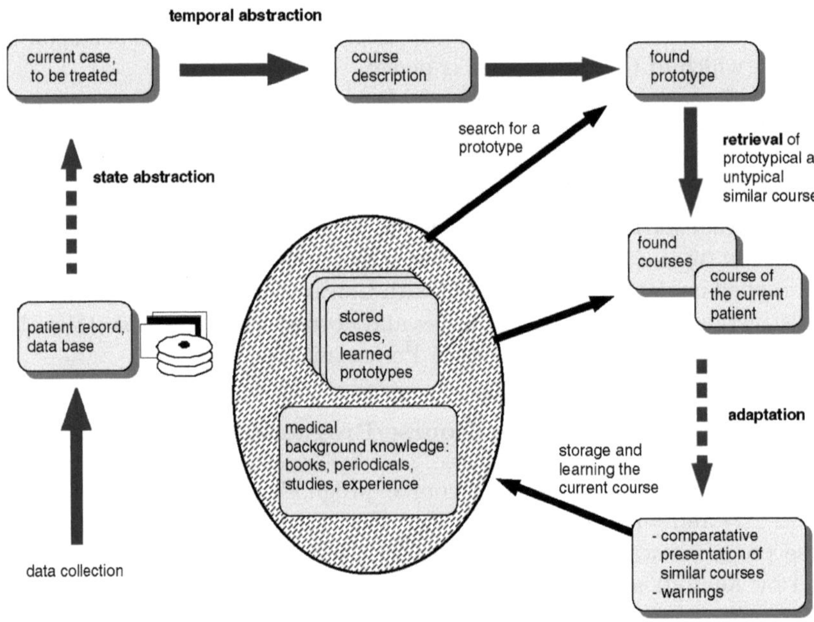

Fig. 8. Prognostic model for temporal courses

solutions does not take place. On the other hand, three steps are added to the original CBR cycle: a state abstraction, a temporal abstraction, and a search for prototypes.

For multiple parameters (as for the kidney function) a state abstraction shall occur. For single parameter courses (as for influenza) this step is, of course, unnecessary. The next step, a temporal abstraction, should provide some trend descriptions, which can not only help to visualise tendencies of courses, but the description parameters can also be used for retrieving similar courses.

In CBR programs, the retrieval often consists of two steps, a pre-selection and a fine selection. Especially in the medical domain, prototypes are an appropriate knowledge representation form to generalise from specific single cases to more abstract ones [5]. Prototypes help to structure the case base, to guide and to speed up the retrieval, and to get rid of redundant cases [24]. So, the search for a fitting prototype is a sort of preliminary selection, before the main retrieval takes only those cases into account that belong to the retrieved prototype.

About the role of prototypes in medical CBR systems see [24]. For details about prototypes for the prognosis of kidney function courses see [10].

In CBR the retrieval is connected with a similarity measure, which determines the similarity between a current query case and the cases in the case base. This measure can either be explicitly applied or it can be implemented in a more sophisticated retrieval algorithm. For the prognosis of kidney function courses a spreading activation algorithm [18] is applied, while for influenza forecast an explicitly defined similarity measure is used [23].

Many medical CBR systems are so-called retrieval-only systems [25]. Sometimes it is appropriate to visualise temporal courses in comparison to similar former ones. For the prognosis of kidney function courses such a comparative presentation was implemented, while for influenza forecast adaptation is performed to decide whether warnings are appropriate or not.

3 Case-Based Reasoning in Medicine

The first international CBR conference was organised in 1993. However, some national CBR workshops took place slightly earlier, especially in the US, already in 1988. From the beginning, medical applications were part of the CBR community. Though later on medical applications were presented at every international CBR conference, medicine never became one of the main application areas of CBR. However, as a result of an increasing interest in CBR in medicine, a first workshop on this topic was organised within the international conference in 2003 [26]. Since then this workshop has been continued on the following conferences [27,28].

When looking at the medical CBR applications in the last nearly 20 years, a tendency can be observed. At the beginning the majority of applications dealt with diagnostic tasks, while in the recent years rather more therapeutic and treatment systems have been developed.

Though an increasing interest in CBR in medicine can be observed, the progress in this field is very difficult to assess, because many research groups developed just one medical CBR system and subsequently went to some other application area. On the one side there are computer scientists working on CBR and looking for various fields of application who occasionally come across a medical problem. On the other side there are scientists in medical informatics working on medical applications that occasionally come across a problem where CBR seems to be appropriate. However, a few research groups have been working in the field of medical CBR systems for quite a long time. Unfortunately, so far there have been just very few fruitful discussions between these groups. The main reason is that these groups are developing different sorts of applications in various medical areas.

One of these research groups is our own one, which was led by Lothar Gierl. We have already presented our work in the last section. In this section we firstly introduce the other main researchers in this field and their work. Secondly, we introduce the other people that presented medical applications at international CBR conferences. Apart from these conferences there are researchers who work on CBR in medicine but presented their work elsewhere. Since we are just aware of a few of them, some work may be not mentioned here. We finish this section with a very specific medical task, namely the interpretation of medical images.

3.1 Three CBR in Medicine Researchers

Apart from our own group there are three research groups who regularly presented their work on CBR in medicine.

Isabelle Bichindaritz, who was one of two organisers of the annual "CBR in the health science" workshops at the international CBR conferences [26–28], developed three medical CBR systems.

ALEXIA [29] deals with diagnosis of a patient's hypertension aetiology. The classical indexing of former stored cases is enriched with a meta-indexation level that is connected with a causal physiological model. The dependency relations expressed through the causal model provide a functional point of view that objectivates the selection of the best analogous.

MNAOMIA [30] provides assistance in psychiatry eating disorders for diagnosis, treatment, and research hypothesis recommendation. It is capable of adapting to different cognitive tasks. The memory model of the system comprises both an experimental and a theoretical memory, expressed in a unified knowledge representation language and organisation. The components of the memory are cases and concepts, in the experimental part, and prototypes and models, in the theoretical part. The reasoning supported by this memory model can be various, and takes advantage of all components, whether experimental or theoretical. It is strongly constrained by some specialised models in the theoretical part of the memory, called the points of view.

CARE-PARTNER [31] is a computerised decision support system on the World Wide Web. It supports home care providers. It is applied on the long-term follow-up of patients having undergone a stem-cell transplant, after their return in their home community. The system combines CBR and rule-based reasoning, its memory consists of patient cases and of ontology that contains disease descriptions, signs, symptoms, medications etc.

Isabelle Bichindaritz did not just develop these systems but provided rather theoretical work based on experiences with these systems. This comprises reflections about CBR for temporal problems [32], solving safety implications [33], a framework for the sharing and for the distribution of case bases, and about CBR in biology and medicine [34].

Since 1998 *Stefani Montani*, who at first worked with Riccardo Bellazzi and Mario Stefanelli in Pavia and later on with Luigi Portinale in Alessandria, in Italy, has regularly presented her work at CBR conferences. Within an EU-research project about management of insulin dependent diabetes mellitus she not just developed a multi-modal reasoning systems that combines case-based and rule-based reasoning [35] but additionally investigated theoretical aspects like retrieval and prototypes [36]. Recently, she developed a retrieval system in the haemodialysis domain where the case features are partly static and partly dynamic (time-dependent) [37]. Based on these experiences she subsequently outlined a framework for case representation and retrieval for domains with temporal dimensions [38]. It incorporates different sorts of temporal abstraction [16], namely into states and into trends.

Peter Funk and his research group joined the "CBR in medicine" community rather recently. At first he presented a framework for performing classification of measurements derived from noisy data [39] and subsequently his approach about how to classify time series data for respiratory sinus arrhythmia [40]. Most recently, at the "CBR in the health science" workshop 2005 he and his colleagues had three contributions on different aspects of time series and about determining stress levels in the domains of heartbeats and respiration [28].

3.2 Further Medical CBR Applications

Apart from the researchers and research groups already introduced above, here we want to summarise all the others. We do not claim on completeness but hope to present all important systems and developments in the community of the CBR in medicine.

3.2.1 Diagnostic Systems

One of the earliest medical CBR systems is CASEY [41], which deals with heart failure diagnosis. The most interesting aspect of CASEY is the attempt to use more general adaptation operators. However, though many useful domain dependent operators could be defined, not all adaptation situations could be solved with them. So, when adaptation fails or when no appropriate similar case can be found, a rule base is used.

Another diagnostic system of the late 1980s is MEDIC [42]. It is a schema-based diagnostic reasoner whose domain is pulmonology. Its interesting aspect is the memory organisation. Schemata represent the problem solvers knowledge. They are packets of procedural knowledge about how to achieve a goal or a set of goals. The memory does not only consist of schemata, but additionally of diagnostic memory organisation packets of individual cases, of diagnoses, and of scenes. A scene represents an instantiation of a schema in a particular case. This memory organisation and retrieval allows a reasoner to find the most specific problem-solving procedures available.

FLORENCE [43] is a system of the early 1990s. It deals with health care planing in a broader sense, namely for nursing which is a less specialised field. It fulfils all three basic planing tasks: diagnosis, prognosis, and prescription. Here diagnosis is not used in the common medical meaning as the identification of a disease but it seeks to answer the question "what is the current health status of a query patient?" Rules concerning weighted health indicators are applied. The health status is determined as the score of the indicator weights.

MERSY [44] is a system for rural health care workers. It has the advantage of relocation of expertise. This is especially important in developing countries where health care workers are rare and are performing with only modest skills. In MERSY the knowledge base can automatically be adapted to special health care problems of a region.

FM-Ultranet [45] and Somnus [46] are primarily diagnostic systems, which were presented at the recent CBR in health science workshops. FM-Ultranet supports ultrasonagraphists in detecting fetal malformations. When a practitioner detects an abnormality during a routine ultrasound screening, FM-Ultranet helps to determine if the abnormality is dangerous. Attributes derived from the scans are used to identify abnormal organs and extremities. Cases are arranged in a hierarchical structure, the hierarchy consists of 39 concepts, which consist of attributes. Similarities between query cases and concepts are calculated by using the attributes. Somnus helps students in a sleep disorder clinic to diagnose and treat obstructive sleep apnoea, a breathing disorder that repeatedly wakes patients from sleep. Somnus combines semiotics, fuzzy logic, and database query techniques with CBR.

A big problem for medical expert systems is to deal with multiple disorders. Recently in the CBR community two approaches have been undertaken to tackle this problem. The first one [47] deals with sonography cases. So far, its results are not very promising, because in its case base only few cases have similar combinations of multiple disorders. The results of the second approach [48] in the same domain are more promising. However, not a pure CBR method is applied but it is a complex combination of CBR and rule-based reasoning.

3.2.2 Therapeutic and Other Support Systems

Most of the therapeutic systems are already mentioned in sections above, because they were developed by Isabelle Bichindaritz (for eating disorders and for stem-cell post-transplant patient care), by the group of Stefania Montani (for diabetes and for haemodialysis), or by our own group. Apart from the ICONS system (for antibiotics therapy advice), which we have summarised in Sect. 2.2.1, we have developed another therapeutic CBR system, namely recently a system called ISOR (in the endocrine domain) [49].

So, here we just mention a few other systems. In TA3-IVF [50], a system to modify in vitro fertilisation treatment plans. Relevant similar cases are retrieved and compositional adaptation [51] is applied to compute weighted average values for the solution attributes. In CASIMIR [52], a system to support decision making for breast cancer treatments, two separate systems, a rule-based and a case-based one, are linked.

More recent systems especially deal with other sorts of health support, namely for prescribing exercise regimen [53], concerning technology needs for the elderly and disabled [54], and for hospital management [55].

3.3 Medical Image Interpretation

Already in the early stages of CBR, systems dealing with medical images were developed. These systems like ProtoISIS [56] and MacRad [25] just performed image retrieval. Users can ask content-based queries and these systems return reference images. In MacRad not only hierarchies for indexing stored images are used for retrieval but additionally constraints specified in the user queries are considered.

However, the early systems did neither perform adaptation nor did they attempt to interpret images. Grimnes and Aamodt [57] developed a prototype of an image interpretation system for computer tomography. It consisted of two layer CBR architecture, a CBR level for lower level segmentation identification and a second layer for higher liver interpretation and understanding. A rather sophisticated image understanding system is SCINA [58]. It automatically derives assessments concerning the presence of coronary artery disease from a scintigraphic image data set. Each image consists of six planes, each plane is divided into 12 segments and the resulting 72 values are considered for retrieval, which is performed by nearest neighbour match. In contrast to the early systems mentioned above, in SCINA adaptation takes place. It is problem specific and it is based on the coronary circulation model.

Later on few presentations (e.g. [59]) about CBR and medical image retrieval were given at CBR conferences. The only prominent researcher in this field, who, since 1998 continuously presented her work at CBR conferences, is Petra Perner. This contains her practical work on, e.g. CT images [60] and fungi strains [61] as well as her theoretical research on various aspects of image interpretation. For readers interested in CBR for image interpretation we especially recommend her invited talk at the international CBR conference in 2001 [62].

4 Conclusion

In this chapter, we have mainly presented the work of Lothar Gierl on CBR in medicine. Additionally, we have reviewed most researches of this area that have presented their work in the CBR community.

As a tendency we see just a slight shift from diagnostic applications to rather therapeutic and other sorts of support systems. Furthermore, we have the impression that the number of medical CBR systems has already increased and we hope that it will probably grow further.

CBR has been applied in various medical application areas. The choice mainly seems to depend on the involved CBR researchers and their personal contacts. Bioinformatics might be a new promising area for CBR techniques, though very few investigations have been undertaken so far.

Acknowledgments

The ICONS project was funded by the German Ministry of Education and Research (BMBF). The work on influenza forecast was partly funded by the German Research Foundation (DFG).

References

1. Schank, R.C., Leake, D.B.: Creativity and learning in a case-based explainer. Artificial Intelligence 40 (1989) 353–385
2. Kolodner, J.: Case-based Reasoning. Morgan Kaufmann, San Mateo (1993)
3. Aamodt, A., Plaza, E.: Case-based reasoning: Foundation issues. Methodological variation and system approaches. Artificial Intelligence Communications 7(1) (1994) 39–59
4. Gierl, L., Bull, M., Schmidt, R.: CBR in medicine. In: Lenz, M., Bartsch-Spörl, B., Burkhard, H.-D., Wess, S. (Eds.): Case-based Reasoning Technology, from foundations to applications. Lecture Notes in Artificial Intelligence, Vol. 1400, Springer, Berlin Heidelberg New York (1998) 273–297
5. Schmidt, R., Montani, S., Bellazzi, R., Portinale, L., Gierl, L.: Case-based Reasoning for medical knowledge-based systems. International Journal of Medical Informatics 64(2–3) (2001) 355–367
6. Nilsson, M., Sollenborn, N.: Advancements and trends in medical case-based reasoning: An overview of systems and system developments. In: Proceedings of the Seventeenth International Florida Artificial Intelligence Research Society Conference, AAAI Press, Menlo Park, California (2004) 178–183

7. Gierl, L., Stengel-Rutkowski, S.: Integrating consultation and semi-automatic knowledge acquisition in a prototype-based architecture: Experiences with dysmorphic syndromes. Artificial Intelligence in Medicine 6 (1994) 29–49
8. Gierl, L., Arias-Lewing, G., Stengel-Rutkowski, S., Jakobeit, M., Lohse, K.: Knowledge acquisition for scheme-based medical expert systems: The dysmorphic syndrome example. In: Riehoff, O., Piccolo, A., Schneider, J. (Eds.): Expert systems and decision support in medicine. Springer, Berlin Heidelberg New York (1988) 347–350
9. Gierl, L., Steffen, D., Ihracky, D., Schmidt, R.: Methods, architecture, evaluation and usability of a case-based antibiotics advisor. Computer Methods and Programs in Biomedicine 72 (2003) 139–154
10. Schmidt, R., Heindl, B., Pollwein, B., Gierl, L.: Multiparametric time course prognoses by means of case-based reasoning and abstraction of data and time. Medical Informatics 22(3) (1997) 237–250
11. Schmidt, R., Gierl, L.: A prognostic model for temporal courses that combines temporal abstraction and case-based reasoning. International Journal of Medical Informatics 74(2–4) (2005) 307–315
12. Schmidt, R., Gierl, L.: Applying temporal abstraction and case-based reasoning to predict approaching influenza waves. In: Surjan, G., Engelbrecht, R., McNair, P. (Eds.): Proceedings of the Medical Informatics Europe, MIE'2002, IOS-Press, Amsterdam (2002) 420–424
13. Tversky, A.: Features of similarity. Psychological Review 84 (1977) 327–352
14. Stottler, R.H., Henke, A.L., King, J.A.: Rapid retrieval algorithms for case-based reasoning. Proceedings of the 11th IJCAI, Morgan Kaufmann, San Mateo (1989) 233–237
15. Wenkebach, U., Pollwein, B., Finsterer, U.: Visualization of large datasets in intensive care. Proceedings of the Annual Symposium on Computer Applications in Medical Care (1992) 18–22
16. Shahar, Y.: Timing is everything: Temporal reasoning and temporal data maintenance in medicine. In: Horn, W., Shahar, Y., Lindberg, G., Andreassen, S., Wyatt, J. (Eds.): Artificial intelligence in medicine. Proceedings of AIMDM'99, Lecture Notes in Artificial Intelligence, Vol. 1620, Springer, Berlin Heidelberg New York (1999) 30–46
17. Haimowitz, I.J., Kohane, I.S.: Automated trend detection with alternate temporal hypotheses. In: Proceedings of the 13th International Joint Conference on Artificial Intelligence, Morgan Kaufmann, San Mateo (1993) 146–151
18. Anderson, J.R.: A theory of the origins of human knowledge. Artificial Intelligence 40, Special Volume on Machine Learning (1989) 313–351
19. DeSarbo, W.S., et al.: TSCALE: A new multidimensional scaling procedure based on Tversky's contrast model. Psychometrika 57 (1992) 43–69
20. Schmidt, R., Gierl, L.: Case-based reasoning for predicting the temporal spread of infectious diseases. In: Damiani, E., Howlett, R.J., Jain, L.C., Ichalkaranje, N. (Eds.): Knowledge-based intelligent information engineering systems & allied technologies, IOS Press, Amsterdam (2002) 21–25
21. Farrington, C.P., Beale, A.D.: The detection of outbreaks of infectious diseases. In: Gierl, L., Cliff, A.D., Valleron, A.-J., Farrington, C.P., Bull, M. (Eds.): International Workshop on Geomedical Systems, Teubner, Stuttgart (1997) 97–117
22. Shindo, N., et al.: Distribution of the influenza warning map by internet. In: Flahault, A., et al. (Eds.): Abstracts of third international workshop on geography and medicine, Paris (2001) 16

23. Schmidt, R., Gierl, L.: Predicting influenza waves with health insurance data. In: Perner, P., Brause, R., Holzhütter, H.-G. (Eds.): Medical data analysis, Lecture Notes in Computer Science, Vol. 2868, Springer, Berlin Heidelberg New York (2003) 91–98
24. Schmidt, R., Gierl, L.: Case-based reasoning for antibiotics therapy advice: An investigation of retrieval algorithms and prototypes. Artificial Intelligence in Medicine 23(2) (2001) 171–186
25. Macura, R., Macura, K.: MacRad: Radiology image resources with a case-based retrieval system. In: Aamodt, A., Veloso, M. (Eds.): Case-based reasoning research and development. Proceedings of the International Conference on Case-Based Reasoning, ICCBR-95, Lecture Notes in Artificial Intelligence, Vol. 1010, Springer, Berlin Heidelberg New York (1995) 43–54
26. Bichindaritz, I., Marling, C.: Workshop case-based reasoning in the health science. In: McGinty, L. (Ed.): Workshop Proceedings of the International Conference on Case-Based Reasoning (2003) 3–88
27. Bichindaritz, I., Marling, C.: Workshop case-based reasoning in the health science. In: Gupta, K.M., Gervas, P. (Eds.): Workshop Proceedings of the European Conference on Case-Based Reasoning (2004) 3–82
28. Bichindaritz, I., Marling, C.: Workshop case-based reasoning in the health science. In: Brüninghaus, S. (Ed.): Workshop Proceedings of the European Conference on Case-Based Reasoning (2005) 3–86
29. Bichindaritz, I., Seroussi, B.: Contraindre l'Analogie par la Causalite. Technique et Sciences Informatiques 11(4) (1992) 69–98
30. Bichindaritz, I.: Case-based reasoning adaptive to several cognitive tasks. In: Aamodt, A., Veloso, M. (Eds.): Case-based reasoning research and development. Proceedings of the International Conference on Case-Based Reasoning, ICCBR-95, Lecture Notes in Artificial Intelligence, Vol. 1010, Springer, Berlin Heidelberg New York (1995) 391–400
31. Bichindaritz, I., Kansu, E., Sullivan, K.M.: Case-based reasoning in CARE-PARTNER: Gathering evidence for evidence-based medical practise. In: Smyth, B., Cunningham, P. (Eds.): Advances in case-based reasoning. Proceedings of the European Workshop on Case-Based Reasoning, EWCBR-98. Lecture Notes in Artificial Intelligence, Vol. 1488, Springer, Berlin Heidelberg New York (1998) 334–345
32. Bichindaritz, I., Conlon, E.: Temporal knowledge representation and organization for case-based reasoning. In: Proceedings of TIME-96, IEEE Computer Society Press, Washington DC (1996) 152–159
33. Bichindaritz, I.: Solving safety implications in case-based decision support system. In: McGinty, L. (Ed.): Workshop Proceedings of the International Conference on Case-Based Reasoning (2003) 9–18
34. Bichindaritz, I.: Memoire: Case-based reasoning meets the semantic web in biology and medicine. In: Funk, P., Gonzalez Calero, P.A. (Eds.): Advances in case-based reasoning. Proceedings of the European Conference on Case-Based Reasoning, ECCBR 2004. Lecture Notes in Artificial Intelligence, Vol. 3155, Springer, Berlin Heidelberg New York (2004) 47–61
35. Montani, S., Bellazzi, R., Portinale, L., Stefanelli, M.: Evaluating a multi-modal reasoning system in diabetes care. In: Blanzieri, E., Portinale, L. (Eds.): Advances in case-based reasoning. Proceedings of the European Workshop on Case-Based Reasoning, EWCBR 2000. Lecture Notes in Artificial Intelligence, Vol. 1898, Springer, Berlin Heidelberg New York (2000) 467–478

36. Bellazzi, R., Montani, S., Portinale, L.: Retrieval in a prototype-based case library: A case study in diabetes therapy revision. In: Smyth, B., Cunningham, P. (Eds.): Advances in case-based reasoning. Proceedings of the European Workshop on Case-Based Reasoning, EWCBR-98. Lecture Notes in Artificial Intelligence, Vol. 1898, Springer, Berlin Heidelberg New York (1998) 64–75
37. Montani, S., Portinale, L., Bellazzi, R., Leonardi, G.: RHENE: A case retrieval system for hemodialysis cases with dynamically monitored parameters. In: Funk, P., Gonzalez Calero, P.A. (Eds.): Advances in case-based reasoning. Proceedings of the European Conference on Case-Based Reasoning, ECCBR 2004. Lecture Notes in Artificial Intelligence, Vol. 3155, Springer, Berlin Heidelberg New York (2004) 659–672
38. Montani, S., Portinale, L.: Case-based representation and retrieval with time dependent features. In: Munoz-Avila, H., Ricci, F. (Eds.): Case-based reasoning research and development. Proceedings of the International Conference on Case-Based Reasoning, ICCBR 2005. Lecture Notes in Artificial Intelligence, Vol. 3620, Springer, Berlin Heidelberg New York (2005) 353–367
39. Nilsson, M., Funk, P., Sollenborn, M.: Complex measurement classification in medical applications using a case-based approach. In: McGinty, L. (Ed.): Workshop Proceedings of the International Conference on Case-Based Reasoning (2003) 63–72
40. Nilsson, M., Funk, P.: A case-based classification of respiratory sinus arrhythmia. In: Funk, P., Gonzalez Calero, P.A. (Eds.): Advances in case-based reasoning. Proceedings of the European Conference on Case-Based Reasoning, ECCBR 2004. Lecture Notes in Artificial Intelligence, Vol. 3155, Springer, Berlin Heidelberg New York (2004) 673–685
41. Koton, P.: Reasoning about evidence in causal explanations. In: Kolodner, J. (Ed.): Proceedings of the Case-Based Reasoning Workshop, Clearwater Beach, Florida (1988) 260–270
42. Turner, R.: Organizing and using schematic knowledge for medical diagnosis. In: Kolodner, J. (Ed.): Proceedings of the Workshop on Case-Based Reasoning, Florida (1988) 435–446
43. Bradburn, C., Zoloznikow, J.: The application of case-based reasoning to the tasks of health care planning. In: Wess, S., Althoff, K.-D., Richter, M.M. (Eds.): Topics in case-based reasoning. Proceedings of the European Workshop on Case-Based Reasoning, EWCBR-93. Lecture Notes in Artificial Intelligence, Vol. 837 Springer, Berlin Heidelberg New York (1993) 365–378
44. Opiyo, E.T.O.: Case-based reasoning for expertise relocation in support of rural health workers in developing countries. In: Aamodt, A., Veloso, M. (Eds.): Case-based reasoning research and development. Proceedings of the International Conference on Case-Based Reasoning, ICCBR-95. Lecture Notes in Artificial Intelligence, Vol. 1010, Springer, Berlin Heidelberg New York (1995) 77–87
45. El Balaa, Z. et al.: FM-Ultranet: A decision support system using case-based reasoning applied to ultrasonography. In: McGinty, L. (Ed.): Workshop Proceedings of the International Conference on Case-Based Reasoning (2003) 37–44
46. Kwiatkowski, M., Atkins, S.: Case representation and retrieval in the diagnosis and treatment of obstructive sleep apnea: A semio-fuzzy approach. In: Gupta, K.M., Gervas, P. (Eds.): Workshop Proceedings of the European Conference on Case-Based Reasoning (2004) 25–34
47. Baumeister, J., Atzmüller, M., Puppe, F.: Inductive learning for case-based diagnosis with multiple faults. In: Craw, S., Preece, A. (Eds.): Advances in

case-based reasoning Proceedings of the European Workshop on Case-Based Reasoning, ECCBR 2002. Lecture Notes in Artificial Intelligence, Vol. 2416, Springer, Berlin Heidelberg New York (2002) 28–42
48. Shi, W., Branden, J.A.: How to combine CBR and RBR for diagnosing multiple medical disorder cases. In: Munoz-Avila, H., Ricci, F. (Eds.): Case-based reasoning research and development. Proceedings of the International Conference on Case-Based Reasoning, ICCBR 2005. Lecture Notes in Artificial Intelligence, Vol. 3620, Springer, Berlin Heidelberg New York (2005) 477–491
49. Schmidt, R., Vorobieva, O.: Adaptation and medical case-based reasoning focusing on endocrine therapy support. In: Miksch, S., Hunter, J., Keravnou, E. (Eds.): Artificial intelligence in medicine. Proceedings AIME-2005, Lecture Notes in Artificial Intelligence, Vol. 3581, Springer, Berlin Heidelberg New York (2005) 308–317
50. Jurisica, I., et al.: Case-based reasoning in IVF: Prediction and knowledge mining. Artificial Intelligence in Medicine 12 (1998) 1–24
51. Wilke, W., Smyth, B., Cunningham, P.: Using configuration techniques for adaptation. In: Lenz, M., Bartsch-Spörl, B., Burkhard, H.-D., Wess, S. (Eds.): Case-based reasoning technology, from foundations to applications. Lecture Notes in Artificial Intelligence, Vol. 1400, Springer, Berlin Heidelberg New York (1998) 139–168
52. Lieber, J., Bresson, B.: Case-based reasoning for breast cancer treatment decision helping. In: Blanzieri, E., Portinale, L. (Eds.): Advances in case-based reasoning. Proceedings of the European Workshop on Case-Based Reasoning, EWCBR 2000. Lecture Notes in Artificial Intelligence, Vol. 1898, Springer, Berlin Heidelberg New York (2000) 173–185
53. Evans-Romaine, K., Marling, C.: Prescribing exercise regimens for cardiac and pulmonary disease patients with CBR. In: McGinty, L. (Ed.): Workshop Proceedings of the International Conference on Case-Based Reasoning (2003) 45–52
54. Davis, G., Wiratunga, N., Taylor, B., Craw, S.: Matching SMARTHOUSE technology to needs of the elderly and disabled. In: McGinty, L. (Ed.): Workshop Proceedings of the International Conference on Case-Based Reasoning (2003) 29–36
55. Lorenzi, F., Abel, M., Ricci, F.: SISAIH: A case based reasoning tool for hospital admission authorization management. In: Gupta, K.M., Gervas, P. (Eds.): Workshop Proceedings of the European Conference on Case-Based Reasoning (2004) 35–44
56. Kahn, C.E.J., Anderson, G.M.: Case-based reasoning and imaging procedure selection. Investigative Radiology 29 (1994) 643–647
57. Grimnes, M., Aamodt, A.: Two layer case-based reasoning architecture for medical image understanding. In: Smith, I., Faltings, B. (Eds.): Advances in case-based reasoning. Proceedings of the European Workshop on Case-Based Reasoning, EWCBR-96. Lecture Notes in Artificial Intelligence, Vol. 1168, Springer, Berlin Heidelberg New York (1996) 164–178
58. Haddad, M., Adlassnig, K.P., Porenta, G.: Feasability analysis of a case-based reasoning system for automated detection of coronary heart disease from myocardial scintigrams. Artificial Intelligence in Medicine 9 (1997) 61–78
59. Jarmulak, J.: Case-based classification of ultrasonic B-Scans. Case-base organisation and case retrieval. In: Smyth, B., Cunningham, P. (Eds.): Advances in case-based reasoning. Proceedings of the European Workshop on Case-Based

Reasoning, EWCBR-98. Lecture Notes in Artificial Intelligence, Vol. 1488, Springer, Berlin Heidelberg New York (1998) 100–111

60. Perner, P.: An architecture for a CBR image segmentation system. In: Althoff, K.-D., Bergmann, R., Branting, L.K. (Eds.): Case-based reasoning research and development. Proceedings of the International Conference on Case-Based Reasoning, ICCBR-99, Lecture Notes in Artificial Intelligence, Vol. 1650, Springer, Berlin Heidelberg New York (1999) 525–534
61. Jänichen, S., Perner, P.: Case acquisition and case mining for case-based object recognition. In: Funk, P., Gonzalez Calero, P.A. (Eds.): Advances in case-based reasoning. Proceedings of the European Conference on Case-Based Reasoning. ECCBR 2004, Lecture Notes in Artificial Intelligence, Vol. 3155, Springer, Berlin Heidelberg New York (2004) 616–629
62. Perner, P.: Why case-based reasoning is attractive for image interpretation. In: Aha, D., Watson, I. (Eds.): Case-based reasoning research and development. Proceedings of the International Conference on Case-Based Reasoning, ICCBR 2001, Lecture Notes in Artificial Intelligence, Vol. 2080, Springer, Berlin Heidelberg New York (2001) 27–44

Assessing the Quality of Care for End Stage Renal Failure Patients by Means of Artificial Intelligence Methodologies

Stefania Montani, Luigi Portinale, Riccardo Bellazzi,
Cristiana Larizza, and Roberto Bellazzi

Summary. End Stage Renal Disease is a severe chronic condition that corresponds to the final stage of kidney failure. Hemodialysis (HD) is the most widely used treatment method for ESRD. The HD treatment is costly and demanding from an organizational viewpoint, requiring day hospital beds, specialized nurses and periodical visits and exams of out-patients.

In order to assess the performance of HD centers, we are developing an auditing system, which resorts to (1) *temporal data mining* techniques, to discover relationships between the time patterns of the data automatically collected during HD sessions and the performance outcomes, and to (2) *case based reasoning* (CBR) to retrieve similar time series within the HD data, in order to evaluate the frequency of critical patterns. In particular, as regards temporal data mining, two new methods for association rule discovery and temporal rule discovery have been applied to the HD time series. As regards CBR, we have implemented a case-based retrieval system, which resorts to a multi-step architecture, and exploits dimensionality reduction techniques for efficient time series indexing.

The overall approach has demonstrated to be suitable for knowledge discovery and critical patterns similarity assessment on real patients' data, and its use in the context of an auditing system for dialysis management is helping clinicians to improve their understanding of the patients behavior.

1 Introduction

Health care organizations (HCO) have nowadays evolved into complex enterprises, in which the management of knowledge and information resources is a key success factor in order to improve their efficacy and efficiency. Rather interestingly, the types of knowledge that have to be managed comprise of both the empirical and experiential (or tacit) knowledge mirrored by the day by day actions of health care providers and the structured and explicit knowledge contained in guidelines and textbooks. Unfortunately, although HCO are

S. Montani et al.: *Assessing the Quality of Care for End Stage Renal Failure Patients*, Studies in Computational Intelligence (SCI) **48**, 89–112 (2007)
www.springerlink.com

data-rich organizations, their capability of managing tacit knowledge is still very poor: the day-by-day collection of patients' clinical data, of health care provider actions (e.g., exams, drug deliveries, surgeries) and of health care processes data (admissions, discharge, exams request) is not often followed by a thorough analysis of such kind of information. Traditionally, it has been considered that the usefulness of those data for evidence-based medicine purposes is very limited, since they do not come from clinical trials and controlled environments and they may be thus affected by several biases.

Thanks to the knowledge management (KM) perspective [1], on the other hand, the crucial role of process data for institution-based organizational learning has been made clear: process data may be effectively used to change organizational settings and to maintain and retrieve unstructured situation-action knowledge [2].

One of the aspects of organizational learning is the assessment of the quality of hospital services. In detail, the goal of a quality assessment system is the one of relying upon process data to: assess the performance of the overall service at hand; assess the performance of the service for each patient that resorts to it; understand the reasons of failures. Technically speaking, such a system should allow to fulfil two (independent) tasks (1) discover relationships between the time patterns of the process data and the performance outcomes; (2) retrieve similar time series within the process data, in order to assess the frequency of critical patterns.

The aim of this work is to show how both tasks can be dealt with, by resorting to classical Artificial Intelligence (AI) methodologies. In particular, we are interested in the development of an auditing system for assessing the efficacy of the treatment delivered by a Hospital Hemodialysis Department (HHD) on the basis of the process data routinely collected during hemodialysis sessions. HHDs manage End Stage Renal Disease (ESRD) patients that undergo blood depuration (hemodialysis) through an extra-corporal circuit. The data accumulated over time for each patient contain the set of variables that are monitored during each dialysis session. In other words, the data collected are sequences (inter-session data) of multidimensional time series (intrasession data). The majority of these process data is typically neglected in clinical practice, since they are synthesized by few clinical indicators observed at the beginning and at the end of each treatment session. Such clinical indicators are usually related to the well-being of patients, and do not contain detailed information about the quality of the treatment, in terms, for example, of blood depuration efficiency or nurse interventions during the dialysis sessions. The goal of this work is, therefore, to fully exploit hemodialysis process data in order to fulfil the two tasks outlined earlier. In particular, *temporal data mining* techniques are applied to discover relationships between the time patterns of the process data and the performance outcomes, while *case based reasoning* (CBR) [3] is applied to retrieve similar time series within the process data, in order to assess the frequency of critical patterns.

The work has involved the Department of Computer and Systems Science of the University of Pavia, the Department of Computer Science of the University of Piemonte Orientale, the HHD of Vigevano (Pavia) and the Limited Assistance Center (LAC) of Mede, a small town located 35 km far from Vigevano. LAC are dialysis services managed by nurses, with a remote supervision of a HHD. The HHD physicians define the HD prescriptions (dialysis duration, ideal weight loss, pharmacological therapy) during periodic control visits, and the day by day management is carried on by nurses.

The paper is organized as follows: details of the application domain can be found in Sect. 2, the data mining facility we have designed and implemented is described in Sect. 3, while the CBR system is described in Sect. 4. Results are presented in Sect. 5, and conclusions are discussed in Sect. 6.

2 Hemodialysis Treatment for ESRD

ESRD is a severe chronic condition that corresponds to the final stage of kidney failure. Without medical intervention, ESRD leads to death. In the US, the incidence of chronic renal failures ranges between 242–348 patients per million inhabitants [4] while in Italy it is of about 120 per million inhabitants [5]. Hemodialysis (HD) is the most widely used treatment method for ESRD. HD relies on an electromechanical device, called artificial kidney or hemodialyzer which, thanks to an extracorporeal blood circuit, is able to clear the patient's blood from metabolites, to re-establish acid–base equilibrium and to remove water in excess. On average, hemodialysis patients are treated for four hours three times a week. The HD treatment is costly and demanding from an organizational viewpoint, requiring day hospital beds, specialized nurses and periodical visits and exams of out-patients [6].

The overall assessment of an HD treatment center is typically made on the basis of some general outcomes parameters, such as mortality, morbidity and rehospitalization. Periodically, it is also possible to aggregate the data coming from the assessment of the HD sessions of single patients, such as the so-called "KT/V" analysis. Such analysis is performed through the assessment of the removal of the protein catabolism products (urea) with respect to the dialysis time. The KT/V analysis is routinely performed only few times per month (typically one), under the (false) assumption that the therapy conditions do not change over time.

Thanks to the advances of the most recent hemodialyzers, it is now possible to tackle with the problem of assessing the performance of HD centers from a completely different viewpoint. Hemodialyzers may nowadays allow for the automatic monitoring of the dialysis sessions, collecting more than 25 variables. This allows the design of systems for an automatic evaluation of the performance of each dialysis session, and, thanks to a suitable aggregation mechanism, for the evaluation of the overall HD center.

In particular, the efficacy of hemodialysis sessions can be assessed [7] on the basis of a few predefined outcomes, obtainable from a subset of the monitoring variables as follows:

- Removal of protein catabolism products (urea, creatinine); this outcome is indirectly evaluated by measuring the blood flow in the extracorporeal circuit (QB), the body weight loss (WL), and the duration of a hemodialysis session (T).
- Efficiency of the extra-corporeal circuit of the dialyzer; this outcome is evaluated by measuring the hydraulic pressures of the circuit: the arterial (AP) and venous (VP) pressures. AP and VP are, respectively, collected before and after the device where solutes and water are exchanged.
- Body water reduction and hypotension episodes. The monitoring of body water and of patients systemic pressure is performed by measuring the body weight (WB), systolic and diastolic pressures (SP, DP), the cardiac frequency (CF), the hemoglobin concentration (Hb), and the hematic volume (HV).

The data collected during each dialysis session we refer to are summarized in Tables 1 and 2. In particular Table 1 lists the variables collected in the form of time series, while Table 2 lists the variables recorded in the form of single data points (one value per session). In the current technical settings, the sampling time ranged from 1 to 15 min.

Table 1. Monitoring variables for hemodialysis efficiency assessment, collected as time series

variable name	abbreviation
venous pressure	VP
blood bulk flow	QB
arterial pressure	AP
systolic pressure	SP
diastolic pressure	DP
cardiac frequency	CF
hemoglobin	Hb
hematic volume	HV
output pressure of dialyzer	OP
dialysate conductivity	DC

Table 2. Monitoring variables for hemodialysis efficiency assessment, collected as single data points

variable name	abbreviation
weight before session	WB
weight loss	WL
dry weight	DW
vascular access	VA
dialysis time duration	T

In this context, data mining techniques appear to be well suited to preprocess the data, and to discover relationships between measured signals and HD failures. On the other hand, through CBR it is possible to look for similar situations, typically patterns corresponding to persistent failures over time; it is then possible to highlight if these patterns are repeated over the same patient or over different ones, and what solutions have been provided in those cases, in terms of dialysis prescription (i.e., the prescribed flow rates at the beginning of dialysis).

Details of how these methodologies have been exploited in our work are introduced in the next sections.

3 Data Mining for ESRD

In order to assess the performance of each dialysis session, we need to compute a suitable summary of the intradialysis time series.

In particular, we decided to resort to the calculation of the more frequent values measured in each session, disregarding the information on the dynamics. Each session is thus synthesized through the median value (50th percentile) of each monitored variable. Such a choice, although arguable for some signals, allows the user to easily interpret the auditing system results. After having calculated the median values, we obtain a new multidimensional time series, in which each point is the vector of the median values of the monitoring variables. We will refer to this time series as the median time series.

On the basis of the median values, it is possible to assess the quality of a session by performing a comparison between a set of reference values and a set of dialysis outcome parameters. In more detail, we consider six outcome parameters: (1) the median levels of VP, AP, that we will denote as VP*, AP*; (2) the difference (ΔQB) between the prescribed QB and its median values (QB*); (3) the difference (ΔT) between the prescribed dialysis time and the observed one; (4) the difference (ΔL) between the prescribed weight loss and the weight loss measured at the end of the dialysis; and (5) the difference (ΔW) between the weight reached at the end of the dialysis and the target weight of the patient.

A general index of success is derived by judging as positive a treatment in which all (logical operator AND) the logic conditions of Fig. 1 are satisfied.

Moreover, a crucial aspect of our work is to be able to provide clinicians and nurses with a deeper insight in the HD temporal patterns, in order to discover the reasons of failures, by deriving associations between monitoring variables and failures that may be interpreted as causal relationships. To this end, we have defined a temporal data mining strategy, based on the median time series of each dialysis session. Such strategy follows two steps: (1) extraction of basic temporal patterns, e.g., trends, from the median time series; (2) search for patient-specific associations between the temporal patterns and the failures; to

Parameters	Condition
ΔQB	Not less than 2% of the prescription
VP^*	Less or equal to 350 ± 3 mmHg
AP^*	Greater or equal to – 250 mg
ΔT	Less or equal than 2% of the prescription
ΔL	Less or equal than 7% of the prescription
ΔW	Less or equal than 5% of the prescription

Fig. 1. Outcome parameters and the corresponding logical conditions for their assessment

this end we have implemented two different algorithms: the first one searches for the contemporaneous presence of the temporal patterns and the failures, while the second one searches for temporal relationships, i.e., precedence, between the temporal patterns and the failures. To extract basic temporal patterns, we have exploited an interesting approach to temporal data analysis and reasoning called Temporal Abstractions (TA) [8].

Through TA, large amounts of temporal information, such as the one embedded in a time series, can be effectively mapped to a compact representation, that not only summarizes the original longitudinal data, but also abstracts meaningful behaviors in the data themselves.

Operatively, the basic principle of TA methods is to move from a *point-based* to an *interval-based* representation of the data [9], where (1) the input points (*events* henceforth) are the elements of the discretized time series; (2) the output intervals (*episodes* henceforth) aggregate adjacent events sharing a common behavior, persistent over time. More precisely, the method described earlier should be referred to as *basic* TA [9].

Basic abstractions can be further subdivided into *state* TA and *trend* TA. *State* TA are used to extract episodes associated with *qualitative levels* of the monitored feature, e.g., low, normal, high values; *trend* TA are exploited to detect specific *patterns*, such as increase, decrease or stationarity, from the time series. The output results of a basic TA depend on the value assigned to specific parameters, such as the granularity (the maximum temporal gap between two events allowed for aggregating them into the same episode) and the minimum extent (the minimum time extent for considering an episode relevant) for state TA, and the slope (the minimum allowed rate of change in an episode) for trend TA.

Complex TA [9] can be defined as well: instead of aggregating events into episodes, complex TA aggregate two series of episodes into a set of higher level episodes (i.e., they abstract output intervals over precomputed input intervals). In particular, complex abstractions search for specific *temporal* relationships between episodes that can be generated from a basic abstraction or from other complex abstractions. The relation between intervals can be any of the temporal relations defined by Allen [10]. This kind of TA can be exploited to extract patterns that depend on the course of several features, or to detect patterns of complex shapes (e.g., a peak) in a single feature.

In the hemodialysis problem, we use basic TA to summarize the dynamics of the median time series of each variable in the monitoring period. Before running the TA mechanisms, the median time series is preprocessed with filtering techniques in order to robustly detect trend TA. Through the extraction of basic TA, we obtain a collection of episodes, that give a compact picture of the profile of each variable. In the same way, we also extract the failure episodes by aggregating the consecutive failures for each specific cause.

Once we have derived the state and trend TA for each monitoring variable, we want to look for possible associations between the TA and the dialysis failure causes. As a first goal, we concentrated our attention on the extraction of rules in which a temporal pattern, i.e., a TA, is contemporaneous to a failure. This means to search for rules of the kind "IF the Trend of Venous Pressure is increasing THEN dialysis fails due to insufficient Weight Loss." The search algorithm described in this section has been inspired by the work of Hoppner [11] and by the well-known PRISM and APRIORI algorithms [12,13]. Let us note that, although the search procedure looks for rules with a predefined set of consequents, and may be, thus, interpreted as a supervised learning problem, its final goal is not to derive predictive rules, but to extract a description of the co-occurrences of abstractions and failures. For this reason, we use the term association rules to denote the outputs of the algorithm. In order to describe the search algorithm we developed, it is necessary to introduce some definitions and notations. Given the median time series M_j of a variable j, the state TA for M_j can be represented as the collection of time intervals in which M_j is either high (H) or normal (N) or low (L), while the trend TA for M_j can be represented as the collection of time intervals in which M_j is either increasing (I), stationary (S), or decreasing (D). Given two or more TA, for example "M_j is N" and "M_i is I," we can easily calculate their intersection as the intersection of their time intervals; the time span ($TS_{ji}(N,I)$) of such intersection corresponds to the number of dialysis sessions in which both TA occur. The intersection can be calculated considering also one or more TA and any failure parameter. In this case, given the abstraction "M_j is S," and the failure parameter $F = F_i$, we denote the time span of their intersection as $TS_{jFi}(S, F_i)$. Let us note that $TS_{jjj}(H,N,L)$ and $TS_{jjj}(I,S,D)$ are equal to zero. Finally, we denote TS_{tot} as the time span of the monitoring period, which corresponds to the total number of dialysis sessions performed. The search procedure aims to define rules of the form $B \rightarrow F_i$ where B is the body and F_i is the head of the rule: in our case B is any conjunction of TA (e.g., "M_i is L" and "M_j is H"), and F_i is a failure parameter (i.e., failure due to ΔL). B is here interpreted as the intersection of TA involved in the conjunction. We define the cardinality of the rule as the number of TA in B. It is, therefore, possible to calculate the time span of B (TS_B) resorting to the definition given earlier. We define the support (SU) of a rule as the ratio between the number of sessions in which the rule holds and the total number of sessions (i.e., $SU = TS_{BFi}/TS_{tot}$) and we define the confidence (CF) of the rule as the conditional probability $\Pr\{F_i|B\}$, which may be calculated as $CF = \frac{TS_{BFi}}{TS_B}$. Resorting to the definitions given earlier, we run a search strategy which constructs rules with the maximal body having $SU > SU_{min}$ and $CF > CF_{min}$, being SU_{min} and CF_{min} suitable threshold values. The strategy works as follows:

(a) *Step 1.* Choose a patient. Choose a failure parameter F_i. Compute the TA for all variables. The TA are in the basic set B_0.
(b) *Step 2.* The TA of B_0 which corresponds to association rules with F_i such that $SU > SU_{min}$ are put in the set B_1. Set the counter k, that represents the cardinality of the rule, to 1.
(c) *Step 3.* Do:
  - Set $k = k + 1$
  - Generate the set B_k from B_{k-1}, in such a way that $SU > SU_{min}$. The generation of B_k is implemented by following the APRIORI itemset generation strategy [13].

  while B_k is not empty.
(d) *Step 4.* Put $B = B_{k-1}$. Filter B in order to have rules with $CF > CF_{min}$. The rule $B \to O_i$ contains the rule with most complex body. Let us note that the algorithm may derive more than one rule for each O_i.

The derived rules with their support can be shown to the users also in graphical form, thus highlighting the temporal location of the sessions in which each rule holds. As an example, Fig. 2 shows the occurrence of an episode with High VP*, Low AP* and High Hb*, corresponding to a series of Blood Flow failures (ΔQB). The method clearly helps to highlight an episode in which the vascular access of the patient was not efficient, thus provoking high absolute values of the pressures in the extracorporeal circuit and, at the same time, an insufficient blood flow through the dialyzer.

Searching for association rules between variables and outcomes allows us to highlight interesting clinical situations, where some temporal patterns are contemporaneous to the presence of a dialysis failure. Another important kind of analysis is to detect temporal rules, where the TA contained in the antecedent of the rules (the body of the rule) have a temporal relationship with the failure. Such rules can be useful to extract failure scenarios, which can be used also for predictive purposes. In computational terms, a way to extract such temporal rules is to map them to a particular kind of complex TA, where a set of contemporaneous patterns (the antecedents of the rule) has a temporal relationship with a failure episode. In our case, we have defined a new temporal relationship, which we have called PRECEDES. Given

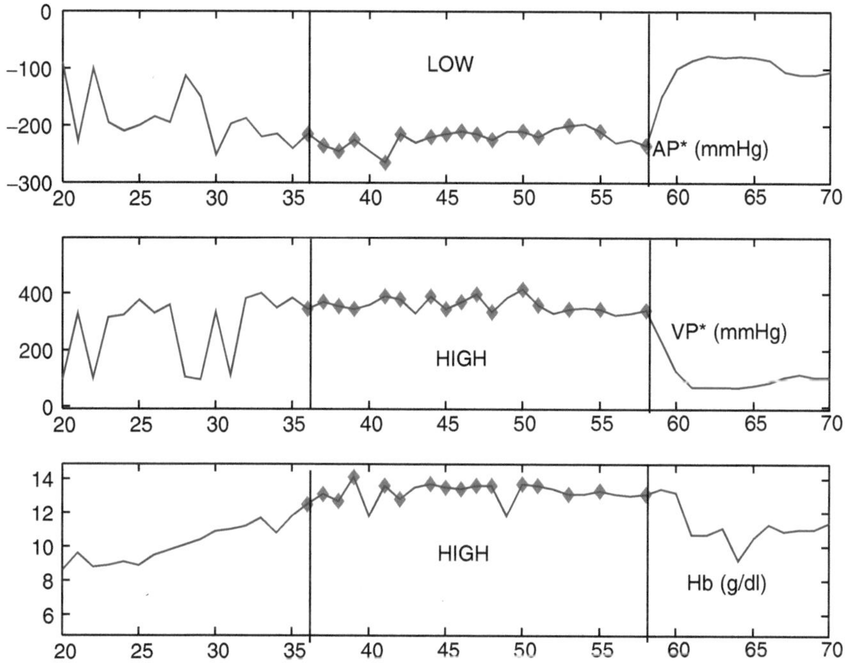

Fig. 2. An example of output of the association rule discovery algorithm. An episode in which a failure for Blood Flow (ΔQB) is contemporaneous to a low value of AP*, a high value of VP* and a High value of Hb*. Such a situation corresponds to an occlusion of the vascular access of the extracorporeal circuit, which was solved after dialysis 60

two episodes A and F, with time intervals $[a_1, a_2]$ and $[f_1, f_2]$, respectively, A PRECEDES F, if $a_1 <= f_1$ and $a_2 <= f_2$.

PRECEDES expresses the intuitive notion that a scenario starts with an episode related to certain monitoring variables and ends with an episode of failure. More precisely, the choice of the PRECEDES operator is motivated by the need of looking for typical temporal scenarios which occur before and may persist during (but not lasting after) the episodes of failure. Therefore, we look for temporal patterns of the kind: "An episode in which variable A is Increasing AND variable B is High PRECEDES Failure F" Let us note that PRECEDES includes the Allen's [10] temporal operators OVERLAPS, FINISHED-BY, MEETS, BEFORE, EQUALS and STARTS (see Fig. 3).

The PRECEDES temporal relationship may be constrained by three parameters: (1) the right shift (RS), defined as the maximum distance between f_2 and a_2; (2) the left shift (LS), defined as the maximum distance between f_1 and a_1; (3) the gap (GP), defined as the maximum distance between a_2 and f_1, when $f_1 > a_2$. The algorithm for extracting the temporal rules is a generalization of the one described earlier.

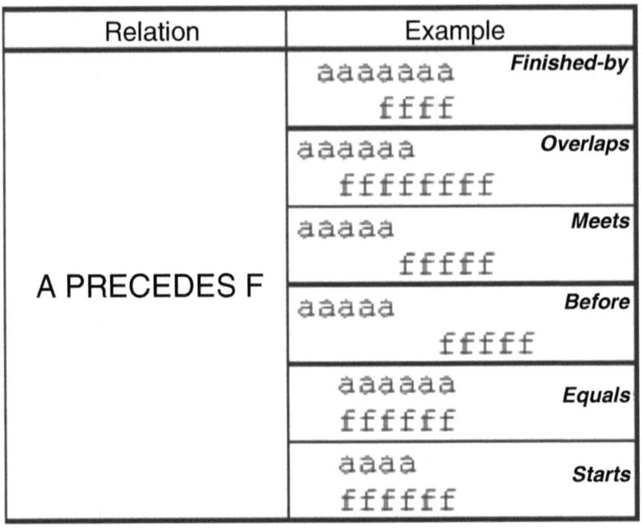

Fig. 3. The PRECEDES temporal operator

Figure 4 shows a complex TA episode extracted from our data by our learning algorithm. The episode is "UF* Low and DP* Low PRECEDES a failure due to insufficient ΔT." Since this temporal pattern is found with confidence 1 and support 0.3 in the overall data (not shown), the rule "UF* Low and DP* Low $\rightarrow$ ΔT" is extracted.

4 Case-Based Retrieval for ESRD

CBR is a problem solving paradigm that utilizes the specific knowledge of previously experienced situations, called cases. It basically consists in retrieving past cases that are similar to the current one and in reusing (by, if necessary, adapting) past successful solutions; the current case can be retained and put into the case library. In the domain of ESRD, we have developed a case-based retrieval system, i.e., a system in which only the retrieval step of the overall CBR methodology sketched earlier is carried out. In our application, in particular, a dialysis session can be interpreted as a case. The case structure involves two categories of features: *static* features and *dynamic* ones. Static features represent general information about the patient (e.g., age class, sex, type of the disease that caused ESRD), long-term varying data, that can be approximately considered as static within an interval of a few weeks/months (e.g., several laboratory exams), and measurements taken only once per session (see Table 2). On the other hand, dynamic features are the information automatically measured several times within a dialysis session, and thus recorded in the form of discretized time series (see Table 1).

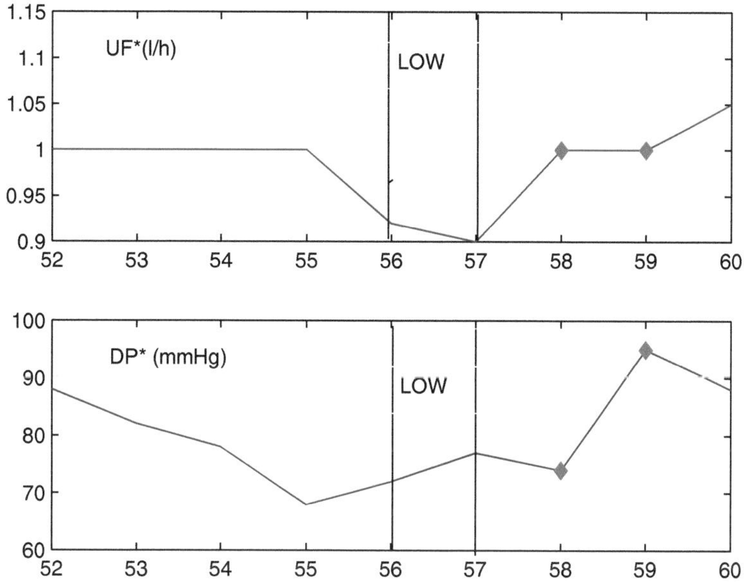

Fig. 4. A PRECEDES relationships between a temporal pattern and a failure extracted by the proposed algorithm from the dialysis data set. In this case, an episode with Low values of UF* and DP* PRECEDES a Failure due to insufficient dialysis time (ΔT)

Since static features provide both a general characterization of the patient and of the dialysis session as a whole, they provide the context under which to evaluate the results of the dialysis, based on the interpretation of all the relevant measured parameters (both static and dynamic). Defining the context for retrieval corresponds to the so-called *situation assessment* step of CBR. Therefore, it is quite natural to structure case retrieval as a two-step procedure, articulated as follows:

1. *Classification.* it is based on static features alone, and it produces the relevant context under which to base retrieval; a classification step can be important if the physician needs to restrict attention only to particular subsets of the whole case base. Classification relies on classical K-Nearest Neighbor (K-NN) techniques.
2. *Retrieval.* it takes place on the restricted case base possibly produced by the classification step. Intraclass retrieval is in turn a two-step procedure:
   (a) First of all, the physician has the possibility of choosing a set of dynamic features (that are in the form of time series) on which to ground the retrieval; this allows her/him to focus the attention on a subset of features that s/he considers relevant for the current analysis s/he's going to perform. The requirement implemented by the system is that the retrieved cases must have a specified level of similarity

for every selected feature. For each one of the selected dynamic features (a subset of those listed in Table 1), we work on *local similarity*, i.e., we look for the most similar cases to the input case relatively to the direction represented by the feature at hand. We perform such a search by executing a range query on the feature distance: a case will be retrieved only if the distance of the considered feature from the corresponding series in the input case is smaller than a given threshold s. The local retrieval process is then applied to all the selected dynamic features and the intersection of the set of cases obtained with each local retrieval is returned.

(b) Since in practice we are interested in *global similarity*, we finally compute the distance from the input case in the space of all the case features, for the data set composed by the cases obtained at step 2(a). In particular, we include all the dynamic features which have not been selected for local retrieval as well as static features. Cases can then be ordered in decreasing order of distance (i.e., in increasing order of similarity) and the best ones can be shown to the user.

The overall methodology is summarized in Fig. 5.

Intraclass retrieval is the core of our methodology, and we will provide some additional details about it.

A wide literature exists about similarity-based retrieval of time series. Several different approaches have been proposed (see the survey in [14]), but most are based on the common premise of dimensionality reduction. As a matter of fact, a (discretized) time series can always be seen as a vector in an n-dimensional space (with n typically extremely large). Simple algorithms for retrieving similar time series take polynomial time in n. Multidimensional spatial indexing also known as spatial access methods (SAM) (e.g., resorting to R-trees [15] or similar structures) is a promising technique that allows sublinear retrieval; nevertheless, these tree structures are not adequate for indexing very high-dimensional data sets [16].

One obvious solution is thus to reduce the time series dimensionality, adopting a transform that preserves the distance between two time series or underestimates it. In the latter case a postprocessing step is required to filter out the so-called "false alarms"; the requirement is never to overestimate the distance, so that no "false dismissals" can exist [14]. A widely used transform is the discrete Fourier transform (DFT) [17].

DFT maps time series to the frequency domain. DFT application for dimensionality reduction stems from the observation that, for the majority of real-world time series, the first (1–3) Fourier coefficients carry the most meaningful information, and the remaining ones can be safely discarded. Moreover, Parseval's theorem [18] guarantees that the distance in the frequency domain is the same as in the time domain, when resorting to any similarity measure that can be expressed as the Euclidean distance between feature vectors in the feature space. In particular, resorting only to the first Fourier coefficients can underestimate the real distance, but never overestimates it. The definition of

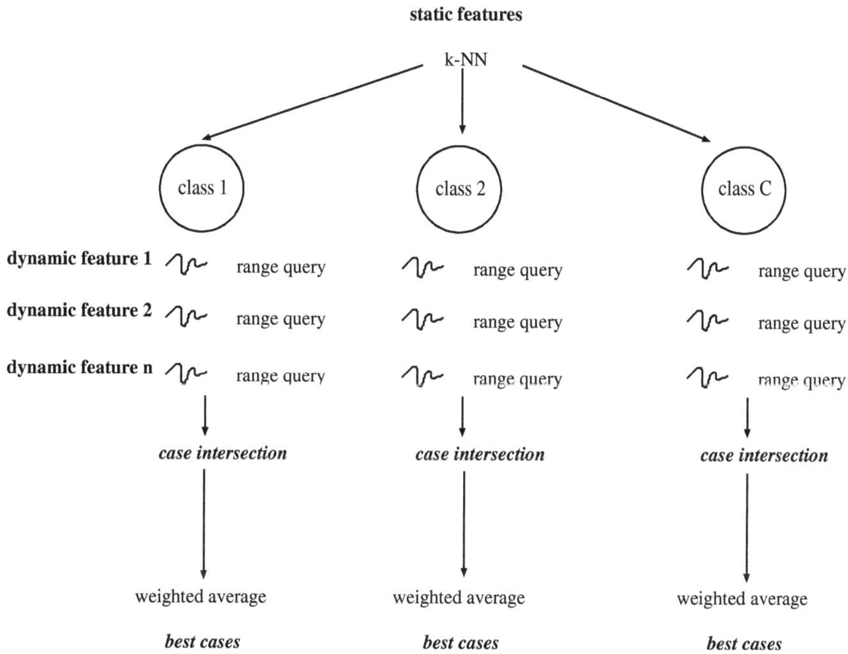

Fig. 5. The overall case retrieval process implemented within our system. Classification exploits k-NN in the static features space. Intraclass retrieval then extracts the most similar cases in each of the n selected dynamic features directions: to guarantee that retrieved cases have the required level of similarity on each selected feature the intersection on the set of returned cases is computed. On this set, global distance is calculated, by computing a weighted average; returned cases are then ordered in terms of overall distance

similarity can also be extended with invariance under a group of transformations, like amplitude scaling and shift (see [19, 20]).

In our system, we are currently implementing DFT as a means for dimensionality reduction, exploiting the Euclidean distance as a similarity measure (in particular, in presence of missing data, we set the distance equal to its maximum value, i.e., to the feature range). The choice of DFT is motivated by the observation that DFT is a standard technique, that is widely reported in the literature and that has been successfully applied in several application domains. Moreover, DFT offers the possibility of relying on well known index structures, without studying ad hoc solutions, and avoiding exhaustive search (which, on the other hand, would be required for methods not relying on coefficients). In particular, we have implemented an index belonging to the family of *k-d trees* and a range query algorithm directly operating on k-d trees themselves [21]. K-d trees are a technique frequently used in CBR systems, both for indexing nonhierarchical cases, and for indexing cases represented through hierarchies of attributes [22].

Given two time series $X = \{x_1, \ldots, x_r\}$ and $Y = \{y_1, \ldots, y_q\}$, a parametric distance measure can be defined by considering an integer parameter p (if $p = 2$ we get the standard Euclidean distance):

$$D(X, Y, p) = \left(\sum_{j=1}^{\min(r,q)} |x_j - y_j|^p \right)^{\frac{1}{p}} .$$

In order to make the distance scale independent with respect to the series values, distance can be normalized over the range $RANGE_f$ of the corresponding feature f as follows:

$$D_f(X, Y, p) = \left(\frac{1}{m} \sum_{j=1}^{m} \left| \frac{x_j - y_j}{RANGE_f} \right|^p \right)^{\frac{1}{p}} = \frac{D(X, Y, p)}{m^{\frac{1}{p}}\, RANGE_f}$$

with $m = \min(r, q)$.

In this way, every distance is in the range $[0, 1]$ independently of the considered feature f and it becomes more natural to characterize a range query. In particular, we exploit a parameter $0 \leq s \leq 1$ used as distance threshold for the range queries concerning the dynamic features of our cases.

Given a query case C_Q, intraclass retrieval starts by considering each single dynamic feature f that the physician has selected for her/his analysis; let T_f be the k-d tree index for feature f, Q_f the query series (i.e., the time series relative to feature f in case C_Q) and s the distance threshold for the range query. The following steps are then implemented: since the dialysis device has starting and ending phases during which monitored data are meaningless, the query series Q_f is first validated by removing head and tail data corresponding to noisy values; in this way all the considered time series are aligned to the first valid point. After that, Q_f is reduced through DFT by considering a predefined number of coefficients[1] (usually 3). We are then able to perform a range query on T_f using Q_f and the threshold s; this returns a set of time series (relative to feature f) having a distance from Q_f that may be less than s (due to Parseval's theorem we are only guaranteed that no indexed time series whose distance is actually less than s has been missed). We then need a postprocessing of the results, where actual distance with respect to Q_f is computed. The whole process is performed for every dynamic feature that has been selected for local retrieval and finally, only cases that have been retrieved in every feature direction are returned (case intersection). Figure 6 depicts this mechanism. Notice that, for each retrieved series, the case intersection step first extracts from the case library the whole case to which the series belongs and then performs the intersection of the obtained set of cases. In this way we are guaranteed that returned cases have a distance less than the threshold for every considered dynamic feature.

[1] The number of DFT coefficients to consider is a tunable parameter of the system.

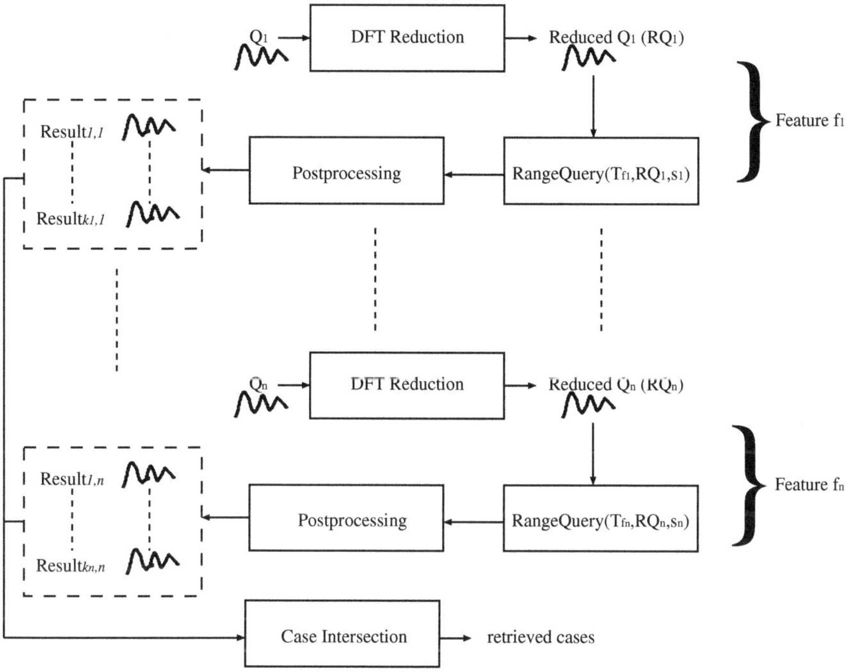

Fig. 6. Block scheme for local retrieval. In the direction of each feature selected by the physician, dimensionality reduction is performed. A range query is then conducted, and the obtained results are filtered through a post processing step, meant to delete false alarms. Finally, all the sets of locally similar cases are intersected, in order to obtain globally similar results

Since we are finally interested in obtaining the best cases in terms of global distance with respect to the query, we compute such a global measure as a weighted average of feature (local) distances for every returned case:

$$D(C, C_Q) = \frac{\sum_{i=1}^{n} w_i D_{f_i}(X_C, Y_Q, p)}{\sum_{i=1}^{n} w_i},$$

where C is a retrieved case, C_Q the query case, X_C and Y_Q are the time series (values) of the feature f_i in case C and C_Q, respectively, and w_i is the weight representing the importance of feature f_i; the former is another tunable parameter of the system available to the physician for biasing the order of presentation with more emphasis on a particular set of features (usually those selected for local retrieval, since they represent features on which to base the analysis of the results).

5 Results

5.1 Testing the Data Mining Facility

The facility for temporal abstractions extraction and association rule discovery described in this paper has been integrated within a more complete software system, called Hemostat. Hemostat also allows the user to define the haemodialysis targets for each outcome parameter for each patient, and to easily calculate the percentage of failures for the overall HHD and for each patient, over any given monitoring time period. Moreover, it provides histograms, pies, charts and text outputs.

The Hemostat software has been installed and used in the LAC of Mede, which treats about 40 patients. It is in routine use since May 2002. Until now, it has been exploited to control the quality of the performance of the dialysis center, by progressively changing and tuning the workflow of the involved nurses. The results obtained are extensively described in [7].

After a period of usage of three years, from 2002 to 2005, a new version of the software was made available to the Department in January 2006. 9,250 dialysis sessions have been collected in the period January 2002–December 2005. The mean number of dialysis session was 230, with a peak of 370 sessions in March 2004. Considering the more reliable collected data, concerning the failures for blood flow, weight loss, dialysis time, and the blood circuit pressure, 3,231 failed dialysis have been collected; this number corresponds to the 35% of dialysis sessions. For what concerns the trend, the percentage of failed dialysis has decreased from 55% (September 2002) to 31% (August 2005). The most frequent cause of failure was ΔL with 1,711 failed dialysis, followed by ΔQb with 1,289 failed dialysis.

The assessment of the rule discovery algorithms described in this paper, on the other hand, has been performed retrospectively, since the integration of Hemostat with the temporal data mining tool has been performed only recently.

The algorithm for extracting association rules was applied to the overall set of dialyses of each patient. The rules have been selected with a minimum confidence equal to 0.9. In order to better assess the algorithm, we run it with different levels of support, thus obtaining different set of rules. Each rule has been evaluated by one of the authors, i.e., by the physician responsible of the Vigevano HHD. The expert judged if the extracted rule confirmed the available knowledge or if it was unexpected but plausible or, finally, if it was not explainable on the basis of the available medical knowledge and of the clinical experience. The results are extensively reported in [7], and briefly summarized in the following.

In particular, we have been able to note that the number of extracted rules decreases with the increase of the minimum support value. Moreover, the percentage of "correct" rules has its maximum values in correspondence to the intermediate support value, while it decreases with a higher support. It is also interesting to see that the number of not explainable rules is relatively low in all the trials and that the average number of rules antecedents (contemporaneous TA) decreases with the increase of the support level. The average number of rule antecedents is nearly constant, and corresponds to a minimum of two antecedents and a maximum of eight. Finally, the algorithm was able to extract rules which satisfy the support and confidence constraints in, at maximum, one third of the patients.

The algorithm that learns temporal rules has been evaluated with a similar approach. In particular, in order to assess the temporal rule learned, we have run the algorithm with different values of the support and of the maximum gap (GP) in the PRECEDES temporal relationship. The extracted rules have been again evaluated in terms of their clinical plausibility. The number of extracted rules is, in the large majority of cases, higher when the support is low and the gap is high; this result is expected, since these conditions correspond to weaker constraints in the search procedure. The sum of the percentages of valid rules, i.e., the ones confirming prior knowledge and of the percentage of the unexpected ones, is higher than the one of not explainable rules. Moreover, also in presence of low support, the algorithm still performs in a satisfactorily way, in particular in presence of gaps of 2 and 3. However, the proportions of not explainable rules are always higher than in the case of association rule discovery. Finally, the number of extracted rules may cover the one third of the patients at maximum, while the average number of antecedents is higher in presence of a gap equal to 1.

5.2 Testing the Case-Based Retrieval System

We restrospectively tested the case-based retrieval system on a set of data coming from the Vigevano HDD. The data set we used comprises ten different patients with more that ten dialysis sessions for each patients and with ten different monitored signals (the time series features of Table 1) for each session.

As an example of the results produced by the system, we considered a situation where the physician wanted to analyze the HV parameter of a dialysis session. In a good session, HV fits a model where, after a very short period of exponential decrease, a linear decrease of the volume follows. Hypotension episodes of the patient under control may influence this kind of behavior of the HV parameter; this may result in a different temporal pattern not fitting the model. Figure 7 shows on the left the signals of a query case (patient #10, dialysis #61) corresponding to a patient with hypotension during dialysis and with a HV profile having a pattern that does not fit the usual HV model; in particular a decrease pattern is followed by an almost stable pattern, followed by another decrease. The right part of Fig. 7 shows the best retrieved case (patient #10, dialysis #68). Retrieval was performed by asking for a high similarity (distance threshold equal to 0.15) with respect to diastolic (DP) and systolic pressure (SP), blood bulk flow (QB), and hematic volume (HV); QB is the first shown signal of the cases in the figure and was considered an important contextual factor of the retrieval, while DP, SP, and

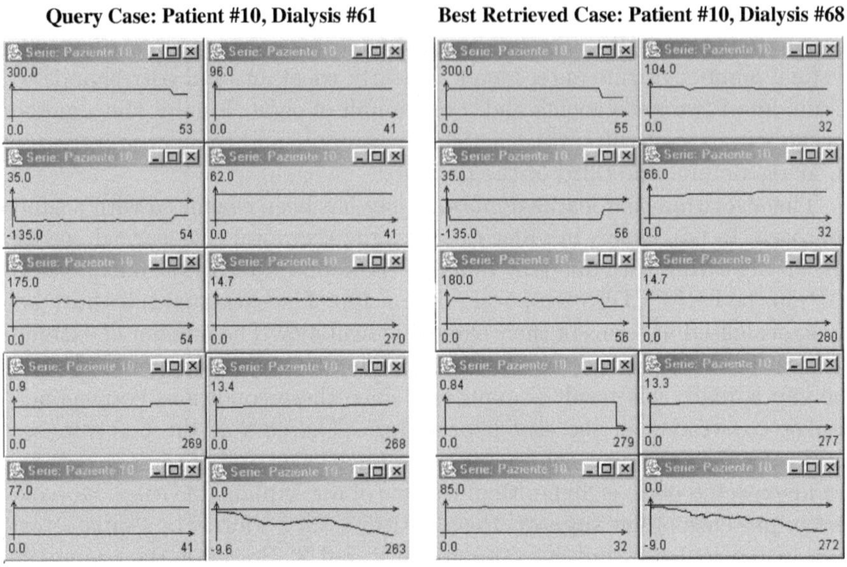

Fig. 7. Example of retrieval of signals of a dialysis session: query case (on the left), best retrieved case (on the right). Numbers on the ordinate of each graphic represent maximum or minimum value of the time series

HV are shown in more details in Fig. 8. We can notice that in the retrieved case some kind of hypotension is still present during dialysis and that HV has the same kind of pattern than in the query case. The same holds for the other retrieved cases; in particular, by asking for the ten best cases, only cases from patient #10 were retrieved. This is not casual, since that patient was the only one having significant hypotension episodes stored in the case base.

Observe that all of these cases were judged as successful by the physician. Actually, it seems that the outcome definition is based just on a macroscopic observation of (a subset of) the features. On the other hand, our system allows to obtain a deeper insight of the situation, highlighting types of anomalies which, if they do not lead to an immediate dialysis failure, could produce poor therapeutic results in the long run.

As a second example, we considered a case (patient #10, dialysis #71) in which some alterations in the extra-corporeal blood circuit took place. This kind of problems (typically due to an occlusion of the patient's fistulae) are indicated by a sudden increase of the arterious pressure (AP) around the end of the session, and by a corresponding decrease of the venous pressure (VP). Retrieval was conducted by requiring a high similarity for AP and VP, and by assigning them the highest weights. Figure 9 details the values of AP and VP for the query case and for the best retrieved one.

Observe that, while the query case was labeled as successfull, the retrieved case resulted in a positive outcome only after nurse intervention. In

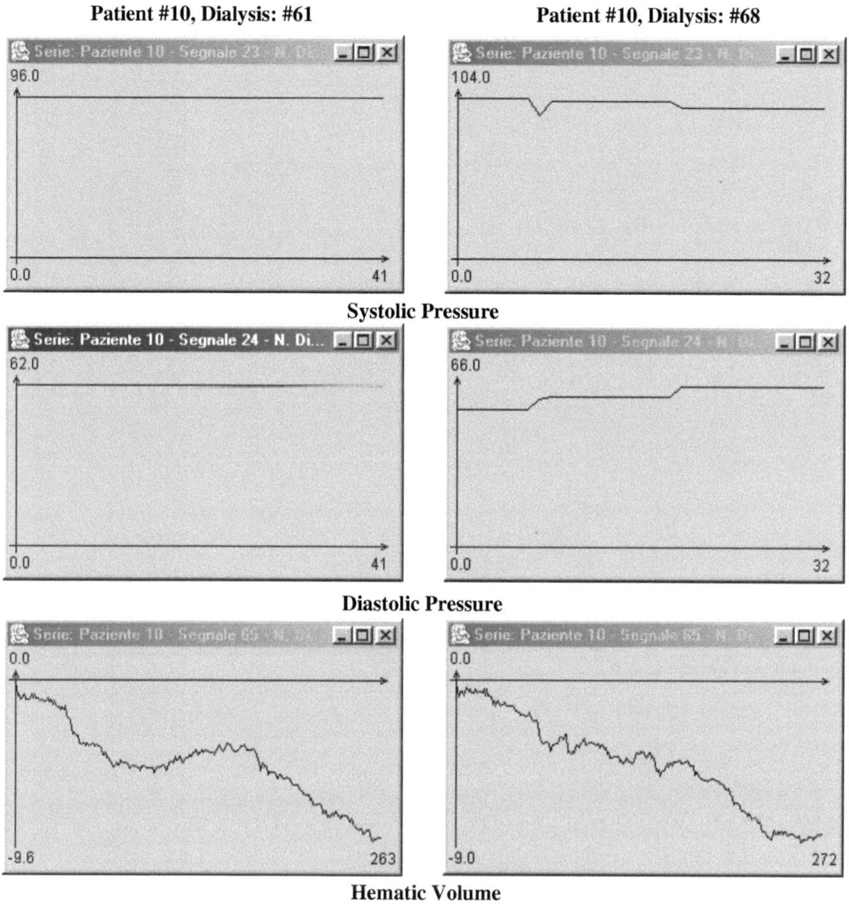

Fig. 8. Diastolic, systolic pressure, and hematic volume retrieval (cfr. Fig. 7)

particular, the nurse provided the patient with a diuretic drug, to compensate hypotension.

This result led us to consider the values of DP and SP (see Fig. 10): as a matter of fact, the values are low in both cases (in particular, the final increase in the retrieved case corresponds to the drug effect). The information provided by the retrieval procedure can thus warn the physician to pay particular attention to hypotension for this patient, since in the past a medical intervention was required, in a situation that is extremely similar to the current one.

Our tool therefore provides results that allow to better assess the dialisys efficiency, and that can indicate directions for further analyses and considerations.

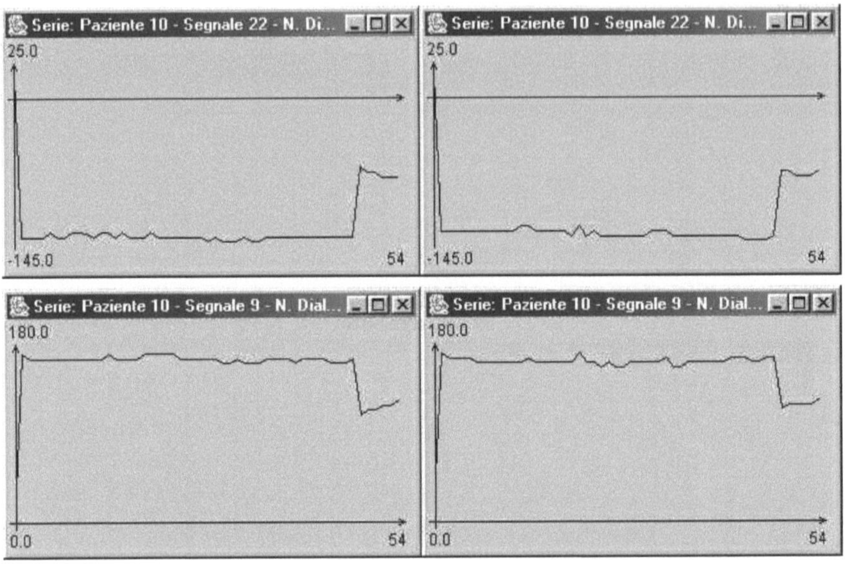

Fig. 9. Arterious and venous pressure retrieval in the second example

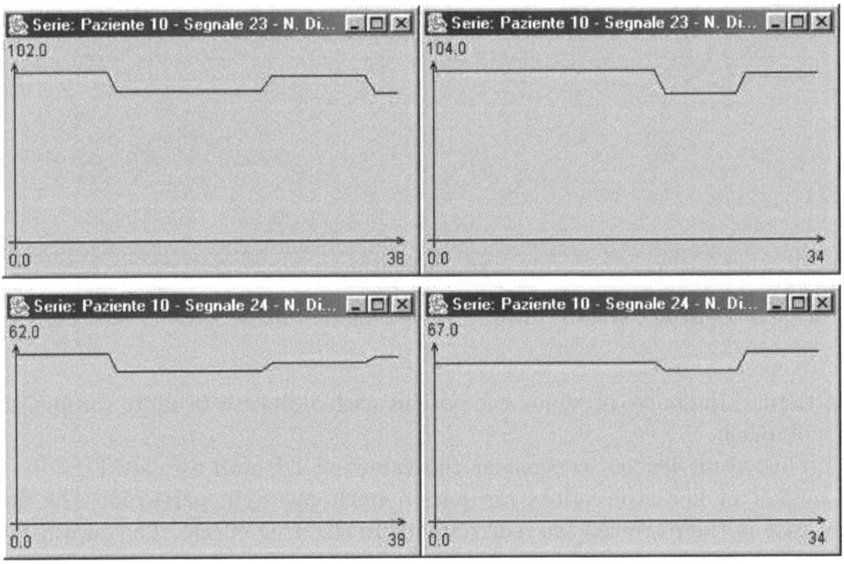

Fig. 10. Diastolic and systolic pressure retrieval in the second example

Finally, we conclude by mentioning the fact that, in the experiments we performed, retrieval has shown to be quite robust to noise; for example, very often patterns of the HV parameters present noise in the form of spikes representing erroneous measures of the dialysis machine. Such spikes seem

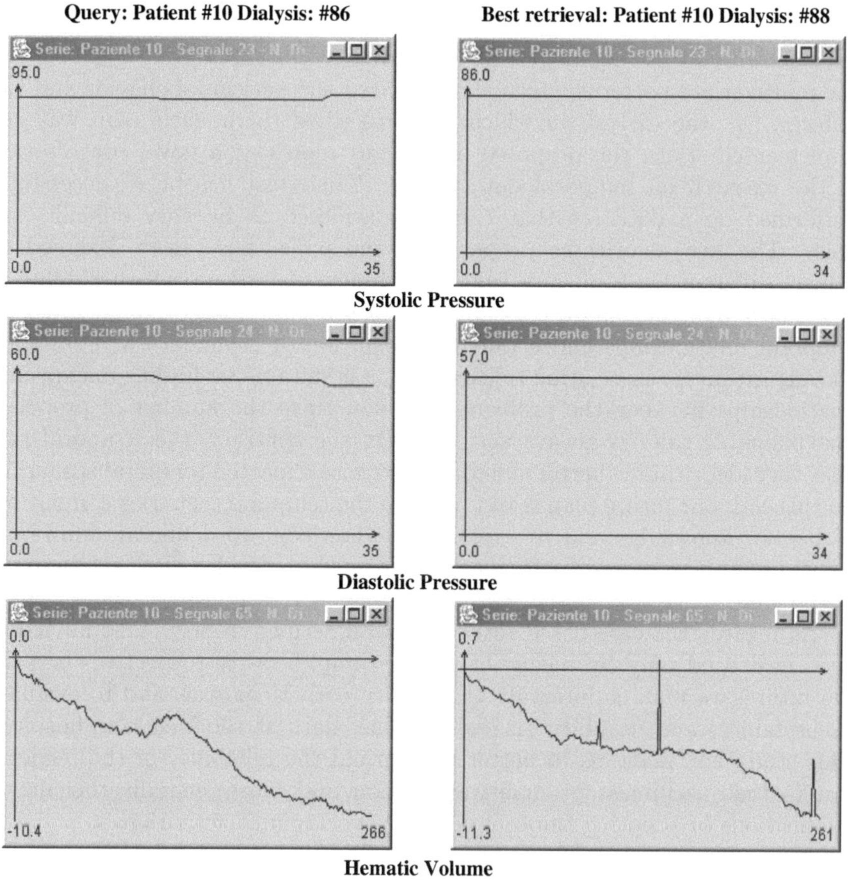

Fig. 11. Retrieval with noise on HV

not to influence very much the retrieval, since the actual pattern (disregarding the spikes) is often captured. An example is shown in Fig. 11.

6 Conclusions

This paper describes a set of AI techniques which have been applied in a system for quality assessment of hemodialysis centers.

The overall intervention is nowadays providing clinical benefits, measured in terms of adherence to the therapeutic prescriptions. Moreover, the availability of such a system is leading to organizational changes in the day by day clinical activities. As an example, the assessment of the single dialysis session given by nurses at the end of the dialysis is now performed on the basis of the data automatically collected by the system.

The role of AI methods in this context is manyfold. In this paper we have shown two methodologies for extracting potential associations between the multivariate patterns which characterized the patients' behavior and the failures, i.e., the dialysis in which the prescribed therapeutic plan was not implemented. Both the proposed algorithms represent a novel contribution in the research on temporal data mining. Their test has been successfully performed on a data set that can be considered to be very difficult and noisy. The two algorithms proposed in the paper have been designed to extract different kinds of rules, and their direct comparison is rather difficult, since, although they share the same search procedure, they exploit different temporal relationships and a different definition of confidence and support. The algorithm for association rule extraction is suitable for finding unexpected relationships between the problem variables, since the number of proposed unexplainable rules is always very low. On the contrary, the temporal rule discovery algorithm is better suited to recognise expected temporal scenarios. To this end, our future plan is to formalize the temporal scenarios compatible with prior knowledge and to exploit this knowledge to define an additional algorithm able to search for frequent and plausible complex clinical situations in the data.

As regards the case-based retrieval tool described in Sect. 4, so far it has been evaluated only by means of some examples on retrospective data. In the future, we plan to integrate the facility with Hemostat, and to evaluate its usefulness and usability on real patients' data at the Vigevano hospital. This study will allow us to better understand the reliability of the retrieval results, their usefulness for quality evaluation, and, more generally, the clinical implications of adopting the tool in the every day unit activities.

As a future development, we also foresee to deal with the "case" definition. We will allow the physician to consider longer monitoring periods, typically all the dialysis sessions of a patient within two weeks. Choosing this enlarged granularity, each session will be synthesized through sufficient statistics indexes, (namely the median and the 10th and 90th percentiles of each monitoring variable). We will then define a case as a two weeks monitoring period, where the case features are the series of the medians and of the percentiles over all the dialysis sessions held in the two weeks at hand. On these features, it will be possible to look for particular patterns (e.g., episodes of increasing values, peaks, etc.) and to retrieve other cases from the library, whose features show an analogous behavior. To make retrieval more efficient, we plan to preprocess the time series resorting to TA in order to immediately highlight meaningful patterns in the data.

This choice is closer to clinical practice requirements, since physicians are often interested in the patient's behavior over longer periods of time, looking for significant trends or alterations in biological signals in the long run. By means of our system, they will be enabled to start with a search for similar cases in the enlarged granularity, and will be allowed to enter the details of single dialysis sessions only when a particularly critical behavior has been outlined. We believe that this choice will augment the tool flexibility, and will make it really usable in practice.

Acknowledgments

This work is partially supported by the grant PRIN 2004 number 2004094558, funded by the Italian Ministry of Education.

References

1. R. Van der Spek and A. Spijkervet. Knowledge management: dealing intelligently with knowledge. In J. Liebowitz and L.C. Wilcox, editors, *Knowledge Mangement and its Integrative Elements.* CRC, Boca Raton, FL, 1997
2. M. Stefanelli. The socio-organizational age of artificial intelligence in medicine. *Artificial Intelligence in Medicine*, 23(1):25–47, 2001
3. J.L. Kolodner. *Case-Based Reasoning.* Morgan Kaufmann, San Mateo, CA, 1993
4. The United States Renal Data System. *http://www.usrds.org*
5. Registro Italiano di Dialisi e Trapianto. *http://www.sin-italia.org*
6. P.A. McFarlane and D.C. Mendelssohn. A call to arms: economic barriers to optimal dialysis care. *Peritoneal Dialysis International*, 20:7–12, 2000
7. R. Bellazzi, C. Larizza, P. Magni, and R. Bellazzi. Temporal data mining for the quality assessment of a hemodialysis service. *Artificial Intelligence in Medicine*, 34:25–39, 2005
8. Y. Shahar. A framework for knowledge based temporal abstractions. *Artificial Intelligence*, 90:79–133, 1997
9. R. Bellazzi, C. Larizza, and A. Riva. Temporal abstractions for interpreting diabetic patients monitoring data. *Intelligent Data Analysis*, 2:97–122, 1998
10. J.F. Allen. Towards a general theory of action and time. *Artificial Intelligence*, 23:123–154, 1984
11. F. Hoppner. Discovery of Temporal Patterns - Learning Rules about the Qualitative Behaviour of Time Series. In *Proceedings of the 5th PPKDD, LNAI 2168*, pp. 192–203. Springer, Berlin Heidelberg New York, 2001
12. I. Witten and E. Frank. *Data Mining.* Academic, New York, 2000
13. R. Agrawal and R. Srikant. Fast algorithms for mining association rules in large databases. In *Proc International Conference on Very Large Databases*, pages 478–499. Morgan Kaufmann, Los Altos, CA, 1994
14. M.L. Hetland. A survey of recent methods for efficient retrieval of similar time sequences. In M. Last, A. Kandel, and H. Bunke, editors, *Data Mining in Time Series Databases.* World Scientific, London, 2003
15. A. Guttman. R-trees: a dynamic index structure for spatial searching. In *Proceedings of the ACM SIGMOD*, pp. 47–57. ACM, New York, 1984
16. S. Berchtold, D.A. Keim, and H.P. Kriegel. The x-tree: an index structure for high-dimensional data. In *Proceedings of the VLDB 96*, pp. 28–39. Morgan Kaufman, San Mateo, CA, 1996

17. R. Agrawal, C. Faloutsos, and A.N. Swami. Efficient similarity search in sequence databases. In D. Lomet, editor, *Proceedings of the 4th International Conference of Foundations of Data Organization and Algorithms*, pp. 69–84. Springer, Berlin Heidelberg New York, 1993
18. A.V. Oppenheim and R.W. Shafer. *Digital signal processing.* Prentice Hall, London, 1975
19. D.Q. Goldin and P.C. Kanellakis. On similarity queries for time-series data: constraint specification and implementation. In *Proceedings of the 1st International Conference on the Principles and Practice of Constraints Programming, LNCS 976*, pp. 137–153, 1995
20. D. Rafiei and A. Mendelzon. Similarity-based queries for time series data. In *Proceedings of the ACM SIGMOD*, pp. 13–24. ACM, New York, 1997
21. V.S. Subrahmanian. *Principles of Multimedia Database Systems.* Morgan Kaufmann, San Mateo, CA, 1998
22. P. Perner. Incremental learning of retrieval knowledge in a case-based reasoning system. In K.D. Ashley, D.G. Bridge, editors, *Proceedings of ICCBR 2003, LNAI, Volume 2689*, pp. 422–436. Springer, Berlin Heidelberg New York, 2003

Mining the Electronic Medical Record to Examine Physician Decisions

Patricia B. Cerrito

Summary. The introduction of the electronic medical record (EMR) makes available more detailed data compared to paper records. In this chapter, we demonstrate how these data can be used to improve care and decrease costs by investigating the variability and timeliness of patient treatments. Several data mining techniques will be demonstrated, including link analysis (association rules) and text analysis. Six months of patient records were downloaded from the EMR from a hospital emergency department (ED). The dataset contained approximately 14,000 patient records and included all patient medications, charges, initial complaints, final diagnoses, initial triage, and length of stay.

Link analysis was used to find the initial and most prominent connections in patient charges, meaning that if a patient A received charge X, then patient A also received charge Y. While not all patients will have that X–Y combination, the combinations found in the link analysis will have the greatest likelihood of occurring in the patient population. Once identified, additional drill down into the data can be used to examine the variability in charges as to when the X–Y combination occurs, and when it does not. Investigations of the variability can lead to a consensus of best practices.

Text analysis is used to compress nominal data with many different levels so that meaningful data analysis can take place. There are so many possible combinations of patient complaints, charges, and medications that standard statistical methods cannot be used. Text analysis can reduce thousands of charges to dozens of classes of charges. Examples of analyses that demonstrate the ability of the methodology to discover ways of reducing costs and improving the quality of care will be demonstrated.

1 Introduction

Retail businesses are using market basket analysis to examine patterns in customer purchases. Most people have at least one shopping card that is used by a retailer to track patterns in customer purchases, or have some familiarity with online retailers such as amazon.com, where purchases are reg-

P.B. Cerrito: *Mining the Electronic Medical Record to Examine Physician Decisions*, Studies in Computational Intelligence (SCI) **48**, 113–126 (2007)
www.springerlink.com

ularly tracked. The premise is that the recognition of patterns can allow the retailer to "know the customer," to anticipate the interests and the needs of each customer. Such businesses use market basket analysis to provide additional purchase suggestions, resulting in increased sales. Others use the analysis for product placement.

This same methodology can be applied to patient use of medical treatments. Unfortunately, medicine is still slow to accept the use of electronic medical records (EMRs), making it difficult to use data mining. Only 9.6% of all US hospitals use electronic physician order entry [1] Healthcare application is somewhat different from retail in that it is not as clear who is the customer and who is the provider. However, the situation is more straightforward in a hospital emergency department where the physician and members of the nursing staff enter a series of procedures, labs, medications, and charges into the patient record with little input from the patient. In this situation, individual members of the healthcare staff can be identified as the customers with the hospital as the provider. In addition, the patient can be identified as a customer, and all charges related to that customer can be tracked.

In a hospital environment, it is possible to examine the relationship between treatment and outcome, and between diagnosis and treatment. It can also be used to examine the variability in practice given patients with similar problems. The objective of data mining is to determine optimal care guidelines using actual data. Similarly, patterns of charges can be examined to look at optimal costs [2, 3].

Each physician practices what he believes is the "best practice." However, without any comparison of outcomes between different physicians, it cannot be determined which decisions lead to better outcomes. Generally, comparisons between physicians are not made because of the difficulty in acquiring data. In a hospital environment, it is possible to collect data across different physicians and to compare outcome results.

In this chapter, we intend to discuss the method of market basket analysis, and how it can be used to "drill down" into the data to examine the different habits of physician practice. The technique gives an idea of how physicians give different orders and charges for patients. Once different practice patterns are identified, they can be compared to patient outcomes to see if there is a relationship between physician decision and outcome, or to see if there is a relationship between physician decision and treatment cost.

2 Method

Several data mining methods will be utilized in the chapter examples, including link analysis (market basket analysis) and text analysis. They will be used in conjunction with more standard methods of statistical exploratory analysis for additional examination, and for validation purposes. The techniques will be briefly described here. For more information, the reader is referred to a new text, Cerrito (2006).

2.1 Market Basket Analysis

Market basket analysis uses association rules that have the form X→Y. It is interpreted that if a customer purchases item X, then that customer also purchases item Y. The pair, (X,Y) forms an itemset. A transaction is a purchase of one or more items. Given a set of items, S, any subset of S is an itemset. The support of the itemset with respect to a set T of transactions is the number of transactions in T that contain all the items in the itemset. A frequent itemset is one where the support is greater than a specified level, α, which is called the minimum support. The confidence of the rule is the ratio: support (XUY)/support(X). The expected confidence is the ratio of support(Y)/support(T). The lift is the ratio of the confidence/ expected confidence. A modification of the association rule is to define itemsets sequentially so that X→Y only if Y is purchased (or charged) after X.

Once all association rules are defined, they can be ranked by any one of the measures of itemset count, support, confidence, expected confidence, and lift. With a large set of items, the number of rules can be quite large, into the thousands and the tens of thousands. The best way to represent these rules is with a link analysis. Itemsets that have support greater than α are represented in the link analysis by a node (rectangular box). They are connected by a line. The width and color of the line indicate the strength of the connection; the number of transactions is represented by the size of the node. Link analysis can also be investigated sequentially to determine the sequence in which patient charges are ordered by the physician. It enables us to examine how one diagnostic test can lead to others based upon results. In this examination, we focus on sequential analysis.

Link analysis has not been much used to investigate clinical decisions, although it has been used to detect fraud in medical billing [4]. Some investigations of patterns in a hospital setting include investigations of nosocomial infection [5–7]. Others include the use of hospital services by patients [8]. Because link analysis can be used to visualize pathways, it can be used quickly and routinely to show patterns that can be examined in detail [9].

Additional statistical techniques were used in combination with link analysis and association rules. These include chi-square analysis, the general linear model, and kernel density estimation.

2.2 Text Analysis

Diagnostic tests are ordered in relationship to patient complaints to determine a course of treatment. However, patients do not use standardized language to specify medical problems. Without that standardization, it becomes difficult to manage the possible number of complaints encountered. Some type of data compression must be done first. A standard practice has been to filter down to a specific number of items. However, such filtering will reduce the potential of the dataset. Another method has been to attempt to compress the items manually. However, when the number of different complaints numbers in thousands, manual compression becomes too time consuming.

Manual compression involves word recognition, and the ability to identify terms that are similar in meaning. Text analysis can be used to automate this compression, and to reduce the number of different patient complaints into a manageable few.

2.3 Data Collection

The EMR is used in an urban hospital's emergency department. Six months of patient records, totaling 14,000+ records, were downloaded and examined. The download included 181,000 charges assigned to the 14,000 patients. In addition, each patient was assigned a physician and a nurse. Charges were ordered by the physician–nurse team. Some preprocessing of the data was required prior to using market basket analysis. Once an identification variable was specified, the charges were ordered with respect to that identification variable and then a sequence variable was assigned to all items with the same identification variable. Once the preprocessing was complete, association analysis was done using the sequenced variable.

Two examinations will be demonstrated here. The first has to do with costs, the second with treatment. For treatment, tests ordered for patients with chest pain are examined. Protocols have been developed to optimize lab choice for chest pain [10–12]. However, it is not clear that these protocols are always followed.

3 Results

To represent the association rules, a link analysis graph was used. Figure 1 gives the link graph with patient as the identification variable. Some of the links in Fig. 1 are rather obvious, as for example, a first and second blood culture or an initial and secondary assessment. It is of interest to determine whether it is the patient length of stay that is related to a second blood draw, or whether it is patient results. In this particular dataset, a second blood draw was related to time in the ED. However, it is not clear whether the second blood draw was because the patient spent more time in the ED, or whether the second draw resulted in increased time.

Special needs (emotional support, etc.) is linked to secondary assessment, and the line connecting the two nodes is fairly wide indicating a high level of support. Also, both are linked to the initial assessment, which is performed on every patient who enters the ED. Because it is such a strong connection, the proportion of patients with these charges was examined. A second set of connections identifies diagnostic tests; combinations of tests ordered will be examined to optimize care.

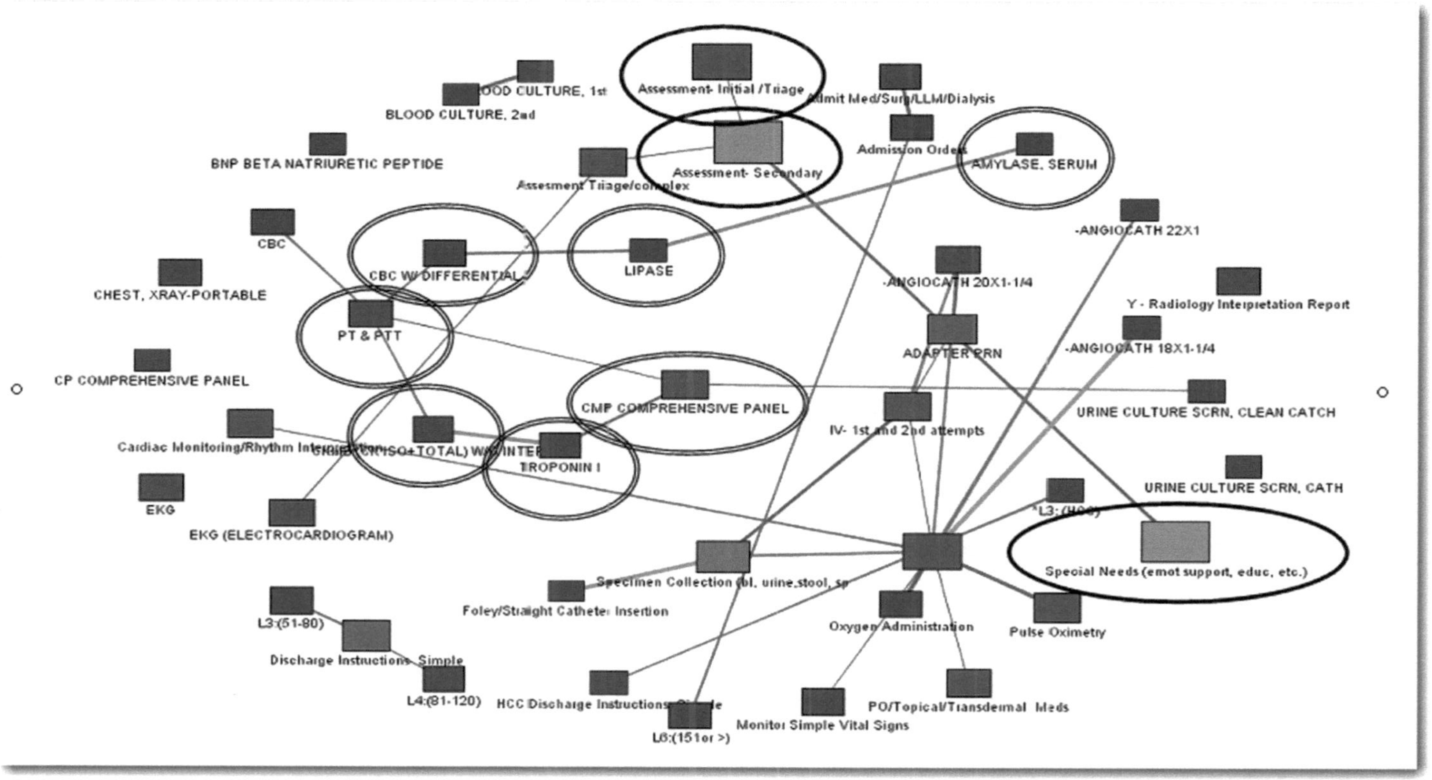

Fig. 1. Link Analysis of Charges by Patient. The values circled in red (single line) represent a set of charges under investigation for cost; the values circled in blue (double line) represent a series of diagnostic tests under examination for treatment optimization

3.1 Examination of Cost Factors

The number of times a nurse entered a charge for special needs was divided by the number of patients assigned to each nurse (that is, the support of special needs/number of transactions = lift (special needs) for each nurse. Therefore, the proportion of patients for which an individual nurse entered a charge for emotional support was computed. Similarly, the lift of secondary assessment was computed. In each case, the proportion of patients was approximately 95% (Figs. 2 and 3). Although not every nurse entered the charge for all patients, most did. Some nurses entered a charge for emotional support more than one time for some patients.

Once the practice has been examined using link analysis and data mining, the hospital can examine it as a matter of policy. Should emotional support be added routinely to a patient's charges and costs in the ED? If not, should some declaration be made that the practice would be discontinued? Is there a real need for emotional support for every patient in the ED? When does the need exist, and when should the charge be entered? Without disclosing the practice, policy decisions cannot be made.

The various charges are assigned a number of points. The point totals are categorized into levels, and reimbursements are based upon level, with the highest level yielding the highest reimbursement. In the EMR, the level, indicating the level for reimbursement, is also entered as a charge. Therefore, the links related to the charge level are also defined in the link analysis. In

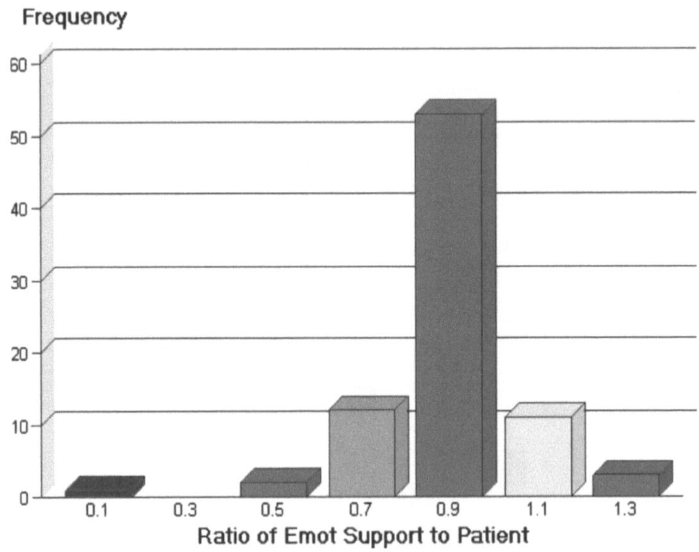

Fig. 2. Bar graph of ratio of special needs to number of patients indicating that over 50% of the nurses routinely charge all patients; over 10% of patients are charged more than once for emotional support

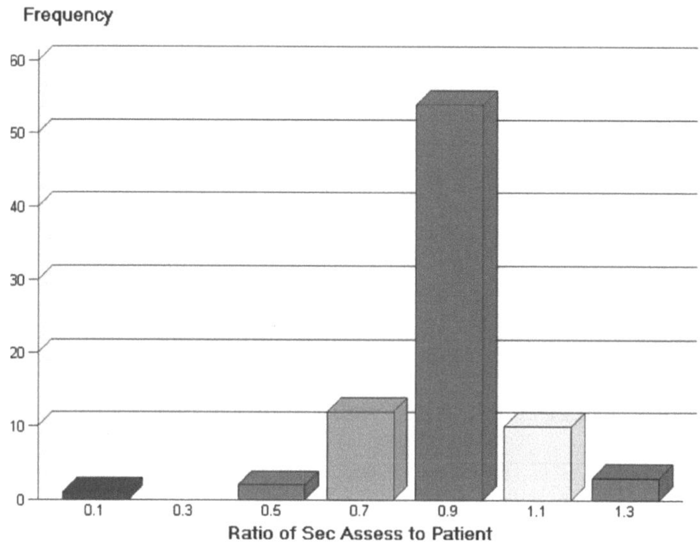

Fig. 3. Ratio of secondary assessment to number of patients again showing that over 50% of the nurses routinely charge all patients with this item; 10% are charged more than once

Table 1. Proportion of patient disposition by level of care

disposition	L1	L2	L3	L4	L5	L6
home	50.71	50.49	71.10	49.79	42.89	25.08
elope	4.48	1.62	1.20	0.94	0.78	0.64
admit	10.18	6.22	7.57	15.88	40.93	51.61
ICU/TCU	1.42	1.15	1.30	2.43	6.23	16.37
transfer	2.46	2.34	2.90	8.49	3.89	4.33
dialysis	30.75	38.18	15.93	22.47	5.28	1.97

Fig. 1, Level 6 (L6) is linked to a charge for admission orders while Levels 3 and 4 (L3, L4) are linked to discharge instructions, indicating that a high proportion of patients in the L3, L4 range are discharged home from the Emergency Department while a high proportion with L6 are admitted. Table 1 shows the relationship between patient disposition and level of care.

Figure 4 indicates that there is a relationship between physician and level. The graph shows that the physicians can differ in the proportion of patients at Level 6 by approximately 30% points. Whether the physicians with a high Level 6 have sicker patients in need of more care, or are shifting patients into higher levels cannot be determined without additional drill down into the data.

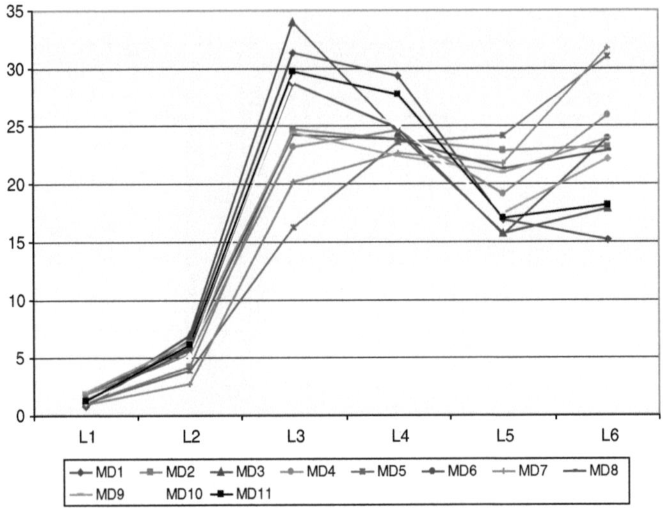

Fig. 4. Line graph of MD by patient levels showing that some physicians (MD 5 and MD 7) have a much higher proportion of patients at Level 6 while others concentrate at Level 3 (MD 3, MD 1, MD 11)

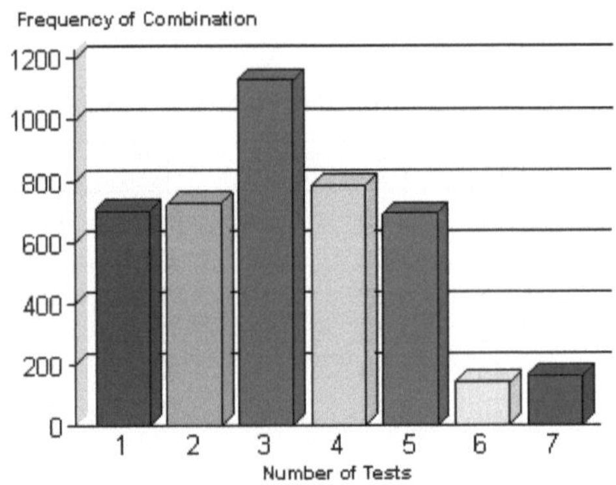

Fig. 5. Number of items by patient showing that there are all possible combinations of patients, but that the peak number is 3 with almost equal numbers for 1, 2, 4, and 5

3.2 Examination of Treatment Combinations

Another series of connections of interest in Fig. 1 is Amylase > Lipase > CMP Comprehensive > CBC with differential > CKMB comprehensive panel > tropinin > PT&PTT. Because there are so many links, it is difficult to examine the combinations in their entirety. Figure 5 gives a summation of the number of items in the link by the frequency of patients. Additional examinations cannot be performed until additional preprocessing is completed. The observational unit must be changed from charge to patient. First, the data are sorted by charge and by patient identifier. Then the data are transposed and concatenated so that all charges under consideration are contained within one text string. Once this is completed, the dataset containing charges is merged with the dataset containing outcomes of interest. There is additional preprocessing required because some tests are ordered in duplicate.

Given a total of seven tests under consideration, there are a total of $2^7-1=127$ possible combinations of tests. A total of 69 different combinations were used in the Emergency Department for a total of 3,464 patients. Figure 6 gives the frequency of combinations that were used for 100 or more patients; Table 2 gives the combinations used for 10 or fewer patients. Those with a large number of combinations should be studied to reach a consensus in terms of standing orders; those with a small number should be studied to determine if these patients had somewhat unique problems.

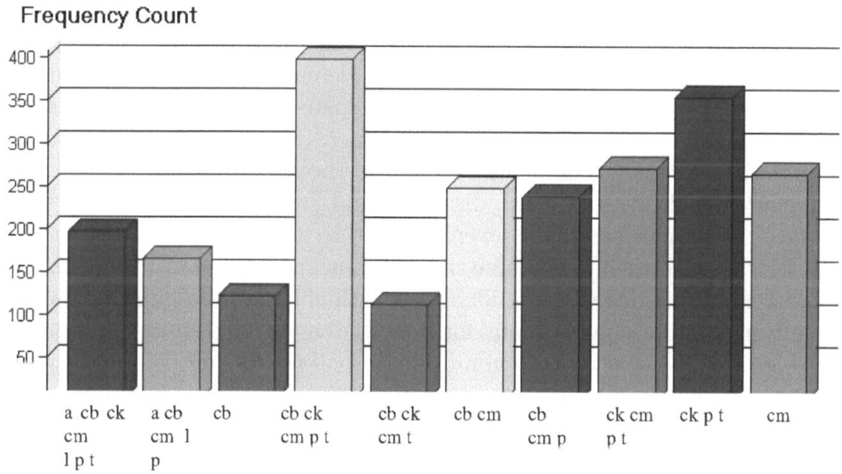

Fig. 6. Test combination ordered for 100 or more patients

Table 2. Test combinations used with 10 or fewer patients

A	a ck cm l p	cb ck cm l p	Ck
a cb ck cm l p	A ck l t	cb ck l p t	ck cm l p t
a cb ck cm l t	A cm l p t	cb ck p	ck cm l t
a cb ck l p t	A cm l t	cb ck t	ck p
a cb ck l t	A cm p	cb cm l p t	cm l p
a cb cm l t	A l	cb cm l t	cm l t
a cb cm p	Cb ck	cb p t	p
a cb l	cb ck cm	cb t	p t
a cb l p			

a Amylase Serum, *cb* CBCw/differential, *ck* CKMB comprehensive panel, *cm* CMP comprehensive panel, *l* Lipase, *p* PT&PTT, *t* Troponin

Given the ten most frequent combinations, the next step is to examine whether there is a general consensus concerning which combinations are used when. These ten test combinations are used for 71.3% (Emergent), 72.11% (Urgent), and 65.77% (NonUrgent) of all patients who receive any combination of these tests, showing that some of the tests are not really reserved for more critically ill patients. Not one of the combinations is used for a majority of the patients in any triage category.

Of the 3,464 patients receiving one or more of these tests, 206 presented to the ED with an initial complaint of chest pain. Of that number, 24% received the combination of ck p t, 14% received cb ck cm p t, and 13% received ck cm p t. No other combination was used more than 10% of the time.

It is very difficult to examine all possible patient complaints to see which ones are related to the tests ordered. However, we can use text analysis to group the complaints. In order to do this, only the seven tests in all combinations listed above were retained in a subset of the data. All complaints in that subset were clustered using text analysis. Table 3 gives the clusters along with the terms used to define the clusters. An entropy weighting was used for the clustering. Chest pain with no other complaint is listed in cluster 5. Chest pain is also prominent in cluster 2, which contains the majority of patient complaints related to the seven diagnostic tests along with shortness of air, back pain, dizziness, and low blood sugar.

Once the patient complaints were reduced to a total of 12 clusters, a table analysis was performed to examine the relationship between tests and clusters. The test combinations that are identified with cluster 5 are given in Table 4. Three test combinations account for 70% of the cluster (cb ck cm p t, ck p t, and cm t). The test for troponin occurs on all combinations. For cluster 2, the test combinations that occur in over 100 patients are a cb ck cm l p t, a cb cm l p, cb, cb ck cm p t, cb cm, cb cm p, ck cm p t, ck p t, cm, and cm p. While it is possible that fewer tests are used because a heart attack can be ruled out early on, it is also possible that physicians have different habits of tests given the patient complaints. The test combinations for cluster 12 related to shortness of air were scattered so that only one combination was given to more than ten patients: cb ck cm p t.

Published protocols suggest 5 of the 7 tests for chest pain and 2 of the 7 for abdominal pain. These protocols do not appear to be universal and are not used in the ED under study [13–15].

3.3 Examination of Antibiotic Use

Because no infection cultures are performed in the ED (requiring 48–72 hours), only broad spectrum antibiotics should be used in the ED. Table 5 gives the number of antibiotic prescriptions for the top eight antibiotics used in the ED. These eight antibiotics account for 96% of all antibiotic prescriptions in the ED. Given these eight, it is possible to determine which are the most generally

Table 3. Text clusters related to diagnostic tests given in Table 2

#	Descriptive Terms	Freq	Percentage
1	abdominal_pain, cardiac_complaints, abd_pain, dizzy, nausea, fall, syncope, vomiting, asthma, neck_pain, cp, _soa, unr espomsive, blood_in_stool, arm_pain-left, cough, stomach_pain, right_arm_numbness	296	0.085450346...
2	soa, headache, cp, chest_pain,_soa, low_back_pain, right_flank_pain, body_aches, lower_abd_pain, mva, epigastric_pain, low_sats, low_glucose, left_leg_pain, bradycardia, high_blood_sugar, loc, dizzy, vaginal_bleeding, chest_tightness, near_syncope	2439	0.704099307...
3	stroke_symptoms, +seizure, cp, rectal_bleeding	54	0.015588914...
4	back_pain	29	0.008371824...
5	chest_pain	252	0.072748267...
6	nausea_and_vomiting, abd._pain	20	0.005773672...
7	decreased_loc, rlq_pain, diabetes_related, left_sided_chest_pain, leg_pain-_right, midsternal_cp, migraine, allergic_reaction, confusion, altered_mental_status, irregular_heart_beat, vomitting_blood, soa, _chest_pain, sore_throat, cp, _midsternal, rectal_bleed, left_chest_pain, possible_uti, gi_bleed	83	0.023960739...
8	shortness_of_breath	73	0.021073903...
9	weakness	40	0.011547344...
10	fever, ab_pain, hip_pain-_right, hypoglycemia, abnormal_labs, coughing_up_blood, left_flank_pain, flank_pain, syncopal_episode, cp_soa, nosebleed, +chill, full_arrest, numbness, epigastric_pain_with_rad._to_back, chest_pressure, hypertension, soa, _cough	87	0.025115473...
11	dizziness	31	0.008949191...
12	soa	60	0.017321016...

Table 4. Test combinations related to cluster 5, chest pain

tests	#	tests	#	tests	#	tests	#
a cb ck cm l p t	23	Cb	1	ck cm p t	49	a cm l	1
a cb ck l t	1	cb ck	1	ck cm t	4	ck cm l p t	1
a cb cm l p t	5	cb ck cm p	1	ck p t	69	cm t	1
a ck cm l p t	3	cb ck cm p t	60	ck t	4	l	1
a ck cm l t	1	cb ck cm t	14	cm	1	p t	1
a ck l p t	5	cb cm t	1	cm p	2	t	2

Table 5. Frequency of antibiotic prescription

antibiotic	Frequency	Percent
azithromycin	317	10
cefazolin	207	6
cefotaxime	318	10
ciprofloxacin	295	9
clindamycin	114	4
levofloxacin	1,285	40
piperacillin/taxobactam	270	8
Vancomycin	252	8

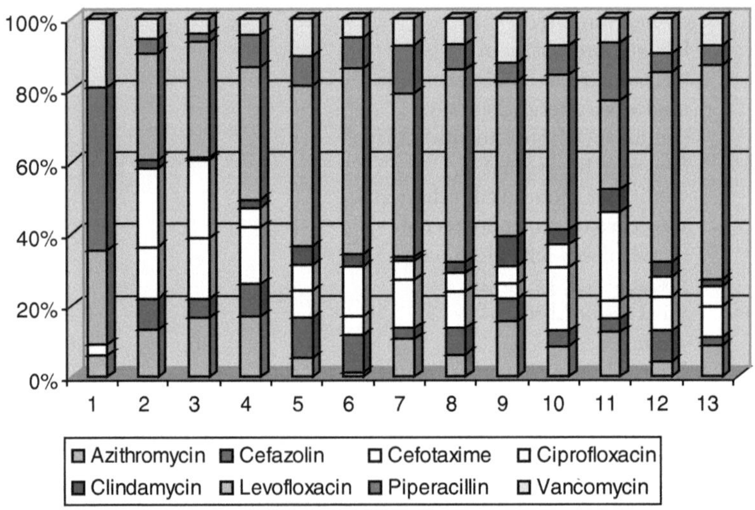

Fig. 7. Antibiotic prescribing by physician. Physician 1 favors Piperacillin while Physicians 5–10,12–13 favor Levofloaxcin. Physicians 4, 11 tend to give equal favor to other antibiotics as well

effective in the absence of a culture, and if any substitutions can be made to reduce cost.

Of the remaining 4%, two of the least used include Linezolid and Tobramycin, both of which are extremely expensive. These 4% can be scrutinized to determine whether such expensive antibiotics are necessary, again in the absence of a culture.

Figure 7 shows that there are physician preferences for antibiotic use. Note, for example, that physician 1 has a preference for Piperacillin/Taxobactam that is not shared by his colleagues. While Levofloxacin is preferred by all others, they also prescribe Ciprofloxacin, which is a very similar antibiotic.

4 Discussion

The availability of the EMR allows the use of data mining to examine variability in physician decision making. Once the variability is discovered, the decisions can be examined in relationship to patient outcomes. The results of such analyses can be used to define protocols and guidelines to improve the quality of care while simultaneously reducing costs.

Without using data mining techniques to "drill down" into physician decisions, it will remain unknown just how much variability occurs, and just what decisions are routinely made in the ED. Data mining allows the unknown to become known.

References

1. W.F. Bria, Applied medical informatics for the chest physician: Information you can use!, Part 2, Chest 129 (2006) 777–782
2. A.M. Berger, C.R. Berger, Data mining as a tool for research and knowledge development in nursing, Computers, Informatics, Nursing 22 (2004) 123–131
3. S. Doddi, A. Marathe, S. Ravi, D. Torney, Discovery of association rules in medical data, Medical Informatics and the Internet in Medicine 26 (2001) 25–33
4. L. Sokol, b. Garcia, J. Rodriguez, M. West, K. Johnson, Using data mining to find fraud in HCFA healthcare claims, Topics in Health Information Management 22 (2001) 1–13
5. S.E. Brossette, A.P. Sprague, J.M. Hardin, K.B. Waites, W.T. Jones, S.A. Moser, Association rules and data mining in hospital infection control and public health surveillance, Journal of the American Medical Informatics Association 5 (1998) 373–381
6. L. Ma, F.-C. Tsui, W.R. Hogan, M.M. Wagner, H. Ma, A framework for infection control surveillance using association rules, Annual Symposium Proceedings/AMIA 2003 (2003) 410–414
7. M.K. Obenshain, Application of data mining techniques to healthcare data, Infection Control and Hospital Epidemiology 25 (2004) 690–695

8. T. Dart, Y. Cui, G. Chatellier, P. Degoulet, Analysis of hospitalised patient flows using data-mining, Studies in Health Technology & Informatics 95 (2003) 263–268
9. S. Stilou, P. Bamidis, N. Magiaveras, C. Pappas, Mining association rules from clinical databases: an intelligent diagnostic process in healthcare, Medinfo 10 (Pt 2) (2001) 1399–1403
10. Anonymous, NACB: Recommendations-Logistics: Chapter 4, in, Vol. 2006 (NACB, 2005)
11. R.X. Davey, Troponin testing: an audit in three metropolitan hospitals, MJA 179 (2003) 81–83
12. S.E. Kahn, The challenge of evaluating the patient with chest pain, Archives of Pathology and Laboratory Medicine 124 (2000) 1418–1419
13. Anonymous, Chest Pain Program Protocol, in, Vol. 2006 (Division of Cardiology, University of Alberta, 2006)
14. Anonymous, Pancreatitis, in, Vol. 2006 (CNN.com, 2006)
15. G. Quin, Chest pain evaluation units, Journal of Emergency Medicine 17 (2000) (237–240)

Capturing and Specifying Multiagent Systems for the Management of Community Healthcare

Richard Hill

Summary. Community Care in the UK relates to the provision of effective support in response to both predicted and unpredicted personal needs. Extensive co-operation between independent care agencies is fundamental to the effective operation of care delivery services, each of which needs to meet its own goals. Typically this results in the unnecessary use of resources as the current systems cannot share relevant information without compromising the security of all the information held. The use of semantics for inter-agent communication enables more effective interoperability between collaborative intelligent agents. Contractual agreements to support the negotiations with community healthcare agencies creates a complex economic environment that must be described in a robust way if agent managed services are to be accepted commercially. This chapter considers the 'Event Accounting' model in relation to the myriad payment transactions within the community care environment, and demonstrates the use of Transaction Agent Modelling (TrAM), a robust transaction-based framework for the requirements capture of agent managed community healthcare systems.

1 Introduction

The delivery of home-based community healthcare services to frail and disabled people provides a complex set of challenges for UK Local Authority Managers. Whilst there are arguments that support the perceived desire for people to remain in their home environment for as long as possible, it is extremely difficult to coordinate and control the wide range of separate care agencies, both in terms of effective delivery and efficient resource utilisation. Since there is a strong motivation to effectively manage the recipients' quality of life, there is a temptation to introduce redundant resources, thus contributing to high levels of cost.

Each care service is provided by an independent autonomous party, a practice that has been encouraged by UK Local Authorities in pursuit of cost savings generated by an open, economic market. Inevitably each party instigates and maintains their own management information system, leading

R. Hill: *Capturing and Specifying Multiagent Systems for the Management of Community Healthcare*, Studies in Computational Intelligence (SCI) **48**, 127–163 (2007)
www.springerlink.com

to a scenario that includes many disparate, heterogeneous repositories. The prospect of integrating these resources seems rather onerous, thus there is a continued reliance upon more informal methods of control.

Beer et al. [1] proposed the development of an architecture to address these issues that utilised collaborative intelligent agents [2] to mediate queries amongst the myriad agencies and platforms. As such it would seem that the reactive, proactive, social and autonomous behaviours exhibited by intelligent software agents have much to offer in terms of designing and developing more effective healthcare management systems.

The abstract qualities of agent technologies makes them an attractive proposition for system designers as it is relatively simple to map stakeholders to intelligent software agents. However, the realities of attempting to accurately capture healthcare system requirements indicates that more assistance is required, particularly during the earlier stages of analysis, over and above a convenient mapping.

In particular, collaborating agents must be able to share and reuse domain knowledge if they are to interact effectively, and therefore the means of capturing and expressing the domain knowledge must be able to accommodate not only complex interactions, negotiation and brokering, but also the complicated, qualitative information that exists in healthcare environments.

This chapter considers the 'Event Accounting' [3] model in relation to the myriad payment transactions within the community care environment, and describes the use of Transaction Agent Modelling (TrAM), a robust transaction-based framework to gather high level requirements, permitting the capture and open expression of pertinent domain knowledge and the relevant semantics for a multiagent system (MAS) [4].

2 Developing an Agent-Based Approach

The use of intelligent agents enables disparate systems to be integrated into a single, collaborative, cooperative system since the social abilities of agents permit conversational exchanges to be made between different agencies. Such an approach makes the job of monitoring the whole system much easier, with tangible benefits for UK Local Authority Care Managers who need to assemble the most effective package of care for each care recipient, without employing redundant resources.

Aside from appropriateness of care, a fundamental goal of a fully integrated community healthcare system is to provide a timely response to care requests, both from the care recipient and the care assessors such as Social Workers (SW) and Occupational Therapists (OT). Such a system should be able to negotiate at many levels if disparate, autonomous care services are to be managed and coordinated, especially since the timeliness of the response must be suited to the nature of the request.

For example the speed of response is more of an issue in the event of an emergency; it follows that there is also an associated cost that is a function of the response time. The system therefore must be able to assess an incident and select the most appropriate response, balancing economic costs against the quality of care delivered. Existing systems are generally limited by the lack of relevant information that is available at any particular time, and there are many instances of care scenarios whereby comprehensive informal systems have evolved to supplement the more formal systems operated by the Local Authority.

For instance, a neighbour may be able to offer assistance based upon their proximity to the care recipient, providing support until a care professional arrives at the scene of the incident. Similarly, help from extended family is often ignored by formal care systems, leading to duplication of resources. This level of cooperation is too advanced for current systems, and demands much more comprehensive exchanges of information between the relevant agencies.

Speed of response is particularly important when the system has to accommodate real world scenarios such as service delivery failures. In such cases, the system needs to be able to recognise faults and offer an alternative course of action. Human agents would generally negotiate a new commitment, or find an alternative supplier. MAS architectures permit individual agents to act in a similar fashion, enabling not only the better provision of services, but also the generation of a history of the reliability of various services, assisting decision-making and subsequent negotiations in the future.

2.1 Event Accounting

Using the notion of economic scarcity as a conceptual basis, Polovina [5] argues that management accounting transactions are a too narrow abstraction of economic reality, referring to the Event Accounting model by Geerts et al. [3]. The transactions in question represent an exchange of monetary and non-monetary resources, thus in the case of community care management this represents a payment, in return for a package of care services.

It follows that transactions need not only represent monetary exchanges, as this notion could be applied to much more qualitative transactions as well. For instance the carers in a community healthcare environment may 'trade' their personal time to study for new care skills, or a recognised qualification. In such instances the carer would consider the balance between reduced leisure time or time with their family, in pursuit of enhanced promotional prospects as a result of successful study. This is an example of the qualitative, rather than purely quantitative, exchange of resources, indicating that there are many more aspects to explore and scrutinise in the community care domain.

Indeed the community care scenario is rich with qualitative transactions. Each transaction concludes when the relevant parties have gained from the participation, and is represented as a 'balance' in that every debit is countered by a credit. The inclusion of a balance within the transaction ensures an implicit validation that the transaction has occurred successfully. The agent transactions evident in community healthcare systems are an example that a desire for robust multiagent systems must be underpinned by a solid transaction foundation.

2.2 Modelling Systems

Bauer et al. [6] describe Agent Oriented UML (AUML) as a notation for the description of agents and their environment. This object-oriented modelling language presents a form of notation for the object-oriented paradigm; it provides system architects working on object analysis and design with one consistent language for specifying, visualising, constructing and documenting the artefacts of software systems, as well as for business modelling. All the models can be constructed, viewed, developed and evaluated during systems analysis and design. It is based on the meta-model that is the Unified Modelling Language [7], which is a notation for expressing object-oriented analysis. Agent modelling requires a greater richness of description, especially since the complex interactions often need to be represented graphically.

Prior work by Beer et al. [1] with the Intelligent Community Alarm (INCA) Demonstrator, illustrated that the design process created a requirement to formally represent various aspects of the agent-managed community healthcare system. AUML facilitated a large proportion of this work, enabling agent models, and the resultant stub-code, to be generated in readiness for deployment with the Zeus Agent-Building Toolkit [8]. Whilst it was possible to produce models of the agents that embodied the required behaviours, and consider the nuances of the community healthcare domain concurrently, it became apparent that some real-world issues were much more difficult to capture. In particular the representation of relatively simple payment transactions proved elusive, as AUML lacked the ability to capture high level qualitative scenarios.

2.3 Designing Community Care Systems

A specification for INCA was initially determined by consulting the ZEUS role modelling guide [8], using this approach to derive the roles of agents, services offered and task descriptions to be described using AUML. These models were then used as an input specification for implementation activities with the ZEUS Agent-Building Toolkit. The abstract input specification was described by a collection of use case, class, interaction and deployment diagrams, which provided a consistent representation of the community healthcare complexities across a number of disparate domains [9].

Whilst this process was remarkably simple in some areas, as the agent architecture mapped directly onto significant portions of the problem domain, a number of areas were identified that proved more problematic. The tasks of selecting the most appropriate care service and brokering service requests were particularly difficult without compromising the accuracy of the model.

It is fundamentally important that agent representations are not unduly compromised if they are to gain acceptance as a resilient and life-like solution to complex management problems, and it was deemed appropriate to investigate the aspects of the community healthcare scenario that did not translate as effectively to an agent architecture.

The payment transactions required for community healthcare do not immediately appear complicated as they are conducted (albeit often quite inefficiently)by human agents, who are familiar with the concept that the agency who requests a service does not always pay for that service, or pays a proportion of the total amount, depending upon a variety of circumstances [10].

Since the INCA Demonstrator did not sufficiently mimic the real-world scenario, then if this aspect could be investigated, it would be possible to establish the requirements of agent managed transaction systems, whilst also evaluating the suitability of agent architectures in the community healthcare domain.

It is also noted that in effect, community healthcare management systems are similar to commercial enterprise systems that manage the delivery of services by controlling and recording transactions. However, although human agents have become accustomed to interact with transactions in a commercial environment, they often question computer delegated transactions, particularly with regard to their robustness.

The allure of reduced resource requirements, improved service delivery and quality assurance, offered by multiagent architectures, combined with the complexities of community healthcare systems, means that we need our agents to assume control of the fundamental transaction workload. Transactions often require goals to be delegated, which is a capability that an agent architecture can offer.

Although the inclusion of human agents implies that issues of 'trust' with regard to agent managed services will arise, it is fundamental that the transactions should be represented in a robust way. It is therefore paramount that any solution, and therefore design process, should include a robust transaction model as its foundation from the outset.

Using the Event Accounting approach, the agent representations of the community care system model have been developed to incorporate a robust transaction design framework that addresses the issues of community care payment complexity and agent managed transactions. In particular, Local Authority agents who tender the services of community care provider agents, is an example agent trading scenario that has a fundamental requirement for a model that is robust and life-like.

Initially AUML representations of auction protocols [9] were included within the INCA demonstrator, but the combination of quantitative and qualitative aspects of transaction management, together with the 'gap' between abstract life-like representations and low-level deployment practicalities directed the research towards an alternative method of representation, to assist the improved capture of qualitative requirements.

2.4 Representing Transactions

In particular it was evident that consideration of the qualitative aspects of community care gave insight into concepts which had not been clear at the outset, thus providing more complexity and a greater need to more accurately map the problem domain. Lucid representations of qualitative and quantitative transactions have been demonstrated by Sowa [11] using conceptual graphs (CGs), not only to accurately record complex transactions, but also to provide a means of eliciting domain facets that are difficult to determine with other, more recognised notations.

Conceptual graphs (CGs) are a means by which otherwise intricate logic can be expressed in a more human readable form, whilst remaining rigorous in their formalism and suitable for exchange between computer systems. They are represented in both text (Linear Form) and graphical format (Display Form), the latter assisting human comprehension during requirements gathering and systems analysis. Using Display Form (DF), concepts and relations are represented by rectangles and ellipses respectively. Relations are linked to concepts by arrows (arcs). The consideration of concepts facilitates the lucid representation of qualitative problem domains [12, 13].

An aspect of the CG approach that is particularly relevant to agent managed community care systems is that the production of a CG, and the resulting predicate logic, can be easily transferred across domains using conceptual graph Interchange Format (CGIF) and Knowledge Interchange Format (KIF) [14]. This assists the rapid generation of domain ontologies, whilst also considering qualitative issues from the initial modelling activities.

This capture of the qualitative transactions allows much broader issues to be modelled, and through an iterative process, representations can 'drill-down' to reveal new aspects. Community care management is an example of a system that has to manage an enormous range of services, and this management inevitably will include the resolution of unsatisfactory service, as well as the provision of satisfactory service, suggesting that CG would assist the modelling of payment transactions.

Multiagent interoperability between disparate agencies necessitates a neutral interchange format, and this has been explored by Harper with the use of CG [14]. It follows that CG models appear suited to accommodate a range of representation vehicles, such as AUML and Entity Relationship (ER) diagrams, enabling the generation of an accurate high level conceptual model.

Community care management has a fundamental requirement that the management system must be sufficiently capable of accommodating disparate software and hardware platforms, in order to be able to effectively command and control the requisite care services. Therefore the use of CG, as a supplement to modelling with other notations, is an important step in the elicitation, specification and implementation of portable, qualitative and quantitative agent managed community care transactions.

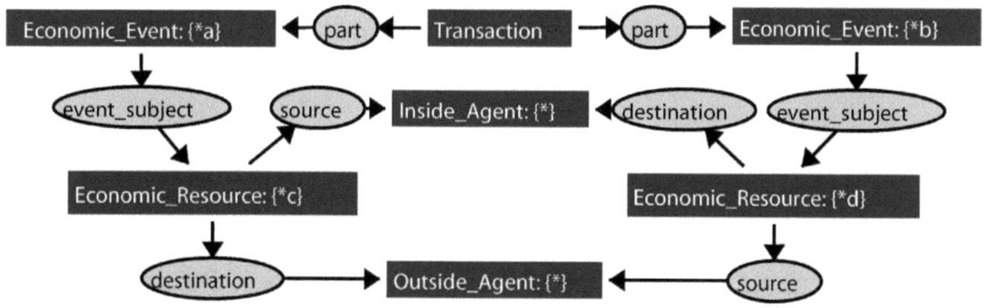

Fig. 1. The transaction model (TM)

2.5 Verifying the Care Model

UML provides robustness diagrams as a means of supporting the process of model checking, by allowing system analysts to examine the collaborations within a model before progressing to sequence models. However, it is possible to derive sequence models directly from use cases as there is no verification discipline enforced within the notation. A model could incorporate verification if the requirements were captured at a much more abstract level. This would assist the whole process by:

- Enforcing a rigour upon the requirements capture stage, to elicit agents, roles and ontological terms from a conceptual perspective.
- Providing a model check much earlier in the process, supporting the design and deployment of robust MASs.

In a MAS trading environment, the goal-directed behaviour of an agent dictates that success occurs when both parties have gained from their participation in a transaction. In essence, the transaction describes a condition where both parties have exchanged resources, resulting in a 'balance'.

Figure 1 illustrates that all transactions comprise two *Economic Events*, denoted by `*a` and `*b`. The transaction is complete when both Economic Events 'balance', which indicates that `*a` always opposes `*b`, representing 'debits' and 'credits'. Additionally there are two related *Economic Resources*, `*c` and `*d`, each having independent *source* and *destination* agents.[1]

[1] Long before the advent of agent oriented computing, Sowa introduced the relation `Agnt` (agent) as a means of relating `act` concepts to `animate` concepts [11]. For example:

```
[Cycle]->(Agnt)->[Person: Richard]->(Loc)->[City: Sheffield]
```

This can be read as: 'There is a person called Richard who is the agent of cycle. This same person is located in Sheffield'. A less unwieldy representation might read thus: 'Richard is cycling in Sheffield'. Whilst there are parallels with agent computing in terms of how Sowa uses 'agent' as a relation, it is important to recognise the distinction as Sowa's agent relation might not include all of the characteristics identified as befitting an intelligent agent. It follows that the presence of an agent relation in a Transaction Model CG also does not necessarily identify an agent, nor indeed a multiagent system.

Prior work by Polovina [5] has shown how CGs have been used to represent the Transaction Model, using the Event Accounting model as a basis.

2.6 Logic and Inferencing

Sowa developed conceptual graphs as an existential notation, permitting direct mappings between graphs and first-order predicate logic [11], the basis of which is the logic of Charles Sanders Peirce (pronounced 'Purse'). This capability enables CGs to be inferenced against, allowing the representation of concepts and reasoning between those concepts. This is particularly attractive for the representation of complex systems since the graphical (Display Form, DF) captures 'visual semantics', whilst also supporting logic and inferencing.

To illustrate, consider the following simple example:

`if Graph A then Graph B`

This can be interpreted as:

'If `Graph A` projects into any graphs in the knowledge base, then `Graph B` can be asserted'.

In Linear Form (LF) this is:

`(Graph A (Graph B))`

Figure 2 illustrates this using DF. It can be seen that the 'Knowledge Base Graphs' dominate both `Graph A` and `Graph B` as they are contained within a negative context (black border). Indeed, `Graph B` is also dominated by `Graph A`, as it is in yet another negative context. The LF example above illustrates that parentheses replace the black borders in DF. If a graph projects into a dominating graph, then it can be *deiterated.* Therefore, if Graph A is projected into the Knowledge Base Graphs the following would occur:

`((Graph B))`

Since each pair of the parentheses represents a negative context, the statement reads logically as:

`not(not Graph B)`, therefore `Graph B` is asserted as true.

Repeating these operations graphically, we derive Figs. 3 and 4. To further illustrate the power of this approach for designing complex healthcare models, let us consider a more pertinent example:

'A resident of Sheffield who is a taxpayer can receive care from the United Kingdom Welfare system if they are ill.'

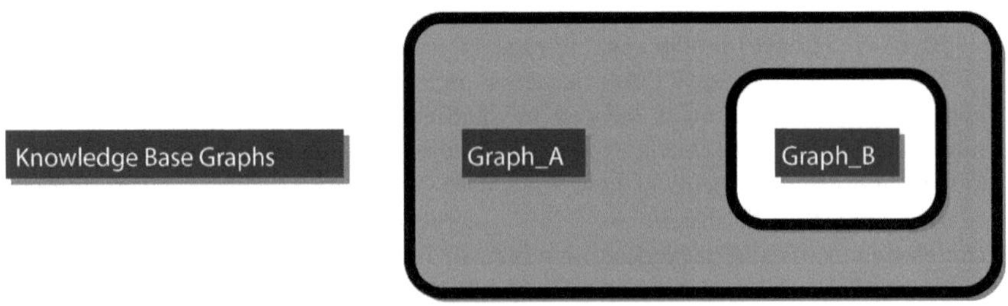

Fig. 2. 'If Graph A then Graph B'

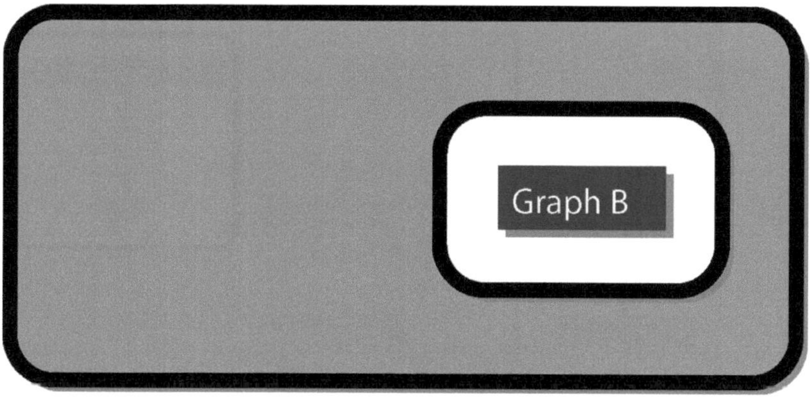

Fig. 3. Deiterated graph

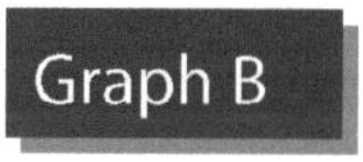

Fig. 4. Denegation

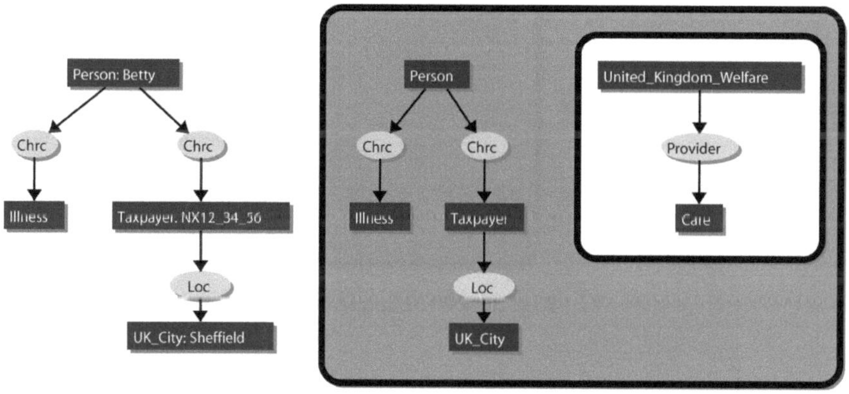

Fig. 5. Original graphs

We also have a particular case, 'Betty', who will be used to test our model. 'Betty is a taxpayer, resident in Sheffield who is ill. Can Betty receive care from the United Kingdom Welfare system?'

Thus these two statements are represented by the initial graphs in Fig. 5.

The first step is to *specialise* the projecting graph with those of the query graph. As shown in Fig. 6, `Person`, `Taxpayer` and `UK_City` are all specialised in the projecting graph to become:

```
Person: Betty
Taxpayer: NX12_34_56
UK_City: Sheffield
```

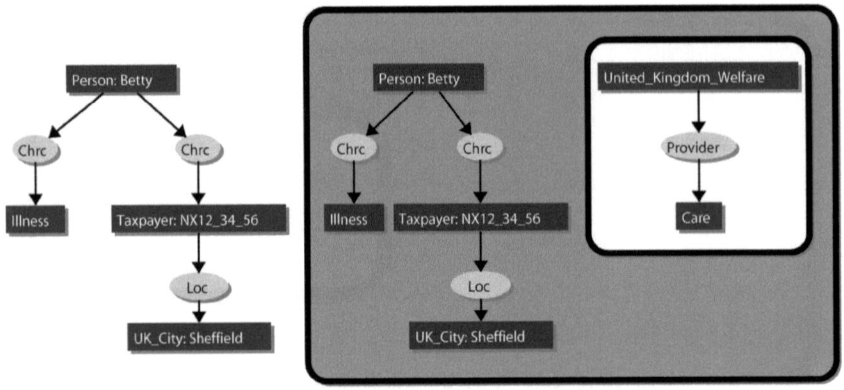

Fig. 6. Specialised graphs

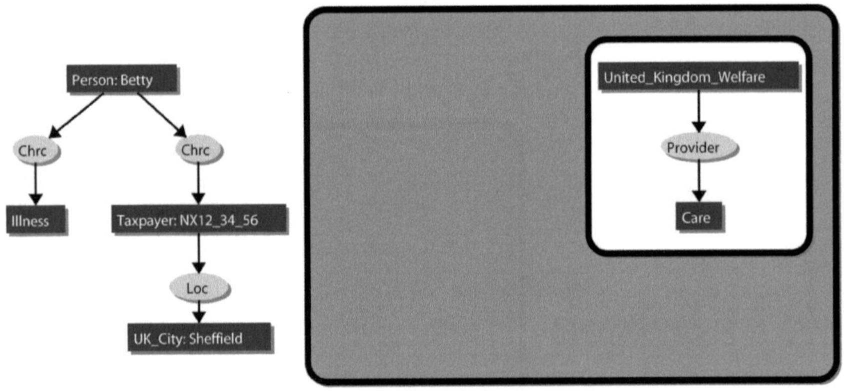

Fig. 7. Deiterated graphs

The projecting graph, once specialised with the query graph, can now be *deiterated*, giving Fig. 7.

Finally the two negative contexts can be removed by *denegation* to leave Fig. 8. Thus Betty does receive care from the United Kingdom Welfare system, since she has the characteristics of 'illness', is a taxpayer and is resident in Sheffield.

The graphical placement of concepts into contexts allows dominating concepts to be identified and the resulting number of contexts to be reduced. This is particularly powerful when combined with agent models, as the initial graphs enable high-level concepts to be captured, yet the inferencing capability permits the models to be queried in a repeatable way.

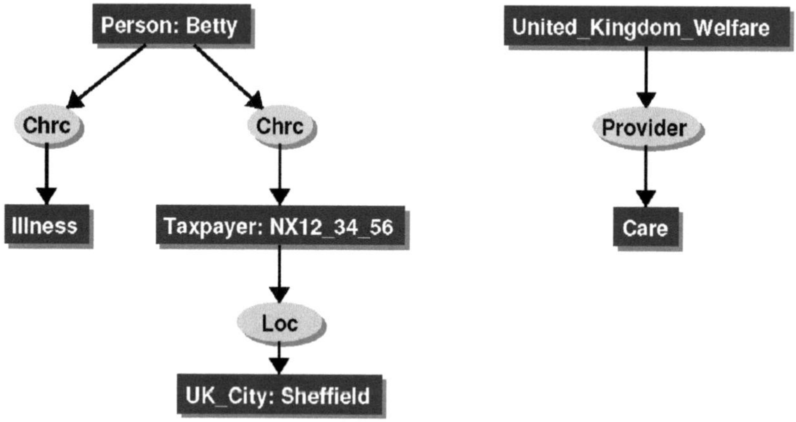

Fig. 8. Denegation

When combined with particular graphs, system specifications that incorporate an established, robust model can be developed. CGs, the Transaction Model (Fig. 1) and Peirce logic, address the difficulties attributed to agent-based models in the following ways:

1. The transactions approach makes model verification implicit as any missing nodes (concepts or relations) render the model out of balance and thus unable to satisfy both sides of the transaction.
2. The richness of CGs permits qualitative issues to be challenged and documented, before refining further by drilling down for more detail. Qualitative reasoning is an important agent capability and the use of conceptual graphs addresses this at the earliest opportunity within the design life-cycle.
3. Roles are identified using the Transaction Model via the 'inside' and 'outside' agents.
4. Ontological terms are derived from the Transaction Model during the process of capturing requirements.
5. CGs are similar to AUML in that there are some obvious mappings from concepts to agents. Prior experiences with AUML illustrated that actors mapped to agents.

A combination of the requirement for a transactions-based model, and a need to represent a community care domain that is inherently complex, has led to the development of Transaction Agent Modelling (TrAM, Fig. 9) [15], a MAS design framework that embodies the notion of robustness, whilst also representing the real-world scenario more faithfully, negating the need to compromise the implementation unduly.

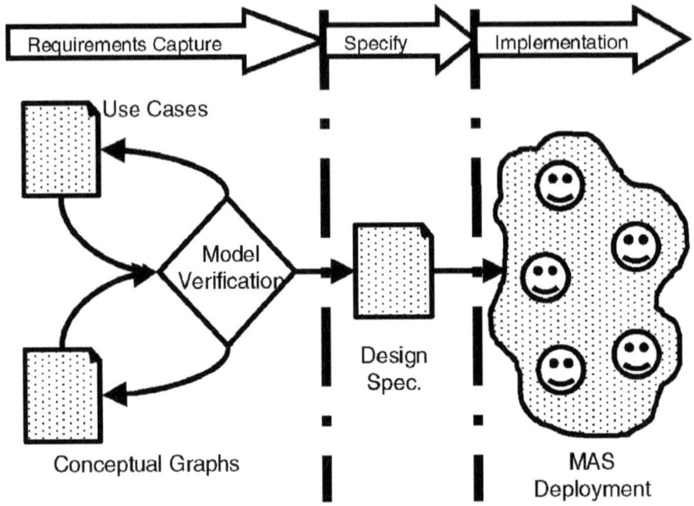

Fig. 9. Overview of TrAM framework

2.7 A Transaction Architecture

For the agents to work effectively within the community care domain, they must be able to ignore the traditional proprietary data formats to permit maximum flexibility. It is not feasible for the multitude of agents to each possess the capability to recognise every data source.

INCA has demonstrated that the management of community healthcare requires much more than the traditional n-tier model. If an organisation or collection of agencies needs to manage its knowledge then it must be able to access all of the heterogeneous repositories on demand. The work on INCA developed a 'Transaction Enabled Agent Layer (TEAL, Fig. 10)' [16], that ignores the cultural issues in data, allowing data sources to be either queried directly or via other interface agents. Requests for data are handled by the transaction layer, which manages the allocation of the most appropriate data source driver, or data access agent.

The architecture thus serves as a specification for a robust, transaction compliant API that exhibits the flexibility required to manage transactions in a multiagent community. Such a layer requires an awareness of general knowledge issues, together with domain specific detail, which can be provided with the appropriate ontologies. This approach goes beyond the presentation/logic/data model of separation by providing the advantages of a highly cohesive, loosely coupled system, that moves towards true encapsulation of data and behaviour, together with the proactive, reactive and autonomous traits of a multiagent system. The adoption of artificial boundaries creates too many compromises for the final model to be realistic, which was a major concern of the early INCA work.

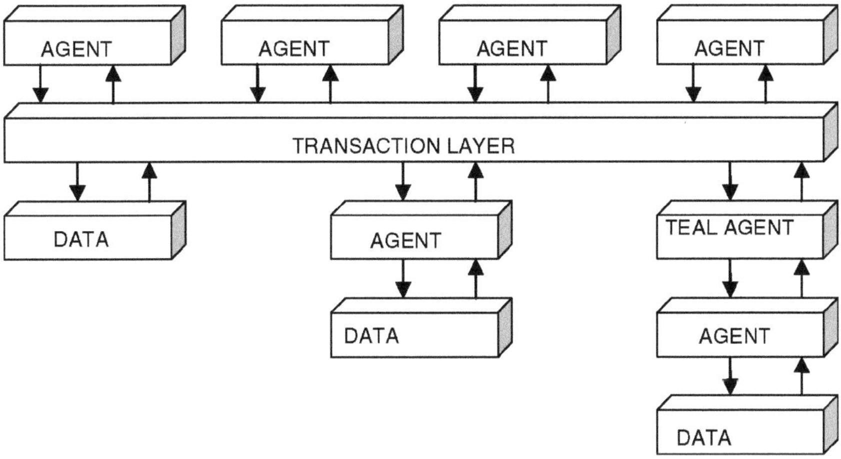

Fig. 10. Transaction Enabled Agent Architecture

3 Agent Interoperability

A key feature of this research is the ability to design and specify a MAS that can facilitate interoperability between the myriad command and control systems that exist within the community care domain. It follows that communication between agents must be able to go beyond that offered by traditional, object-based approaches to software development, by supporting an open infrastructure that comprises many different existing systems. Whilst agents can be represented as objects in terms of their ability to pass and receive messages, it is the increased abilities of agents that permit more flexible communication methods.

Essentially both the object or agent representation of a system describe state; it is the means by which this state is described and manipulated that provides one of the key differences between the two paradigms. Objects describe themselves with attributes, relations and methods (behaviours). If the attributes, relations and methods are public, then they can be manipulated by other objects. Objects pass messages in order to directly invoke the methods of a receiving object, therefore the 'sender' object determines when the 'receiver' object's methods are called.

In contrast to this, agents represent their state in terms of their beliefs (facts about the agent itself and its environment) and intentions (plans). Thus the concept of public methods is redundant, and in the case of two agents communicating, the 'sender' agent could make a request to call a 'receiver' agent's methods, however the receiver agent would autonomously reason with its beliefs about itself and its environment, against its desires and plans, before deciding upon a course of action [17].

Thus the control of the method is retained by the agent that owns the method; if execution of the method does not suit the self-interest of the receiving agent then the request will not be fulfilled. It follows that agents can only exert action through communicative acts. However, these acts are based upon an agent's beliefs, which must embody an explicit representation of agent and domain knowledge.

3.1 Syntactic Interoperability

As discussed above, an agent communicates a representation of its mental state to a receiving agent, rather than directly manipulating the receiver's methods. This means that the responsibility for the outcome of an action is transferred to the receiving agent, rather than lying with the sender in an object environment.

This enables an agent to delegate responsibilities (and by implication its *goals*) to other agents, in the same way that responsibilities are delegated by human managers in a typical hierarchical management structure [18]. Since agent architectures facilitate delegation, the following issues are addressed:

- It is easier to capture and specify the requirements of hitherto complex systems, thus embodying autonomy, delegation and proactivity.
- The resulting software models represent the domain more faithfully.

The imperative message passing approach of objects results only in receiving objects being forced to perform actions in a particular way, whereas agents can make requests without specifying how that request might be achieved. The fact that objects need to specify how something is performed, has led to the development of messaging protocols that rely on syntactic arguments; an object message specifically orders the execution of a method.

Such an approach delivers systems that need developers to program to the appropriate interface, using the correct syntax. It also means that the receiver has no information as to the intended outcome of the request, other than the specific method invocation, thus the receiver cannot reason about how an outcome might be achieved.

Whilst interoperability can be achieved between systems using specific syntactics, this is somewhat restrictive if the systems to be integrated are disparate, and certainly prevents the potential capabilities of agent architectures for open systems, since every agent needs to understand every other agents' communication syntax.

3.2 Semantic Interoperability

If the semantics of a request are considered, an immediately more attractive scenario is presented:

- Communicating agents would not have to rely on restrictive syntactic messages, and would be able to interpret those messages within the context of the agent's own belief-base.

- Agents could delegate responsibilities to achieve goals without specifying how those goals should be achieved.
- Environments of semantically-able agents could be assembled automatically, safe in the knowledge that they could interoperate and cooperate independently of syntactical restrictions, whilst maintaining loose coupling and agent autonomy.
- Communication is simplified as agents only have to communicate the goals that they wish to achieve.

Agent Communication Languages (ACL) such as FIPA-ACL [19] define syntactic and semantic standards for inter-agent communication in terms of *speech acts* [20]. Speech acts are a collection of utterances that appear to have some influence over a physical world. Austin [20] identified a number of speech acts that can be represented by *performative* verbs, and defined three aspects of the acts:

1. *Locutionary.* 'Please wash the dishes.' The act of making an utterance.
2. *Illocutionary.* 'She asked me to wash the dishes.' The action that was performed in response to the utterance.
3. *Perlocutionary.* 'She got me to wash the dishes.' The resulting effect of the act.

The performative verbs are a means by which the action of the speech act is described. Examples include *request*, *inform*, and *promise*. Successful completion of the performative was classified as three *felicity conditions* [20]:

1. There must be an accepted conventional procedure for the performative, and the circumstances must be as specified in the procedure.
2. The procedure must be executed correctly and completely.
3. The act must be sincere, and any uptake required must be completed, insofar as is possible.

Searle [21] extended this work to include a much more rigorous specification of the domain in which the conversation takes place. For instance we must consider whether the 'hearer' can hear the 'speaker', or if the domain has specific characteristics that might affect the comprehension of a speech act. We would expect that an agent that receives a speech act instructing the murder of someone would be able to differentiate between the domain context of a theatre play and the real world.

In particular, FIPA-ACL has a rich set of performatives that formally specify meaning for communication primitives, based upon speech acts, enabling agents to interpret messages correctly and act accordingly. Thus agents that can understand the meaning of a communication, by interpreting its semantics, stand a much better chance of reacting properly, thereby facilitating much more flexible systems for open environments.

If an agent wishes to know the time it would need to express a communicative act that represents 'What is the time?'. Using FIPA-ACL this would look like:

```
(Query-ref
        :sender Agent_A
        :receiver Clock_Agent
        :content '((any ?t (time ?t)))'
)
```

However, the following statement is also valid: 'I want to know the time'. This would result in the `Inform` performative being used.

```
(Inform
        :sender Agent_A
        :receiver Clock_Agent
        :content '((I Agent_A (exists ?t (B Agent_A (time ?t)))))'
)
```

In essence, both of these communicative acts should result in the same message, even though the original language is grammatically different. An agent with semantic capability can interpret both of these messages and use the following communicative act as a reply:

```
(Inform-ref
        :sender Clock_Agent
        :receiver Agent_A
        :content '((any ?t (time ?t)))'
)
```

This approach simplifies agent construction considerably as the agent system designer can concentrate upon developing cooperative and domain-specific features instead of attempting to capture (or predict) every variant of conversation with the associated message handling protocol.

Community healthcare is a domain that is rich with diversity and inconsistency, particularly since it is composed of many disparate heterogeneous systems. Such an environment demands flexible communications, and applications that rely upon syntactic exchange of knowledge cannot offer the potential of a semantic agent approach.

3.3 Communicating Intentions

Having established that a semantic approach to agent communication is desirable for the community healthcare domain, it is necessary to consider the means by which the agent intentions (communicative acts) can be constructed. The process of capturing requirements gathers together, amongst other artefacts, the business rules by which an organisation operates. If agents are to operate as a flexible MAS, then it is important that the business processes, rules and protocols are captured in order that they can be utilised by a MAS. Indeed, the following list is applicable not only for community healthcare, but for organisations in general:

1. Domain rules should be written by the individuals who perform the tasks, not necessarily domain experts.
2. Each role within the domain may require a bespoke interface for composing context dependent rules.
3. Domain rules should ideally be dynamically generated by interacting with the system.
4. Rules are likely to be incomplete and will be refined over a period of time.

The complexity of community healthcare is such that a large proportion of the knowledge is held with the users of the various systems. This, in turn, leads to informal processes and protocols that have evolved over time to accommodate deficiencies in the existing command and control systems. Sowa [22] proposes Controlled English as a formal language for description, which could be used to facilitate the generation of ACL message content whilst maximising semantic interoperability.

However, organisation protocol rules can be convoluted, and it is probable that rule generation can become an overwhelming task. Compton [23, 24] describes 'Ripple-Down Rules (RDR)', a method of 'rules maintenance' whereby rules are created or edited within the context of a specific task, resulting in easier comprehension and more stable rule building. A key part of this approach is the realisation that the post-conditions of a task in a particular context need capturing and expressing if a representative rule is to be generated.

For example, the Local Authority (LA) Agent needs to assess the financial status ('means test' in UK) of a potential Care Recipient, via the Care Recipient (CR) Agent. This rule can be expressed simply as:

```
If care_recipient has assets > 6000 Then
   care_recipient is billed full amount
```

However, this blanket rule takes no account of other circumstances, such as whether the Care Recipient has dependent children living at the same address. Since the overall rule has been created, modification is required rather than composing a new rule.

```
If care_recipient has assets > 6000 Then
   If care_recipient has dependents Then
      care_recipient is not billed
   Else
      care_recipient is billed full amount
```

Whilst the nesting of these statements will undoubtedly result in large rule trees, it is necessary only to consider each rule within the context of the particular case of use, and therefore the justification for a change is localised. Such an approach therefore enables agents to update their belief sets as they encounter new scenarios, by tailoring general rules with new specific variants.

4 Building the Model with TrAM

Having considered the various methods of representing the complexity of the community care environment, this section illustrates by way of an exemplar, how Transaction Agent Modelling (TrAM), can be utilised to gather system requirements and produce a model.

4.1 Capturing Care Scenarios and Early Requirements

Beer et al. [25] describe five scenarios that a community healthcare system would be required to manage. The following section illustrates how a MAS approach can be used to accommodate such scenarios within an integrated community care system. These scenarios are summarised as thus:

1. The creation and maintenance of an Individual Care Plan (ICP) for each care recipient that details the package of care services that are required to address the specific needs of an individual.
2. The provision of positive care to maintain and improve the quality of life of a care recipient [26].
3. Using the ICP as a reference, the delivery of regular, routine care in order to support daily living.
4. The provision of emergency care in response to some unexpected event, such as an accident or medical emergency.
5. Quality assurance management, by monitoring the delivery of care, managing exceptions and interventions to the ICP when required.

The first step of the approach is to identify the key stakeholders in the system, represent them as UML actors and describe the roles that they undertake. Once the actors have been discovered, system interactions can then be described with the aid of written use cases and use case models.

4.1.1 Maintaining the Individual Care Plan (ICP)

The Individual Care Plan (ICP) is created by taking information from one or more assessments of the potential care recipient. This activity is managed by the Local Authority and typically employs the services of an Occupational Therapist (OT) for an initial assessment. Once the need has been assessed, the ICP is created to specify the package of care services that are required to meet the needs of the care recipient. In-home assessments enable all aspects of the home environment to be taken into account, though they do require a significant amount of resource to execute. Since a community care system

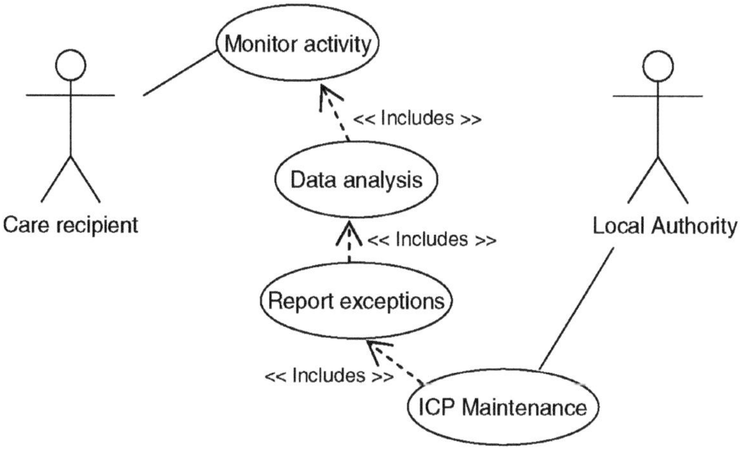

Fig. 11. Use case model for maintaining the ICP

like INCA can monitor the activities of each individual, there is a wealth of information available for analysis. Figure 11 illustrates the use case model representing this scenario.

4.1.2 Improving Quality of Life

The argument for improving quality of life is compelling, and it is often the case that when the delivery of care breaks down for some reason, the reaction is to over-allocate resource to the scenario until the situation returns to normal operating conditions. Successful delivery of the ICP not only includes the effective allocation of resources, but also the inclusion of care services that at least maintain and preferably improve the care recipient's quality of life.

Such actions are referred to as 'positive care'. Positive care aims to improve the psychological and social well-being of the care recipient, by supporting and promoting:

1. Enhanced social interaction between the care recipient, Local Authority and care providers.
2. The provision of information surrounding leisure activities and opportunities for new experiences.

Such information needs to be tailored to the specific needs and preferences of the care recipient. Figure 12 shows the use cases required to facilitate positive care.

4.1.3 Providing Daily Care

The objective of daily care (Fig. 13) is to provide each care recipient assistance with eating, washing, bodily functions, or any other care need. Maintenance of an accurate ICP is paramount and it is important to monitor the actual

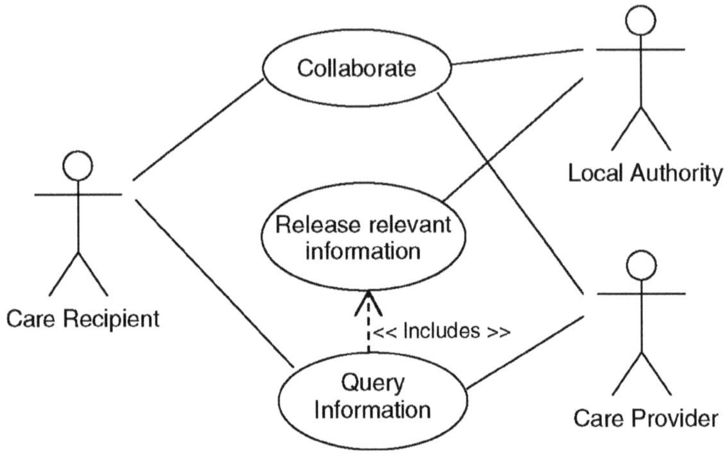

Fig. 12. Use case model for positive care

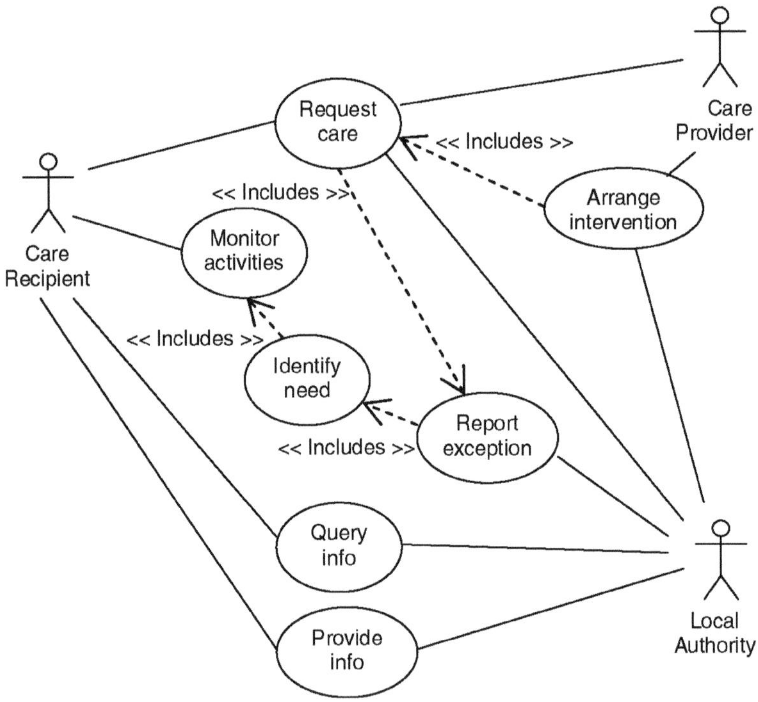

Fig. 13. Use case model for daily care

delivery of care services and report back any exceptions. Unfortunately, towards the end of a care recipients' life, the rate of deterioration is much greater than the responsiveness of the care management system.

This is less of an issue in a hospital or residential home environment as the care is delivered on demand. However, in-home care delivery is provided in relation to a strict schedule to minimise logistical arrangements. This results in a care service that is inflexible, which cannot accommodate exceptions, unless there are informal carers who are able to provide the assistance required.

4.1.4 Emergency Support

Support for emergency situations presents a challenge for community care systems. Whilst it is feasible that monitoring of the care recipient would enable a more proactive approach to care management, an emergency scenario is unpredictable and therefore the system must provide the most appropriate response in a timely manner. The use of agents to collaborate and coordinate their activities means that the results of all interventions can be monitored, and therefore used to update the dynamic ICP. These interactions are shown in Fig. 14.

4.1.5 Quality Assurance

After creation of the ICP, it is necessary to monitor the requirements of the care recipient in order that the ICP can be updated to reflect any changes. Figure 16 shows the Local Authority as the manager of this role. The concept of a dynamic rather than static ICP is fundamental to community care management, if quality of life is to be improved whilst also minimising duplication of resources.

It is also important to ensure that all the care specified in the ICP is delivered at a satisfactory service level, at the appropriate time, standard

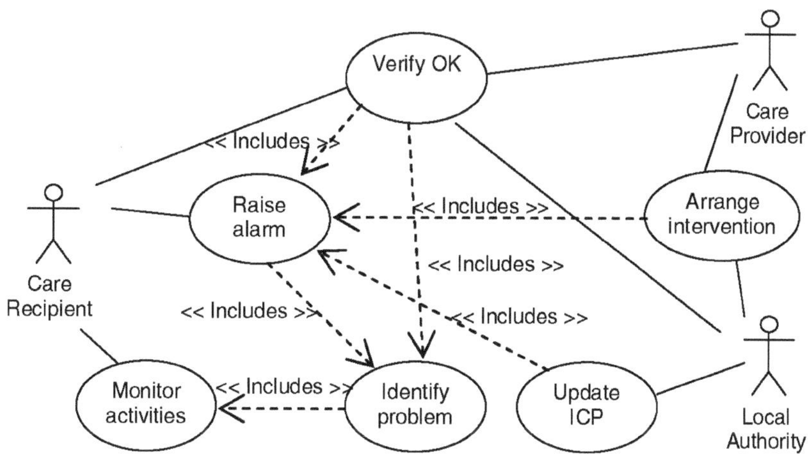

Fig. 14. Emergency scenario use case model

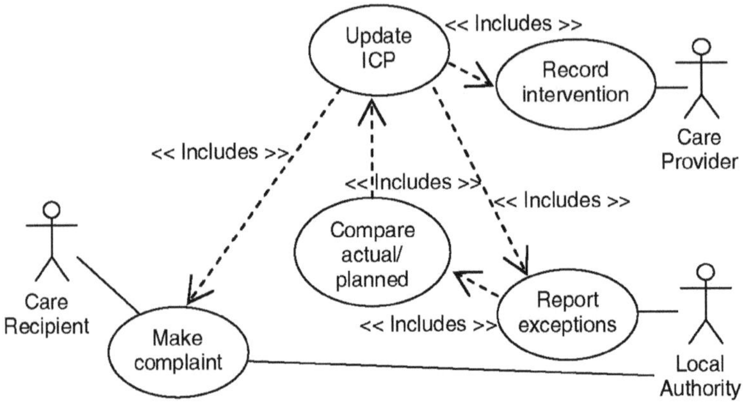

Fig. 15. Quality assurance use case model

and in the correct place. The monitoring of care staff is problematic in the community context, as direct supervision is difficult. The community care system needs to facilitate effective monitoring in two ways:

1. Care providers should log their interventions directly into the system at each visit. These can then be compared directly with the contents of the ICP. Any deviations can then be investigated and either the ICP can be updated or other appropriate action undertaken.
2. Complaints procedures can be based upon direct communication with the Local Authority, improving monitoring and responsiveness.

Figure 15 shows the interaction involved in quality assurance procedures. Now that the early requirements have been gathered, the next stage is to produce an agent model, identify and allocate tasks to each of the agents and then scrutinise the transactional nature of inter-agent communication.

4.2 Identify Agents

After the individual use cases have been captured, the next stage is to identify the agents that will be required to complete a model of the eventual system. Prior work [16] has shown that actors can be mapped straight to actors. Thus, using Fig. 16 as an exemplar overview model, the following agents can be quickly derived:

- Care Recipient Agent (CR Agent)
- Occupational Therapist Agent (OT Agent)
- Local Authority Agent (LA Agent)
- Care Provider Agent (CP Agent)

However, whilst the agent characteristics of reactivity, proactivity, autonomy, intelligence and social ability assist the representation of human agent roles,

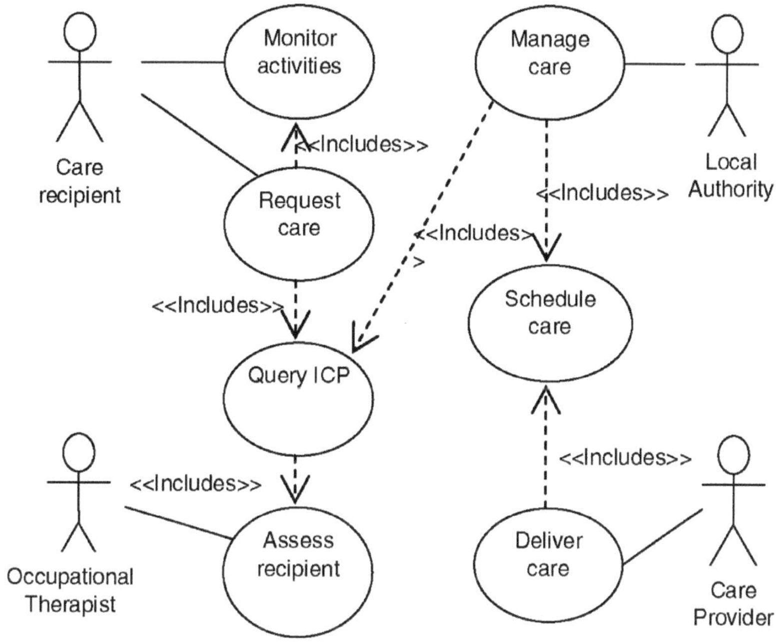

Fig. 16. Overview of care model

there still exist a number of entities that do not possess such characteristics, such as knowledge bases and databases.

One such example is the use case 'Query ICP' from Fig 16, which will need to access a repository to read the contents of a particular ICP. Similarly the use case 'Schedule care' will also require access to a database so that care delivery can be managed. In these cases, each information repository is assumed to map to an 'information agent', who manages the access to each data source. Figure 17 illustrates both the actor to agent mappings, plus the information agents who marshal each data source.

One of the key facets of an agent-based community care management system is the ability to harmonise all of the disparate data sources together without resorting to the drastic action of re-writing existing legacy code. Therefore in this example it is suitable to introduce information agents, thus reducing interference with existing systems.

4.3 Allocate Tasks to Agents

Once the agents have been identified, the next step is to identify and allocate tasks to each of the agents. Each task is taken from the use case descriptions and assigned to the perceived owner of that task, or the agent who is deemed to be responsible for its satisfactory completion. Table 1 shows the initial task allocation.

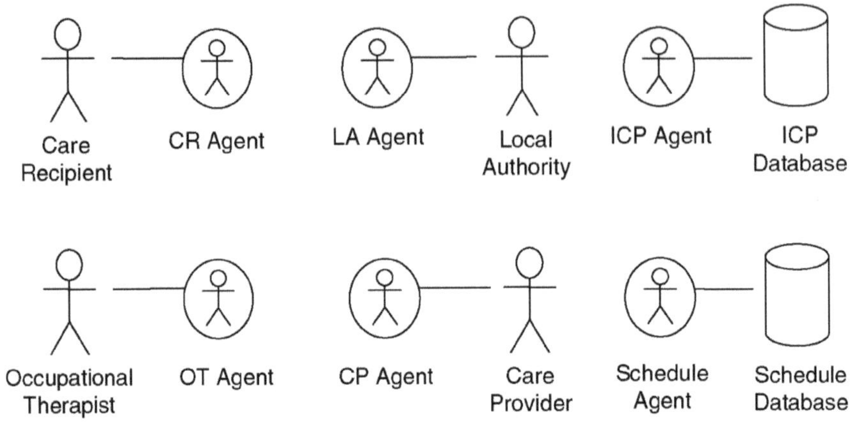

Fig. 17. Initial actor to agent mappings

Table 1. Agent types and allocated tasks

agent type	task
Care Recipient Agent (CR Agent)	1. Make request for care
	2. Raise Alarm
	3. Interact with home monitoring unit
Occupational Therapist Agent (OT Agent)	4. Assess Care Recipient
Care Provider Agent (CP Agent)	5. Deliver care to Care Recipient
	6. Query schedule information
Local Authority Agent (LA Agent)	7. Query Individual Care Plan (ICP)
	8. Schedule care services
	9. Monitor ICP

4.4 Identify Collaborations

It is now possible to examine the collaborations between the agents. Each allocated task is considered in terms of identifying the agents that will be involved in the collaboration. As each task is mapped to an instance of collaboration between two agent types, each potential conversation is considered and new tasks are derived. Figure 18 shows the agent collaboration model, together with the tasks allocated from Table 1.

This process is iterative and it is likely that several refinements are required before a comprehensive model is produced. For brevity the results of only one iteration are shown in Table 2, each additional task being shown in italics. Once the tasks have been discovered, they are added to the overall agent collaboration model as in Fig. 19.

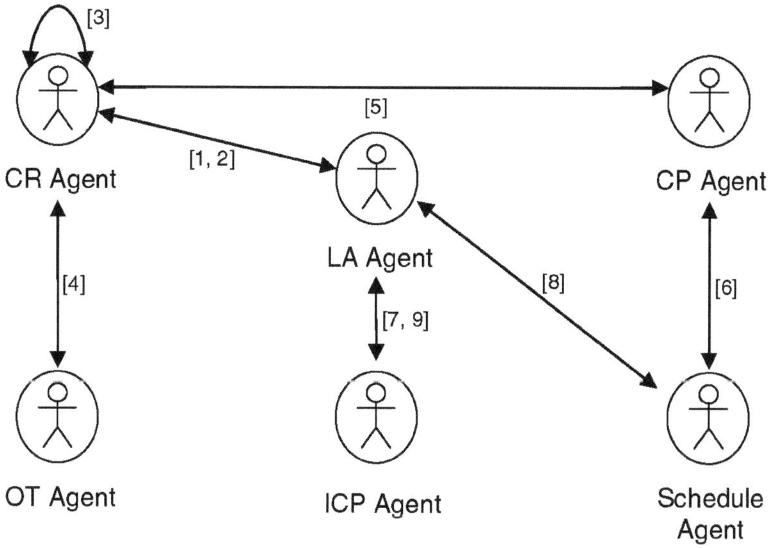

Fig. 18. Agent collaboration model

Table 2. Iterated agent types and allocated tasks

agent type	task
Care Recipient Agent (CR Agent)	1. Make request for care
	2. Raise Alarm
	3. Interact with home monitoring unit
Occupational Therapist Agent (OT Agent)	4. Assess Care Recipient
	10. *Update ICP*
Care Provider Agent (CP Agent)	5. Deliver care to Care Recipient
	6. Query schedule information
Local Authority Agent (LA Agent)	7. Query Individual Care Plan (ICP)
	8. Schedule care services
	9. Monitor ICP
	11. *Select care provider*

4.5 Apply Transaction Model

After identifying the set of overall collaborations from the use cases and subsequent task allocation stage, the model should now undergo further scrutiny in order to ensure robustness. Using the Event Accounting model described earlier, and a particular graph, the Transaction Model (TM), the community care scenario is scrutinised in terms of specific transactions. In such a complex environment it is clear that many transactions exist. For the purposes of this explanation, only one transaction will be demonstrated.

As discussed earlier, prior work with INCA demonstrated that existing representations such as AUML could not successfully express the complexities

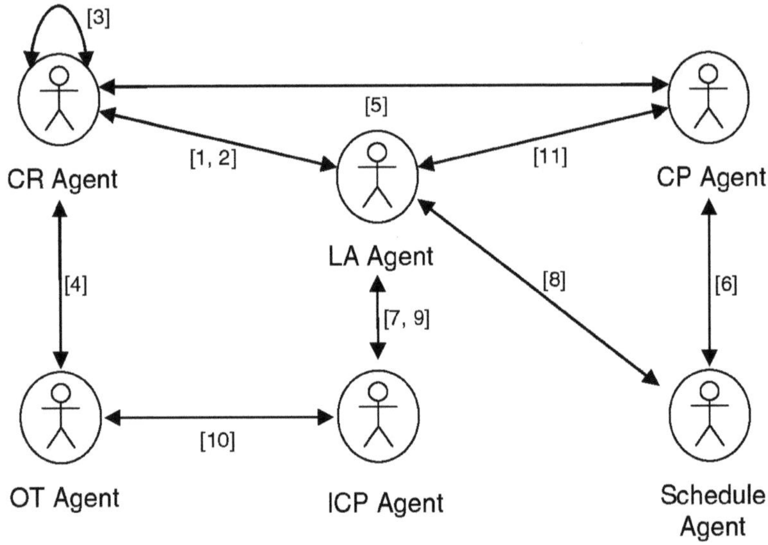

Fig. 19. Iterated agent collaboration model

of community care payment management, particularly with regard to qualitative transactions. To demonstrate the power of a transactional approach to modelling a MAS, the following exemplar will describe how the payment modelling was finally resolved.

4.5.1 Model Concepts

Initially, the whole care scenario is represented as a Conceptual Graph (CG) 20. This notation is utilised as it permits the lucid representation of qualitative as well as quantitative concepts. As described in previous work [4, 15] the Transaction Model (TM) is a useful means of introducing model-checking to the requirements gathering process. The specialisation of the generic TM of Fig. 1 onto the community healthcare scenario is illustrated by the CG in Fig. 20. This specialisation serves two fundamental objectives:

1. The concepts identified within the care scenario are 'balanced' and therefore represent a completed transaction.
2. Since each concept is classified in terms of type, a hierarchy of types for an ontology can be derived.

The overall model (Fig. 21) does not explain which party pays the bill for the care, or who is the 'source' of the money. The UK Welfare System has three particular scenarios:

1. The Local Authority pays for the care in full.
2. The Care Recipient pays for the care in full.

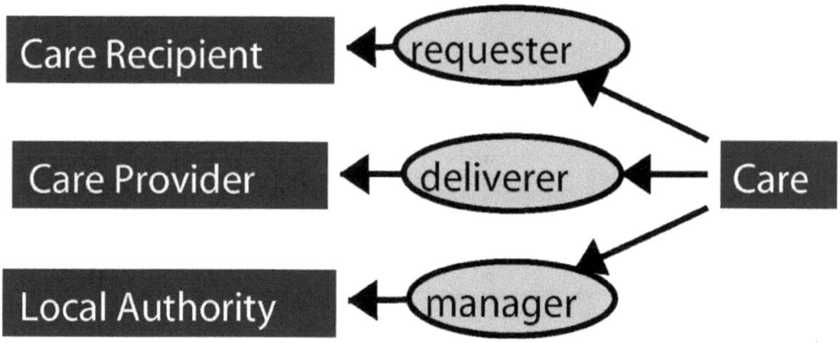

Fig. 20. Conceptual graph (CG) model of care scenario

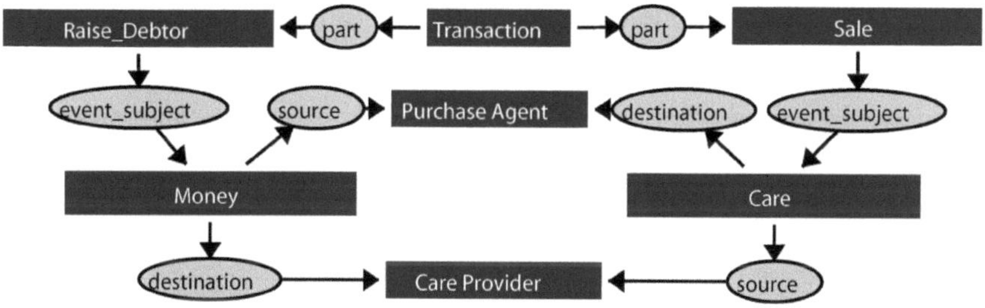

Fig. 21. Overall transaction model of care scenario

3. The Local Authority and the Care Recipient make 'part payments' that amount to 100% of the care cost.

'Purchase Agent' is derived as the supertype of 'Local Authority' and 'Care Recipient' in order to satisfy the TM.

The most significant contribution of this stage is the implicit 'balance check' that immediately raises the analysts' awareness of the need for appropriate terminology. Figure 22 illustrates the hierarchy of types deduced from Fig. 21. Once the generic model has been created, it is tested with some general rules. First, the specific scenario (Fig. 23 whereby a Care Recipient has been assessed and is deemed to be eligible to receive care at zero cost is explored.

Figure 24 shows that the 'source' of the money to pay for the care is the Local Authority 'Sheffield City Council (SCC)', who also manages the provision of the care.

However, the care package is not delivered by the Local Authority, who buys services from designated Care Providers. For this example, the Local Authority is managing a 'Meals on Wheels' service. The party which incurs the cost of the care package is represented by the 'destination' concept.

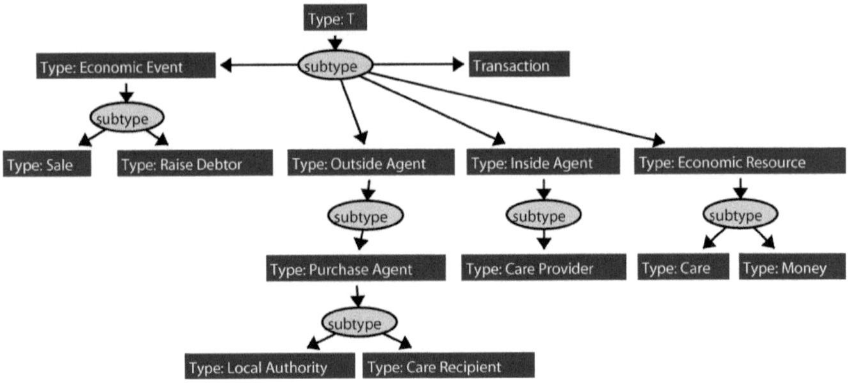

Fig. 22. Initial type hierarchy of care scenario

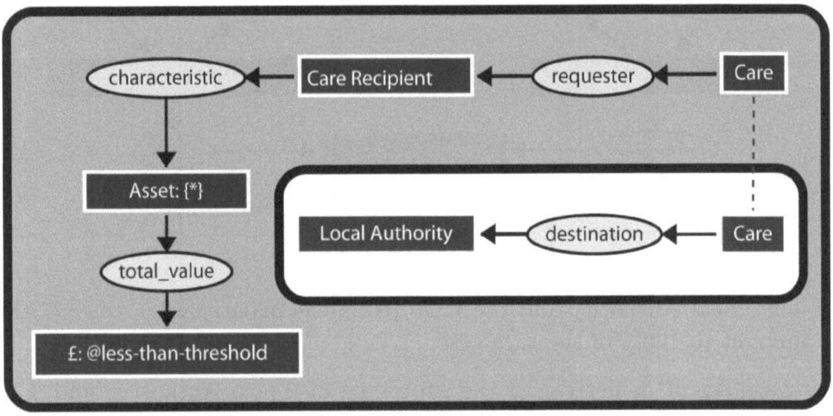

Fig. 23. Local authority pays for care in full

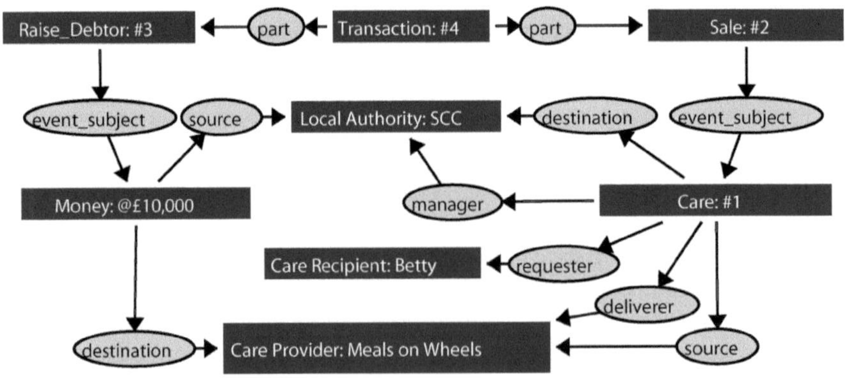

Fig. 24. TM showing care recipient receiving care package at zero cost

Alternatively the Care Recipient may be deemed to have sufficient assets, and is therefore ineligible for free care.

Figure 24 illustrates this, where it can also be seen that the care package is still managed by the Local Authority. In both cases, whether the care recipient has sufficient funds to pay for the care (Fig. 24) or not (Fig. 26), the original relationships of Fig. 20 are included. This ensures that these relevant aspects of the transaction are retained and can be recognised in subsequent development.

4.5.2 Inference Model with Queries and Validate

From the prior figures the general CG pattern in Fig. 27 emerges. To evaluate this scenario we query the model. Firstly, we examine the case where the Care Recipient's ('Betty') 'Assets' are deemed to be less than a particular threshold set by the Local Authority. In such a case, the Local Authority (Sheffield City Council) would be the destination of the care, and would therefore be liable for the bill. Figure 23 shows this particular query graph, which states:

```
If requester of Care is Care Recipient whose
   characteristic is assets < threshold Then
       Local Authority is destination of Care
```

Updating the TM with this gives Fig. 24.

Alternatively, the Care Recipient may be deemed to have sufficient assets to be able to afford the care package. Figure 25 illustrates the relevant query graph, showing the 'less-than-threshold' asset test being set in a negative context (false):

```
If requester of Care is Care Recipient whose
   characteristic is assets > threshold Then
       Care Recipient is destination of Care
```

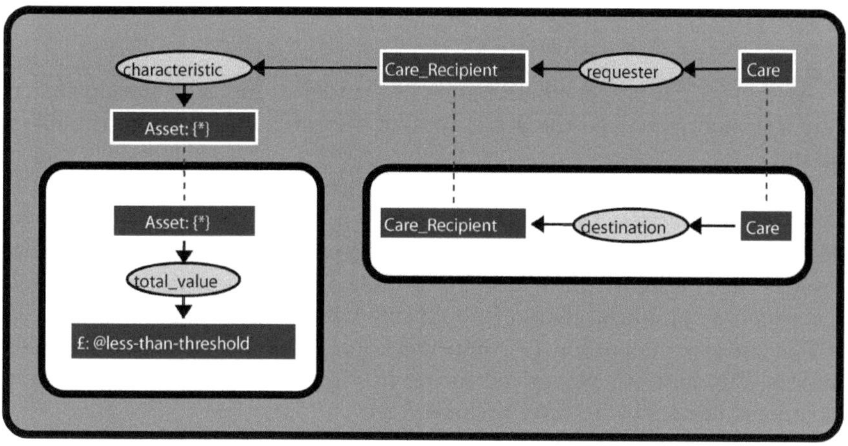

Fig. 25. Care recipient pays for care in full

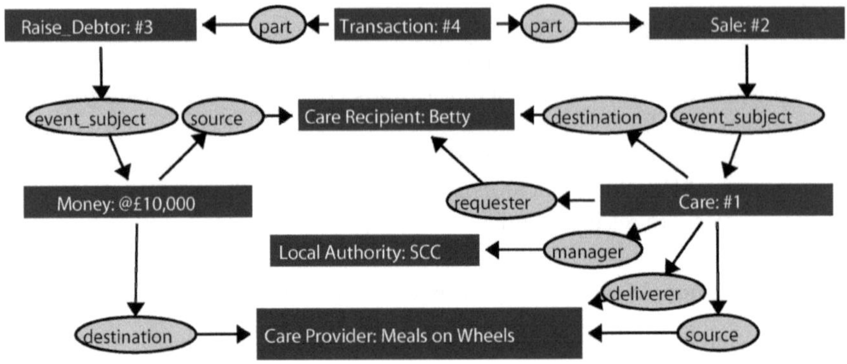

Fig. 26. Updated TM showing care recipient receiving care package at full cost

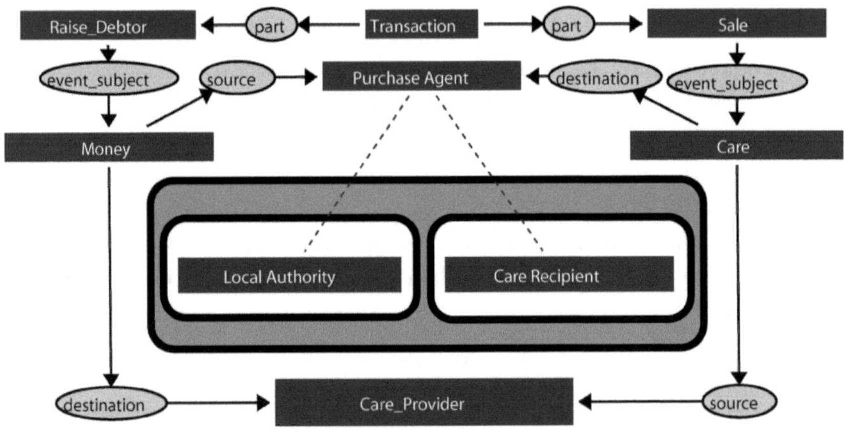

Fig. 27. Emergent CG model

Again the TM is specialised and is illustrated in Fig. 26, showing that the Care Recipient is indeed the destination of the care, and therefore is liable for the full cost.

So far the opposing scenarios whereby either the Local Authority or the Care Recipient settles the bill for the care in full have been explored; for completeness the part-payment scenario, whereby each party makes a contribution towards the total cost, must also be examined. As before, the generic model of concepts is produced, before specialising with an individual scenario. The part-payment model in Fig. 27 comprises Local Authority and Care Recipient, plus the Purchase Agent derived earlier in Fig. 22. However, Fig. 28 does not allow joint parties to be the Purchase Agent.

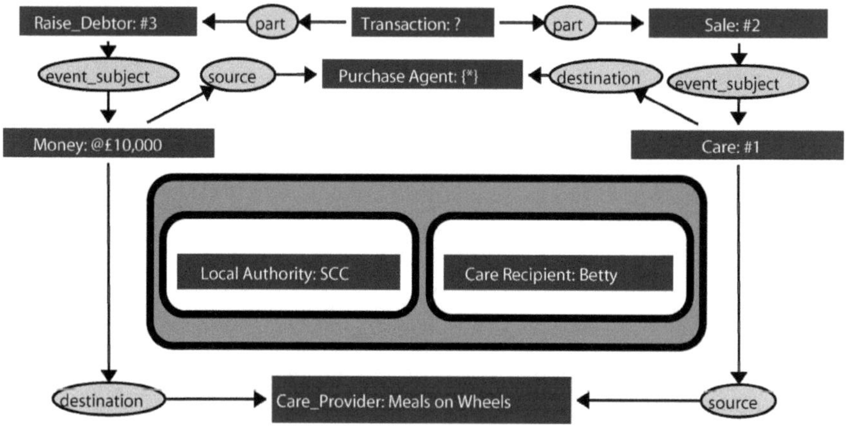

Fig. 28. Incomplete TM

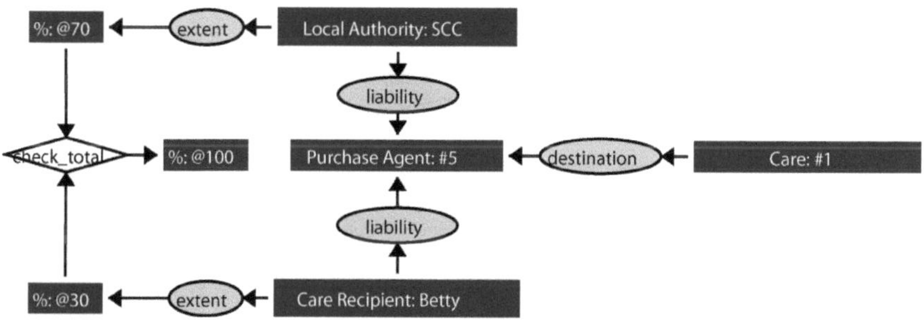

Fig. 29. Part payment scenario with shared liabilities for care cost

First we consider the scenario whereby the Local Authority and Care Recipient have a split liability for the care costs. The liability is apportioned in relation to the amount of assets that a Care Recipient is judged to have. Figure 29 illustrates that the Care Recipient and Local Authority Agents are no longer sub-types of the Purchase Agent as originally illustrated, but are instead associated via 'liability' relations.

In order to correct the original type hierarchy (Fig. 22), the case whereby Care Recipient and Local Authority Agents are sub-types of Purchase agent is false. Thus a rule is created that informs the eventual ontology that such a type relation is also false. Figure 30 demonstrates this rule, which is negated by setting in a negative context. Having elicited this information, the type hierarchy is modified to reflect the new insight, and is illustrated in Fig. 31. Subsequently the TM is also updated with the liability relationship (Fig. 32) in order that the model can now accommodate all three payment scenarios.

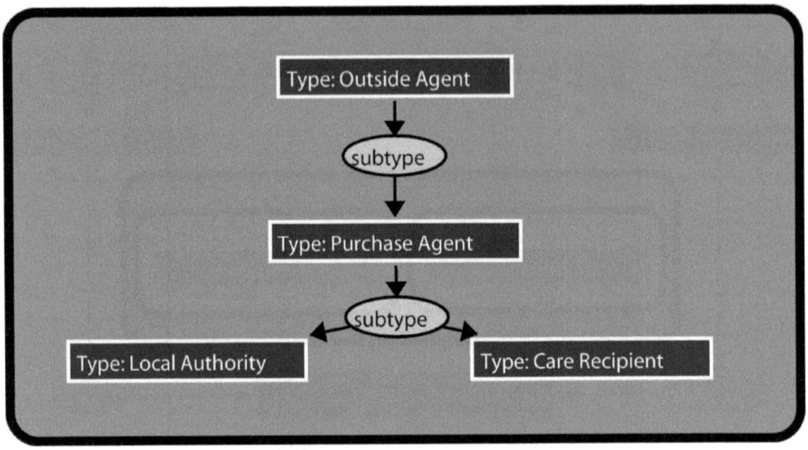

Fig. 30. New rule for ontology

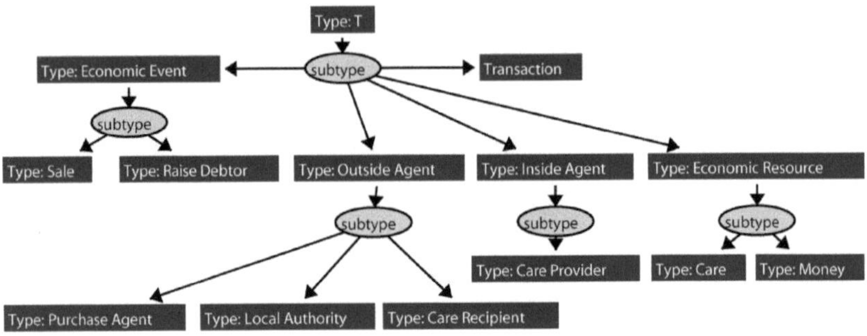

Fig. 31. Revised type hierarchy

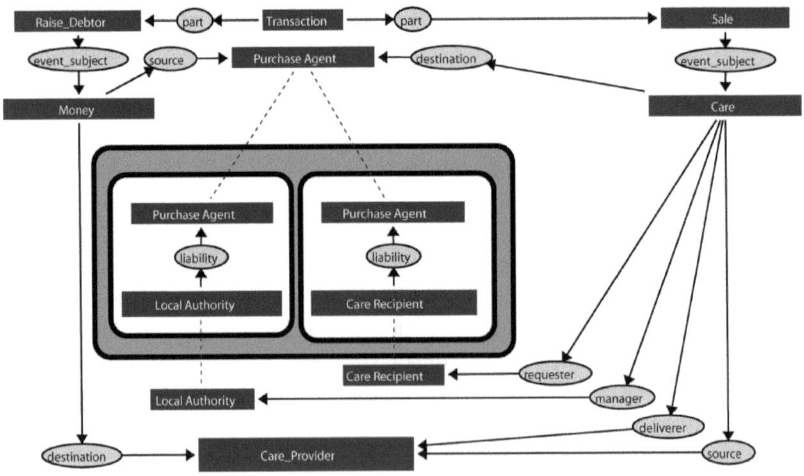

Fig. 32. Refined payment model

5 Conclusions

The management of community healthcare is problematic in that there are many disparate command and control systems, that rely upon informal processes and protocols to provide the necessary integration. Agent-based architectures provide the semantic interoperability capabilities to accommodate these scenarios, enabling delegation, brokering, negotiation, co-operation and co-ordination to take place across the myriad systems. The notion of economic transactions provides a framework by which agent systems can be designed and implemented by addressing the following:

1. Gathering healthcare system requirements can be difficult, and the lack of model verification (even though use case models enable the various actor representations to be established), presents a significant risk that some details are missing from the first modelling iteration [27].
2. A successful MAS must include the ability to reason about the qualitative issues that exist in the community healthcare domain, and system designers must be able to challenge the issues from a business process perspective.
3. The capture and modelling of roles is a crucial step in the MAS modelling process [28], yet there is little guidance as to how roles should be allocated for best performance [29].
4. Ontological rules and terms enable semantic interoperability, however, system designers tend to rely on the process of eliciting use cases from existing processes to obtain the majority of the agent's behaviours.
5. The convenience of actor-to-agent mappings means that the assignment of agent behaviours is often arbitrary and based on current working practices. Whilst the capture of current working practices is vital to the proper analysis of the existing system, this approach restricts the potential of an interoperable MAS solution. Additionally there is no implicit check as to the validity of a role, nor is there an audit trail of how the roles were delegated.

The TrAM approach has enabled the early elicitation of community care domain knowledge, and subsequent ontology specification, whilst incorporating a robust transaction model from the beginning. This has allowed representations of agent-managed transactions to be assembled at a much faster rate, especially since there is greater confidence that the underlying design is based upon a solid framework. The key features of this approach are as follows:

1. CGs represent the problem in a more abstract way, and provide a foundation for modelling the knowledge exchange within a system. The abstraction is such that high-level, qualitative issues such as 'quality of health care received' are addressed, so it is feasible that the system is questioned from the point of view of concepts, rather than relying on an individual's prior experience.

2. CGs are similar to AUML in that there are some obvious mappings from concepts to agents, however there are also subtleties that CGs reveal more consistently.
3. The inherent balance check of the model ensures that ontological terms are agreed upon before the model is complete.
4. The transactions approach makes model verification implicit as any missing nodes (concepts or relations) renders the model out of balance and thus unable to satisfy both sides of the transaction.

The TrAM approach allows agent-based systems to be designed that exploit many different aspects of agent technology. In particular:

1. The development of conversation semantics to characterise interaction between home and carer agents [1].
2. Matching capabilities of carers with current needs using negotiation protocols [10].
3. Building scalable communities of healthcare agents [30].
4. Defining semantic economic models to represent the complex relationships that exist between carers, care providers and those being cared for [31] in an interoperable way.
5. Implementing agent architectural models that promote carer autonomy and privacy whilst ensuring that commitments are realised.

The production of conceptual graph models enables higher-order issues to be captured, scrutinised and considered in an abstract way. This complements use case analysis, and promotes early discussion. The use of a particular graph, the Transaction Model, means that these concepts can be evaluated in a way akin to transactional analysis; the implications of 'duty of care', 'debt to society' and other high level concepts typically would attract little interest as they are difficult to model and even consider. The richness of conceptual graphs firstly allows these concepts to be represented lucidly.

Secondly, the application of the TM enables opposing concepts to be represented. Often one side of the transaction is clearly evident, but the opposing concept or concepts are not always clear. The application of the TM forces such hidden concepts to the fore, promoting discussion and consideration from the outset.

Thirdly, the ensuing discussion results in the generation of the most suitable term to represent each concept. This definition assists the documentation of an ontology, lessening the requirement for a domain expert. Indeed the process steers the system designer so that at least the most pertinent questions can be asked of the expert, rather than requiring the system designers to be domain experts themselves.

Also, the ability to query the representation allows the models to be tested and validated much earlier in the agent system design process. The use of a collaborative agent architecture for a community care system illustrates how agent cooperation can accomplish the provision of health care services and resources for both routine emergency scenarios.

This approach demonstrated that the utilisation of agent-based technologies could be undertaken in order to achieve distributed demand and supply issues within an integrated domain, whilst retaining existing actors and agencies.

Additionally, each actor's autonomy is still retained. Integrating external data sources by the use of information agents enables MAS models to be assembled rapidly and show that it is possible to integrate disparate data sources as part of an overall agent-based system, especially those associated with the various health care organisations.

Acknowledgments

This project is in receipt of an AgentCities Deployment Grant from the European Union AgentCities.rtd Project (IST-2000-28385). The author would also like to thank the participants of the AgentCitiesUK (GR/S57617/01), 'e-Health' Challenge Day 1, who explored a healthcare case study.

References

1. Beer, M.D., Bench-Capon, T., Sixsmith, A. (1999). "The Delivery of Effective Integrated Community Care with the aid of Agents", Proceedings of ICSC'99, Hong Kong, December 1999. (Lecture Notes in Computer Science 1749, Springer, Berlin Heidelberg New York, pp. 303–398)
2. Wooldridge, M.J., Jennings, N.R. (1995). "Intelligent Agents: Theory and Practice," *The Knowledge Engineering Review*, 10(2), pp. 115–152
3. Geerts, G., McCarthy, W.E. (1991). "Database Accounting Systems", in Williams, B. and Sproul, B.J., Information Technology Perspectives in Accounting. An Integrated Approach. Chapman and Hall, London, pp. 159–183
4. Hill, R., Polovina, S., Beer, M.D. (2006). "Improving AOSE with an enriched modelling framework", in üller J.P.M., Zambonelli F., 6th International Workshop on Agent-Oriented Software Engineering (AOSE 2005), Utrecht, The Netherlands, 25–26 Jul 2005, in Agent-Oriented Software Engineering, Lecture Notes in Computer Science, vol. 3950, ISBN 0302-9743, Springer, Berlin Heidelberg New York
5. Polovina, S. (1993). "The Suitability of Conceptual Graphs in Strategic Management Accountancy" (PhD thesis)
6. Bauer, B., Muller, J.P., Odell, J. (2000). "Agent UML: A Formalism for Specifying Multiagent Software Systems", in Ciancarini, P. and Wooldridge, M.J., "Agent-Oriented Software Engineering", Lecture Notes in Computer Science 1957, Springer, Berlin Heidelberg New York
7. OMG, (2004). "Unified Modeling Language Resource Page", vol. 2004, http://www.uml.org/
8. Nwana, H., Ndumu, D., Lee, L., and Collis, J. (1999). "ZEUS: A Toolkit for Building Distributed Multiagent Systems", *Applied Artifical Intelligence Journal*, 13(1) pp. 129–186

9. Huang, W., Beer, M.D., Hill, R. (2003). "Community Care System Design and Development with AUML", 9th International Conference on Information Systems Analysis and Synthesis (ISAS '03), July 31–August 2 2003, Orlando, Florida, USA
10. Beer, M.D., Anderson, I., Huang, W. (2001). "Using agents to build a practical implementation of the INCA (intelligent community alarm) system", in Proceedings of the fifth international conference on autonomous agents, pp. 106–107
11. Sowa, J.F. (1984). "Conceptual Structures: Information Processing in Mind and Machine", Addison-Wesley, Reading, MA
12. Polovina, S., Hill, R., Beer, M.D. (2005). "Enhancing the Initial Requirements Capture of Multiagent Systems through Conceptual Graphs", in Pfeiffer H., Wolff K.E., Delugach H.S., Conceptual Structures at Work: Contributions to ICCS 2005 (13th International Conference on Conceptual Structures), LNAI, Springer, Berlin Heidelberg New York
13. Polovina, S., Hill, R., Crowther, P., Beer, M.D. (2004). "Multiagent Community Design in the Real, Transactional World: A Community Care Exemplar", in Pfeiffer, Heather; Wolff, Karl Erich; Delugach, Harry S., Conceptual Structures at Work: Contributions to ICCS 2004 (12th International Conference on Conceptual Structures), Shaker Verlag (ISBN 3-8322-2950-7, ISSN 0945-0807), pp. 69–82
14. Harper, L., Delugach, H.S. (2003). "Using Conceptual Graphs to Capture Semantics of Agent Communication", in de Moor A., Lex and B. Ganter, Conceptual Structures for Knowledge Creation and Communication: Proc. 11th Intl. Conf. on Conceptual Structures (ICCS 2003), vol. 2746. Springer, Berlin Heidelberg New York, pp. 392–404
15. Hill, R., Polovina, S., and Shadija, D. (2006b). "Transaction Agent Modelling: From Experts to Concepts to Multi-Agent Systems". In "Proceedings of the Fourteenth International Conference on Conceptual Structures (ICCS '06): Conceptual Structures: Inspiration and Application", volume 4068 of Lecture Notes in Artificial Intelligence (LNAI), pp. 247–259. Springer-Verlag, Aalborg, Denmark
16. Hill, R., Polovina, S., Beer, M.D. (2004). "Towards a Deployment Framework for Agent-Managed Community Healthcare Transactions", The Second Workshop on Agents Applied in Health Care, 23–24 August 2004, Proceedings of the 16th European Conference on Artificial Intelligence (ECAI 2004), IOS, Valencia, Spain, pp. 13–21
17. Georgeff, M.P., Pell, B., Pollack, M.E., Tambe, M., and Wooldridge, M. (1999). "The Belief-Desire-Intention Model of Agency", in ATAL '98: Proceedings of the 5th International Workshop on Intelligent Agents V, Agent Theories, Architectures, and Languages, 1999, pp. 1–10
18. Castelfranchi, C. (1998). "Modelling Social Action for AI Agents", *Artificial Intelligence*, 103(1)
19. Foundation for Intelligent Physical Agents (FIPA). "FIPA Agent Communication Language Specification". Accessed: 2006, 10/06. 2000. http://www.fipa.org/repository/aclspecs.html
20. Austin, J.L. (1962). How To Do Things With Words. Oxford University Press, Oxford
21. Searle, J.R. (1969). "Speech Acts: an Essay in the Philosophy of Language". Cambridge University Press, Cambridge

22. Sowa, J.F. (1999). "Controlled English". Available at http://www.jfsowa.com/clce/specs.htm
23. Compton, P., Peters, L., Edwards, G., and Lavers, T. (2006). "Experience with Ripple-Down Rules". In A. Macintash R. Ellis, and T. Allen, eds., "Applications and Innovations in Intelligent Systems XIII: Proceedings of the Twenty-fifth SGAI International Conference on Innovative Techniques and Applications of Artificial Intelligence", pp. 109–121. Springer, Cambridge, UK ISBN 1-84628-223-3
24. Compton, P., Jansen, R. (1990). "A Philosophical Basis for Knowledge Acquisition", Knowledge Acquisition 2, pp. 241–257
25. Beer, M.D., Hill, R., Huang, W., Sixsmith, A. (2002). "Using Agents To Promote Effective Coordination In A Community Care Environment", in "Agent Supported Collaborative Work", Book chapter, Co-editors: Ye, Y., IBM T.J. Research Centre, Churchill, E.F., FX Palo Alto Laboratory, Inc., Kluwer, Netherlands, Winter 2002
26. Sixsmith, A., C. Hawley, J. Stilwell, J. Copeland (1993). "Delivering 'Positive care' in nursing homes". *International Journal of Geriatric Psychiatry*, 8(5), pp. 407–412
27. Mellouli, S., Mineau, G.W., and Pascot, D. (2002). "The integrated modeling of multi-agent systems and their environment", in Proceedings of the first International Joint Conference on Autonomous agents and Multiagent Systems, pages 507–508. ACM, New York. ISBN 1-58113-480-0
28. Depke, R., Heckel, R., and Kuster, J.M. (2001). "Improving the agent-oriented modeling process by roles". In "Proceedings of the Fifth International Conference on Autonomous Agents (AGENTS-01)", Montreal, Canada, pp. 640–647. ACM Press.
29. Dastani, M., Dignum, V., and Dignum, F. (2003). "Role-assignment in open agent societies", in Proceedings of the Second International Conference on Autonomous Agents and Multiagent Systems, pp. 489–496. ACM, New York. ISBN 1-58113-683-8
30. Beer, M.D., Hill, R., Sixsmith, A. (2003). "Building an Agent Based Community Care Demonstrator on a Worldwide Agent Platform", in Agents and Healthcare, Barcelona, February 2003, pp. 19–34, published in the Whitestein series on Multi-agent Systems
31. Hill, R., Polovina, S., Beer, M.D. (2005). "Managing Community Health-care Information in a Multi-Agent System Environment", Multi-Agent Systems for Medicine, Computational Biology and Bioinformatics (MAS*BIOMED), AAMAS'05, Utrecht, Netherlands, July 2005, pp. 35–49

Assistive Wheelchair Navigation: A Cognitive View

U. Cortés, C. Urdiales, R. Annicchiarico, C. Barrué, A.B. Martinez, and C. Caltagirone

Summary. A key issue in autonomy assistance is mobility, as mobility impairment has proven to cause a downward trend in quality of life. Assistive devices mostly differ on user interfaces, sensory–motor hardware, and algorithms to share control between the user and the device. This work reviews current approaches to assisted wheelchair navigation. It also presents experimental evaluation of the performance of different users presenting different pathologies depending on how much control they exert over their wheelchair, as shared control is of capital importance. Results are correlated with their pathologies to extract conclusions about the benefits of assistive navigation.

1 Introduction

Population today is progressively aging in developed countries. The increase in the proportion of older persons (60 years or older) is being accompanied by a decline in the proportion of the young (under age 15). Nowadays, the number of persons aged 60 years or older is estimated to be 629 million and expected to grow to almost 2 billion by 2050, when the population of older persons will be larger than the population of children (0–14 years) for the first time in human history [1]. This tendency also implies an increasing number of people affected by chronic diseases, such as heart disease, cancer, and mental disorders. Chronic diseases may frequently lead to disability. It is estimated that the costs of health care could rise from $1.3 trillion to over $4 trillion for these reasons [2].

It is assumed that a person's independence is threatened when physical or mental disabilities make it difficult to carry out the basic activities of daily life such as bathing, eating, using the toilet, and walking across the room, as well as shopping and meal preparation. Under these circumstances, either home assistance has to be granted or the person needs to be institutionalized. In nursing facilities, though, costs are higher and the quality of life is often reduced [3].

U. Cortés et al.: *Assistive Wheelchair Navigation: A Cognitive View*, Studies in Computational Intelligence (SCI) **48**, 165–187 (2007)
www.springerlink.com

Lack of human resources to assist elder people leads naturally to create systems to do it in an autonomous way (e.g., [4, 5]). Studies on the use of assistive devices in a general population in Swedish descriptive cross-sectional cohort studies [6] reported that one-fifth at the age of 70 and almost half the population at the age of 76 had assistive devices, usually in connection with bathing and mobility. Another study of 85-year olds in a general elderly population found that 77% of them had one or more assistive devices, also more frequently for bathing and mobility. The same pattern has been found in other general population studies, although the prevalence rates vary from 23 to 75% according to population studied, age group, and type of assistive devices. To sum up, prevalence rates vary, but the use of assistive devices is very common among the elderly, particularly bathing and mobility devices, and their use increases with age. At the age of 90, assistive devices in bathing and mobility were the most frequently used, and the same results have been obtained in persons of 70 and 76 years of age. It is consequently of extreme importance to create a new generation of tools to assist people with disabilities, so that their independence and autonomy are improved.

Regarding mobility, the most usual assistive devices are wheelchairs and walkers. Both devices have been robotized to assist people with disabilities to move in houses, residences, and hospital. Hardware modifications basically consist of adding sensors and processing units to detect what the device is doing with respect to the environment state and to provide commands to the motors that can either replace or complement the user's input. It is necessary to note that assistive robotics differ from conventional robots in several basic aspects. Mainly, the goals of the agent controlling the robot are continuously affected by the user's goals or needs. Consequently, optimization or intensive deliberation is not advisable in these cases. Besides, in this case robotic agents tend not to act completely autonomously, nor continuously. Instead, when the user performs an action, its outcome may be affected by the actions of the assistive agent. Regarding assistive devices, it is important to establish a clear distinction between walkers and wheelchairs. From a practical point of view, walkers must provide both balance and support and, hence, imply a highly collaborative profile: if the walker motion differs from the user's expectations, a fall can result. Most works on walkers [7–9] focus, consequently, on kinematics, whereas wheelchair works focus on navigation, defined as the task of safely reaching a given destination and is, therefore, less dependent on technology specifics. In order to keep this paper as general as possible, it is centered on wheelchairs.

Experience with new technology, though, has shown that increased computerization does not guarantee improved human–machine system performance. Poor use of technology can result in systems that are difficult to learn or use and even may lead to catastrophic errors [10]. This may occur because, while there are typically reductions in physical workload, mental workload has increased [11]. Also, in this particular field, the recommended action might go against the user's wishes and cause him/her stress.

Besides, excessive assistance may lead to loss of residual capabilities, as no effort is required on the user's part. Cognitive research provides insight and guidance in areas such as the effects of practice on performance, rational decision-making, and expert problem-solving in the user interface. In order to achieve a cognitive assistive device, engineering must be coupled with medical research.

Section 2 in this chapter focuses on the medical point of view on assistance and disabilities, especially regarding disability quantization and evaluation, which is basic for engineers building assistive devices. Section 3 provides a review on current assistive technologies. Section 4 evaluates agent technology as an option to handle the problem complexity. Finally, Sect. 5 shows some results on a real experiment on assistance. Conclusions are given in Sect. 6.

2 Age-Related Disability: A Clinical View

Age-related disability is generally thought of as a common endpoint, through impairment in physical, cognitive, or sensory domains, of the chronic diseases and conditions that affect aging persons. According to prevailing models of the disablement process, disability results when these diseases and conditions, via specific impairments and functional limitations, lead to limitations in the ability to perform basic social roles. As defined by World Health Organization (WHO), in the International Classification of Functioning, Disability and Health, known as ICF: "disability serves as an umbrella term for impairments, activity limitations, or participation restrictions" [12]. Hence, disability is usually defined as the degree of difficulty or inability to independently perform basic activities of daily living (ADL) such as bathing, eating, using the toilet, or other tasks essential for independent living, without assistance. It is generally recognized, however, that disability is not merely a function of underlying pathology and impairment, but involves an adaptive process, which is subject to a host of individual (psychosocial) and ecologic (environmental) factors.

Currently, this complex syndrome is known as functional disability (FD). In fact, FD has to be intended as the result of the interaction of different individual components of compromised functions: physical, emotional, and cognitive aspects usually interact to produce a comprehensive disability which is more than the simple addition of the single impairments, affecting the patient's global function and his self-dependency [13].

2.1 Disability Evaluation

However, disability has no clear limits, and defining different levels in different patients is very difficult, particularly when referring to FD. The scientific community lacks consensus on how to measure disability and how to individuate subgroups of disabled individuals [14].

Since disabled population is highly heterogeneous, functional assessment plays a fundamental role in defining disability profiles, depending on specific sort and degree of disability. Such profiles reflect on different approaches to new technologies.

Many assessment scales have been proposed to correctly define disability since Katz introduced the ADL in 1963. The field grew rapidly and by 1986 Feinstein [15] identified 43 different indexes of ADL for use patient care and population research. Clinicians' most widely used approach is to produce an absolute or relative score for each assessed patient [16, 17] to classify him/her or his/her disability on a scale or a range of values. In these terms, the disability scores of each scale constitute an increasing or decreasing continuum of values related to individual degree of self-dependency.

Rehabilitation is fundamental in disabled population in order to improve and/or to maintain their quality of life. Furthermore, functioning and health must be considered as associated with a condition but also as associated with personal and environmental factors and context. To solve such a complex syndrome as disability, several approaches have been proposed; the most comprehensive approach is represented by the intervention of a multiprofessional rehabilitative team in order to solve medical, social, and psychological aspects.

A multidisciplinary involvement in comprehensive rehabilitation programs has proven effective [18], and the positive interaction of mental and physical training has been studied [19]. In recent years it has been proposed the use of technological assistive devices. In fact, assistive devices are made available to disabled and older people to help them overcome barriers and remain independent despite disease. The positive effects of assistive technologies on quality of life of elderly disabled people [20] have been proven. The growing numbers of disabled people will increase the demand for assistive devices in the elderly population.

2.2 Autonomy and Disability

As discussed above, in order to quantify residual autonomy and level of disability of individuals, it is commonly accepted to talk in terms of functional disability and functional status. In fact, functional status is usually conceptualized as the "ability to perform self-care, self-maintenance, and physical activities."

Behind that, physical and mental functions, conditions, and diseases affecting such functions are to be taken into account as well.

It is well documented that global declines and alterations in motor coordination, spatial perception, visual and auditory acuity, gait, muscle and bone strength, mobility and sensory perceptions of environmental stimuli (heat, cold) increase with age, as well as chronic diseases and their disabling sequels [21].

Multiple chronic degenerative diseases (stroke, arthritis, hypertension, cancer, degenerative bone/joint disease, and coronary artery disease) may lead to either sensory loss or physical impairments that limit mobility, impair cognition, or reduce the ability to perform daily activities.

Evidence shows that older and/or disabled populations are made up by individuals who present widely different and heterogeneous functional profiles. Impairments range from extremely mild (people able to walk with a cane or affected by such a mild memory loss that allows them to live on their own) to extremely severe (persons bedridden or completely unable to understand a simple instruction).

The simultaneous presence of cognitive and mobility impairments has a multiplicative effect, worsening global function more than expected by the sum of the single conditions.

Cognition and mobility heavily affect the capacity of daily planning. For an activity to be effective, the person must be capable of performing it when he/she wants to or when it is necessary: the possibility of successfully performing daily life connected activities implies the chance of remaining or not in the community. Some people, due to their memory problems or their inability to relate concepts, are not able to formalize a set of goals. They may also have the ability to generate the goals, but be unable to generate a cognitive plan to execute them due to their inability of problem-solving or external information processing. It is also possible that a person has most capabilities, but due to problems in attention and sensitive stimuli processing, is unable to relate the environment through he/she is navigating with the mental plan he/she wants to follow.

As a consequence, the capacity of performing ADLs becomes an important indicator of self-dependency or disability, it is used as a comprehensive measure in disabled people, and it can be chosen as a marker of functional status.

It is then mandatory to take into account age-related functional status impairment among senior citizens when developing devices to improve disability, and to judge their effectiveness in maintaining and improving self-dependency in terms of ADLs.

Section 3 covers the different options in assistive wheelchairs, including the various shared control options required to assist both physical and cognitive disabilities.

3 Autonomous Assistive Devices

Most work on assistive devices is still in the research stage, but there are some companies that manufacture such products. KIPR (http://www.kipr.org/), for example, has designed a controller that can be attached to conventional power wheelchairs in its Tin Man series. Applied AI Systems (http://www.aai.ca/) manufactures TAO-7, mostly to researchers, though. Active Media Robotics (http://www.activrobots.com/) has also announced development of its independence-enhancing wheelchair (IEW).

Research has given much attention to assistive devices. Sensor-aided intelligent wheelchair navigation system (SENARIO) [22], VAHM [23], Wheelesley,

SIAMO, Rolland, Navchair, and Smartchair are wheelchair autonomous navigation systems [24, 25]. All these systems share some common features: a set of sensors, some processing units, and a control software to decide what to do at a given moment and circumstances. Still, extensive testing with real users has to be performed to probe the concept.

In the following subsections, we separately cover the hardware and software modifications required in a conventional wheelchair to achieve an autonomous assistive device.

3.1 Sensory Hardware and User Interfaces

Autonomous wheelchair navigation relies on the same principles as mobile robotics does. Navigation is roughly defined as the ability to reach a destination point in a safe way. In order to do so, onboard sensors are used to detect obstacles in the way and also to calculate the position of the mobile in the environment. It is necessary to note that wheelchair navigation tends to be assistive rather than to totally replace the user's commands. Consequently, the user's interface in these cases may be considered as an additional sensor representing the user's will.

The most frequent user interfaces in wheelchairs are joysticks, which simply allow the user to direct the mobile toward a given direction. Joysticks are cheap and fairly intuitive, but they only provide direction information and speed is usually quantified. In order to grant safety, force feedback joystick [26] has also been used. These joysticks make it difficult to move toward obstacles, as they present more resistance depending on how close they are with respect to the mobile (Fig. 1).

In some cases, though, users may be unable to use a joystick, either due to cognitive or physical disabilities. Some approaches rely on touch screens that present a map of the environment. Using them, a goal can be set by simply putting the finger on the desired position [27–29]. In other cases, a voice interface is used [30]. These devices, as joysticks, are commercially available

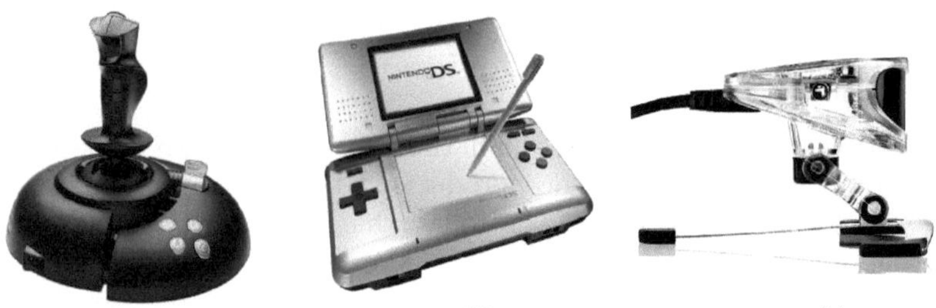

(a) (b) (c)

Fig. 1. Control devices: (**a**) Microsoft Sidewinder Force Feedback Joystick, (**b**) Nintendo DS Touchscreen, (**c**) TrackIR3 Pro

(Fig. 1). Voice control, however, can be problematic because a failure to recognize a voice command could cause the user to be unable to travel safely. Also, it is almost impossible to make frequent small adjustments to the wheelchair's velocity [31].

Voice can be complemented or replaced by other physical interfaces controlled by heat, feet, chin, shoulder switches, electromiographic sensors, or ultrasonic head tracker, which are fairly common (Fig. 1). In more critical situations, even simpler, specific interfaces can be used. The Telethesis project [32], after studying the needs of a patient stricked by amyotrophic lateral sclerosis (ALS), used an on/off switch to choose an option in a screen that continuously renovated. In the worst case, invasive interfaces may offer an option. EagleEyes uses electrodes to measure the electro-oculographic potential (EOG), which corresponds to the angle of the eyes in the head [33].

Regarding computer-controlled motion, traditionally, range sensors (Fig. 2) have been the most profusely used in wheelchair navigation. These sensors – in decreasing order of cost, weight, and range – include laser, sonar, infrared, and bumpers. Range sensors basically offer the distance to the closest obstacle in the direction of the sensor. These distances can be either used on its own to avoid close obstacles by heading the wheelchair in a free direction or combined in time and space to produce a model of the environment. A very common approach in wheelchairs is to use occupancy grids [34]. Grids are built by dividing the environment into cells and statistically modeling the range sensor into a function. The probability of being occupied of the area of the grid where the sensor detects no obstacle is decreased whereas the probability of the detection area is increased (Fig. 3b). Readings may be combined in space to produce local grids or in time and space to produce global grids (Fig. 3c).

Video cameras have also been used for navigation, but usually in combination with range sensors to grant safety and fast responses [35] or in environments where artificial landmarks are clearly defined [36,37]. This happens because artificial vision in unstructured real environments is complex,

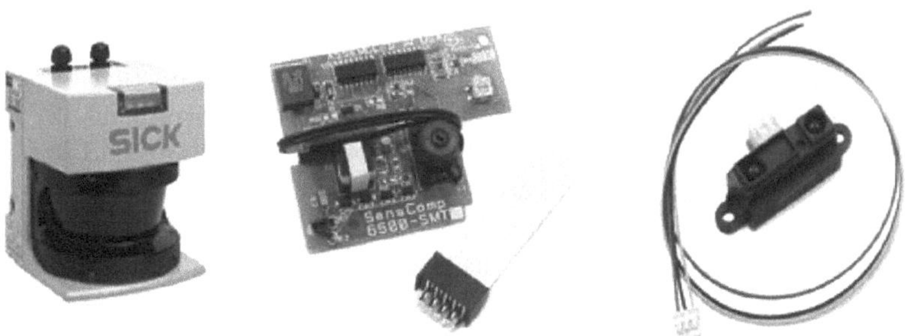

(a) (b) (c)

Fig. 2. Range sensors: (**a**) SICK laser, (**b**) Polaroid sonar, (**c**) SHARP infrared

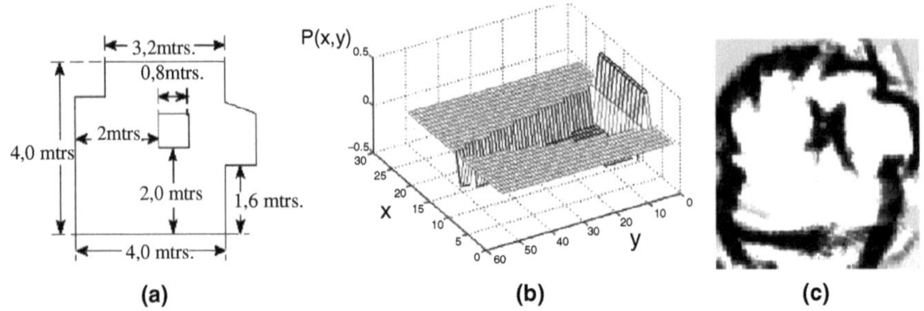

Fig. 3. Occupancy grids: (**a**) room, (**b**) local sonar grid, (**c**) global sonar grid

computationally exhaustive, very problem-oriented, and prone to errors. Special cases are omnicameras, whose optics has been designed to ensure that all points in the world are projected through a single center of projection [38]. Hence, they capture 360° fields of view in a single frame and usually extract fairly reliable landmarks from the picture.

3.2 System Architectures and Shared Control

After a given sensory input is available, processing control architectures provide a suitable command to the motors. In order to handle the problem complexity, different structures have been proposed.

Early control architectures were based on deliberative processing, according to the traditional *sense–plan–act* scheme (SPA): given a model of the environment, SPA relies on classic processing algorithms to calculate a safe path to the goal (Fig. 4a). In order to model the environment, mobiles are usually equipped with range and odometric sensors. The readings of these sensors are statistically combined in time and space to produce a diagram of the free and occupied space that can be either geometric (Fig. 5a) [34] or topological (Fig. 5b) [38]. Since odometry is prone to errors and maps heavily rely on correct localization, some corrective techniques like Kalman Filters [39] or Monte Carlo localization [38] are frequently used in these systems.

SPA usually presents (a) a top-down hierarchical structure with well-defined functions for each level; (b) predictable and deterministic control flow; and (c) strong dependence on representations of the environment. SPA control, unfortunately, presents serious drawbacks (1) all modules had to be fully functional to perform a basic test; (2) a single failure provokes a collapse in global functioning; (3) it has poor flexibility; and (4) it cannot act rapidly because information is linearly processed by every module. Besides, in dynamic environments, the system response may not be valid if the model does not adapt rapidly to changes.

In order to solve the SPA drawbacks, the subsumption architecture tried to emulate simple low-level animal behaviors to work in highly dynamic

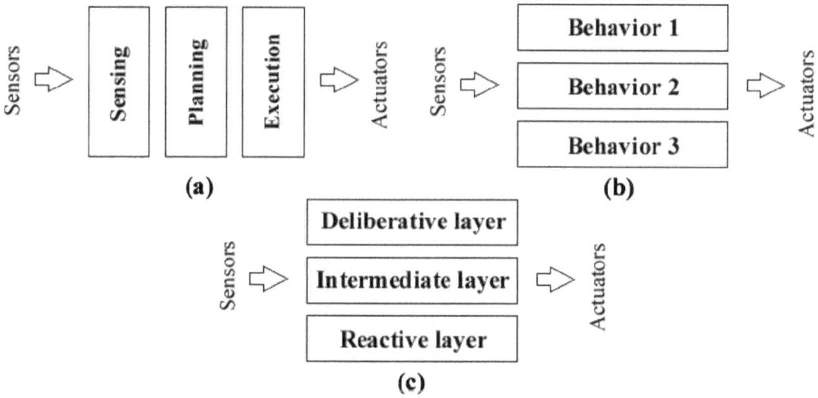

Fig. 4. Control architectures: (**a**) SPA, (**b**) reactive, (**c**) hybrid

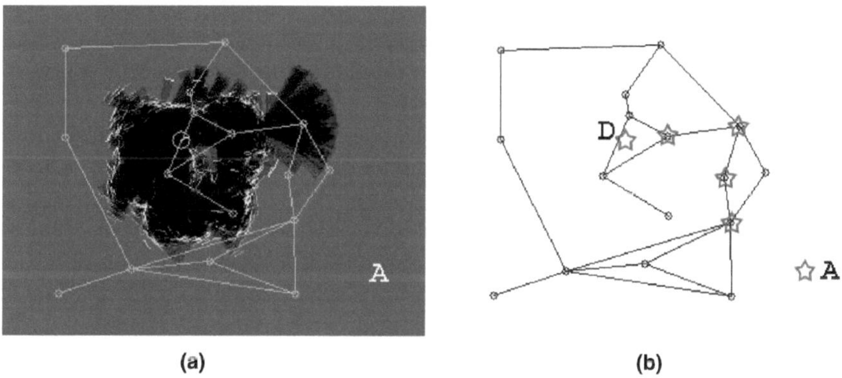

Fig. 5. Hybrid planning: (**a**) topological map built over a grid, (**b**) path planning from D to A at topological level

unpredictable environments. The subsumption architecture is also hierarchical, but in a bottom-up way. Simple behaviors are the result of coupling sensor readings and actions. The combination of several basic behaviors running concurrently produces a complex one, known as emergent behaviors (Fig. 4b). Reactive schemes (1) can easily deal with several sensors and goals; (2) they are quite robust against sensor errors and noise; and (3) they adapt to changes in hardware or tasks. The main problem of reactive architectures is that resulting global behaviors are unpredictable and, hence, not necessarily efficient and that they may be sensitive to local traps.

A later development, hybrid schemes, consisted of combining both reactive and deliberative paradigms to achieve the best possible performance (Fig. 4c). The hybrid style facilitates the design of efficient low-level control connected to high-level reasoning. Hybrid architectures typically consist of a *reactive system*, a *control system*, and a *deliberative system* for high-level planning. The reactive system consists of a set of basic behaviors whose combination may produce complex ones. These behaviors must be fast, robust, and not depend on any environment representation. The control system supervises behavior triggering and cooperation to achieve a higher level plan, which is provided by the deliberative system (Fig. 1). This plan provides global guidelines or partial goals to the reactive system, which is supposed to follow the plan as much as possible while avoiding unexpected obstacles at the same time.

Most wheelchair control schemes follow a hybrid scheme. In order to provide a rough classification, the technique employed to share control between the user and the system is going to be considered.

The first autonomous wheelchairs, like Mr Ed [40], offered a basic set of primitives like *AvoidObstacle*, *FollowWall*, and *PassDoorway*. These primitives can be used to assist the person in difficult maneuvers, either by manual selection or automatic triggering. This allows the operator to guide the robot directly, or to switch between various autonomous behaviors. In these so-called behavior-based systems the high-level planner would be that person, as assistance is only used to deal with complex situations. Figure 1 shows an example of this technique, which is mostly based on the subsumption architecture (Fig. 6). Detected events trigger one or several behaviors that are chosen either automatically or by the user and merged into an emergent behavior that is finally executed.

Mobile aid for elderly and disabled people (MAID), NavChair [30], TinMan [41], and Smartchair [42] follow this approach for assisted navigation. The main difference among them is how behaviors are implemented. MAID, for example, relies on an occupancy grid to model free space [34]. Each cell of the grid presents a probability value of being occupied which is updated depending on the sensor readings. A prediction algorithm is used to avoid collisions with mobile obstacles. NavChair uses a modification of the vector field histogram (VFH) [43], also based on a local grid inside an *active window* in front of the mobile. Each cell applies a virtual repulsive force toward the vehicle, proportional to its occupancy value, and inversely proportional to the power of 2 of its distance to the vehicle. The resultant repulsive force vector and a constant-magnitude virtual attractive force are combined into a resulting force vector, which is used to steer the chair. It is necessary to note that all these behaviors present the common feature of handling only local models of the environment.

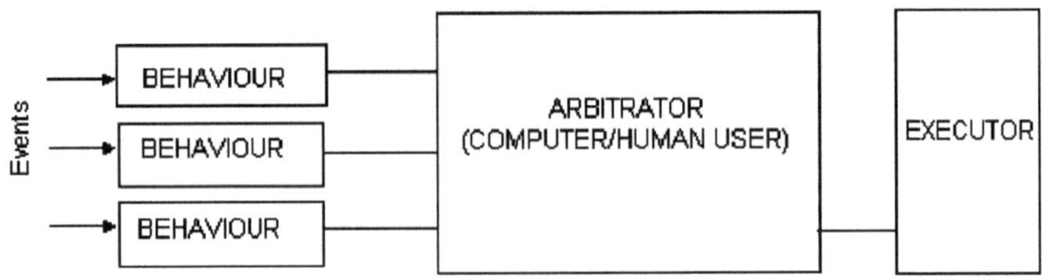

Fig. 6. Subsumption-based architecture for full/shared control

This was expectable, as the user is in charge of determining the global course of action. It is nevertheless interesting to observe of these modern systems, also provides a fully autonomous mode, usually built by adding a deliberative layer to the underlying system. SENARIO [44], for example, also uses a variation of the VFH called the active kinematics histogram, where kinematics are specifically regarded, but this local navigation layer is controlled by a high-level planner based on a topological representation of the environment. This planner takes into account several risk assessments and even the user condition.

Some other systems work like a conventional autonomous robot. The user simply provides a destination and the wheelchair is totally in charge of getting there [45–47]. Even though this might be the only option for people with severe cognitive or physical disabilities, many users may not feel comfortable with this approach, as they do not feel in control. Hence, other systems within this group rely on letting the user override control whenever he/she wants to [41]. For safety reasons, in some cases the wheelchair may also override the human used and select a behavior on its own, either by probabilistic reasoning [30] or by suppression mechanisms [48]. VAHM [23] relies on a subsumption like architecture, where free space is represented by a set of rectangles and obstacles are defined by their boundaries. Using this model, an A^* algorithm is applied to obtain a trajectory free of obstacles to the goal. At any point, the user may override automatic control and take over. Wheelesley [24] also relies on the subsumption architecture, where the deliberative level is controlled by the user via EagleEyes and the reactive one is a simple obstacle avoidance module.

Gribble et al. [49] models the environment by means of Kuiper's spatial semantic hierarchy (SSH) [50], where the world is represented using a topological model of the environment annotated with geometric information to keep it grounded. While high-level planning is performed at topological level, where the environment is represented by a reduced set of nodes, the geometric level preserves relevant data like distances, directions, shapes, etc.

TAO [48] uses two CCD cameras to detect the deep and size of free space in front of the robot but also to detect visual landmarks. These landmarks are stored into a topological map and the robot can reach a destination by traveling from one to another.

Rolland III [38] uses a dynamic window approach (DWA)-based reactive algorithm [51] to solve local navigation. This algorithm evaluates a cost function which minimizes the distance to the goal and the length of the path to execute and maximizes the distance to the obstacles along the selected path at the same time. Unlike the DWA, paths are composed of clothoids and circular arc segments to preserve curvature. Deliberative navigation relies on a laser-based evidence grid from which a Voronoi diagram is extracted. Voronoi diagrams are partitioning of the grids into convex polygons such that each polygon contains exactly one generating point and every point in a given polygon is closer to its generating point than to any other, and they are fairly common in robotics to reduce the path planning problem instance [52]. Similarly, SIAMO relies on modeling the environment by means of Visibility Graphs processed by an A^* algorithm. Paths are designed through the interaction of two modules: a potential fields based one and a reactive one. Resulting paths are tracked via a fuzzy control strategy.

In brief, it can be concluded through the different works on robotics wheelchairs that in most cases research focuses either on interfaces to support different disabilities or in control architectures mostly based on previous robotic research. It would be desirable to develop intelligent modules capable of adapting to the specifics of each user and to the evolution of his/her condition.

4 Agent-Based Personalized Assistance

Through the previous sections, it can be noted that to determine which type of assistance and how much of it should be provided to each user given a set of external circumstances is probably the hardest problem to solve. Specially, systems must be designed to offer generic assistance to be commercial, but need to be adapted to specific cases to be really useful. It is consequently necessary to find a technology that (1) deals with dynamic environments, often unpredictable inputs; (2) adapts to different users and conditions; and (3) can manage a large complexity.

Software intelligent agents are entities that interact with a virtual environment, obtaining information and exchanging it with other agents. An agent must present the following abilities [53] (1) to act autonomously to some degree, depending on events and changes within their environment; (2) to pursue their own individual set goals; (3) to react to external events and adapt its behavior to carry out its task in the best possible way; (4) to behave socially, to interact and communicate with other agents; (5) to negotiate with other agents to achieve a degree of cooperation; and (6) to improve performance over time.

The agents reasoning capabilities allow them to perform complex tasks such as allocating resources, coordinating the action of heterogeneous systems, or integrating information from different sources. In medical scenarios where many individuals are involved in a decision-making process or when their decisions and actions have to be coordinated, agent-based technology (software systems composed of intelligent software agents) is getting an increasing role to (a) model the processes, and (b) model the decision-making processes [54].

Agents are well suited for use in applications that involve distributed computation or communication between components. Multiagent systems are also suited for applications that require distributed, concurrent processing capabilities. Also, since agents maintain a description of their own processing state and the state of the world around them, they are ideally suited to automation applications.

4.1 Agents in Medicine

Most of the actual agent-based technologies in medicine could be classified as [55]: patient-centered information management; cooperative patient management; patient monitoring and diagnosis; and remote care delivery. In Vazquez-Salceda et al. [56], they are used to help manage the allocation of human tissues for transplantation stored in hospital tissue banks. Another example is to control the use of antibiotics within a hospital pharmacy department [57]. Vicari et al. [58] propose agents to support training of diagnostic reasoning and modeling for domains with complex and uncertain knowledge. In Xu et al. [59], they provide mediation services between different applications to support patient management.

However, all these applications are centered in the information dimension of the health care management. Until now, in the case of senior citizens or elderly people, applications of software agents have been directed toward the integration in society of this population subset via the use of virtual communities, trying to make Internet technology accessible to them (e.g., [60, 61]). This agent-based technology could easily be used to help solve other problems that at a first glance might seem minor but that in reality have a big impact in the quality of life of senior citizens. A good example is given by cognitive problems such as trying to remember where the patient placed some item (the remember what-but-not-where issue). In restricted environments such as a house or a hospital, a software agent may help to trace the location of the desired object by keeping track of the usual places where this object should be or of the last time it was used and/or placed. This may require a shared memory between the intelligent agents and the environment, in a way that allows the agent to use some pointers in the environment to remember how things were the last time without having a complete memory of the whole scenario. Another important area of application is safety management of technologies applied to health care.

The proactiveness of software agents could be used to perform an active safety management layer by the introduction of guardian agents, as in [54], that in a proactive way look for possible hazards and anticipate an answer or send an alert signal to the manager. For example, an intelligent wheelchair must never obey an order asking it to drive the user to the stairs nor to allow the composition of a plan to do that. However, it may override other conditions if the manager asks for it or in the case of an emergency, i.e., the agent should be able to recognize an emergency state or to ask for help in the case of an impasse. To do this, it is necessary to build safety plans and to be able to reason about them.

4.2 Autonomy and Agents

Autonomy is often cited as an important property of agents, although it is difficult to define in this context. Franklin and Graesser [62] define the autonomous agent as "An autonomous agent is a system situated within and a part of an environment that senses that environment and acts on it, over time, in pursuit of its own agenda and so as to effect what it senses in the future." Russell and Norvig [63] define "An agent's behavior can be based on both its own experience and the built-in knowledge used in constructing the agent for the particular environment in which it operates. A system is autonomous to the extent that its behavior is determined by its own experience" and also "The word 'autonomous' has also come to mean something like 'not under immediate control of a human' as in 'autonomous land vehicle'."

The notion of autonomy has many shades of meaning associated. Steels [64] refers to autonomy in the context of robotics and agents as the control autonomy or automatism, where the agent has some way to percept the environment and acts over it, for instance changing its own position or moving an object. For Steels, the autonomy concept in the biological context and by extension to the context of intelligent autonomous agents goes further on. Tim Smithers defines autonomy as: "The central idea in the concept of autonomy is identified in the etymology of the term *autos* (self) and *nomos* (rule or law)." It was first applied to the Greek city states whose citizens made their own laws, as opposed to living according to those of an external governing power. It is useful to contrast autonomy with the concept of automatic systems. The meaning of automatic comes from the etymology of the term cybernetic, which derives from the Greek for self-steering. In other words, automatic systems are self-regulating, but they do not make the laws that their regulatory activities seek to satisfy. These are given to them or built into them. They steer themselves along a given path correcting and compensating for the effects of external perturbation and disturbances as they go. Autonomous systems, on the other hand, are systems that develop, for themselves, the laws and strategies according to which they regulate their behavior: they are self-governing as well as self-regulating. They determine the paths they follow as well as steer along them. So far an autonomous system must be an automatic system and also must be able to build and adapt its behavior while operating in the environment. For that reason most AI systems and robots are automatic but are not autonomous – they are not independent from their designers. In essence autonomous agents have goals generated by themselves in place of adopting them from other agents (human or software). These goals are generated from the agent's motivations, high-level components that characterize the agent's nature, that may be related to their desires or preferences that influence a reasoning process or a behavior. Agency feeds of goal adoption and that goal autogeneration is the responsible of autonomy, thus defines autonomous agents as the agents capable of generating their own goals based on their motivations.

Autonomy is in some way a psychological characteristic and for that reason changes from agent to agent, depending on their personality. Beavers and Hexmoor [65] state that there are leading characters and characters that prefer to follow. On previous works, for instance [66], they state that autonomy can be understood in terms of social independence, but although this vision is satisfactory for simple agents, it gets more inadequate as the agents get enriched with psychological characteristics, in particular, when agents are considerate to have personality.

A third area of exploration is social regulation and the agent's behavior toward laws, norms, and values in the agent's environment as well as the ones present on agent organizations, institutions, and agent society in general. The authors understand that an intentional agent may have different autonomy degrees determined by how much local and nonlocal influence they are perceiving in their decision-making process. Local limitations in decision-making include restrictions on its physical and intentional abilities, while the nonlocal ones can be exerted through social values for instance avoid damaging other agents interests, norms like driving on the right side of lane, legal constrains like not exceeding a speed limit, and the need for cooperation. Castelfranchi defends that autonomy and dependence are opposite concepts, but it is possible that an agent depends on another one and at the same time remains autonomous. Beavers and Hexmoor think that when individuals are immersed into groups, organizations, and institutions their individual autonomy is modified by the group properties. These effects can appear as consequence of membership, as enacting a role of group representative in front of other agents or joining a collective behavior. Membership restrict decision-making and provide them a series of behaviors, duties, rights, and obligations governed by a set of norms and laws. Therefore, agent's individual autonomy can be limited or empowered by membership and this influence depends on the degree of commitment and loyalty toward the group they belong to. When an agent represents a group, it assumes the group's entity and its autonomy, empowering or limiting its own one. A representative must be the carrier of the essential components of the group and must use them when reasoning about the group's autonomy.

4.3 Shared Autonomy

The shared autonomy concept is scarcely explored in literature and often is misunderstood as shared control (e.g., [67,68]). Shared control mostly focuses on how to distribute the autonomy between a person and a sensor-assisted controller. This includes to solve questions like what can the person do and what or when should the controller take over as pointed out in Sect. 3.2. This problem is mostly related to the degree of disability of the person and his/her state. Shared autonomy in the case of people with disabilities focuses on extending the person's autonomy as much as possible with the help of available intelligent and adaptive software and hardware components. Shared-autonomous implies getting assistance from another agent, or reliance on some environmental elements such as tools or resources, or offering help to some other agent who will be the primary executioner of the goal [69].

In the personal autonomy and disability context, two different scenarios of the shared autonomy can be separated. People presenting mainly physical impairments are able to define their own goals, but due to their restrictions they usually are not able to execute them, suffering a limitation in their autonomy. In this scenario the contribution of assistive technologies focuses on physical devices, mostly mobility hardware that allows them to reach their objectives. These devices may be controlled by multiagent systems or through an agent supervised shared control if the user motor capabilities are not severely damaged. Obviously, user interfaces are very important to detect the user intention, which is critical to define goals for the wheelchair to be able to assist him/her.

People presenting mostly cognitive impairments may require a different assistive technology, which may lead even a more relevant role in the sharing of personal autonomy. In this scenario the user probably does not have very clear goals or is not capable of achieving them because he/she cannot remember how to do it. In these cases, assistive technology may empower and complement their autonomy using agents that offer them a set of services, like reminding them what kind of activities they can or should perform at a certain moment of the day or pointing them out how to achieve these activities. The main idea is to offer the users a set of cognitive aids, either rational or memory based, that can ease their daily living.

5 Case Study

Maintaining the autonomy options of senior citizens is a growing societal concern. On the behalf of granting more autonomy and self-dependency to the users suffering from physical or cognitive disabilities, it is crucial to ease their mobility problems. One important issue is to train persons that suffered a vascular accident to get adapted to their new situation and to take advantage from the ICT-based technologies including robotic wheelchairs. Other scenarios are also possible as just train a senior citizen to take advantage of the new technologies. A possible loss, for example could be complex reaction time may slow somewhat, and may not necessarily be recovered by practice or cognitive exercise. When driving a wheelchair this ability is important for safe driving and is the kind of service that can be supplied by the agent-based system.

To illustrate our own approach to this problem (see [70]) we developed some robotic wheelchairs provided with agent-based control [71] and we have been performing some real world experiments with real patients from IRCCS Santa Lucia (Rome). The wheelchair that we used is the one depicted in Fig. 7.

All subjects gave written informed consent for participation to the study, and the protocol was approved by the IRCCS Fondazione Santa Lucia ethical committee. In the following we will explain the general idea of those experiments, more detailed explanation can be found in Barrué et al. [72].

The experiment consisted on the pursuit of a simple straight line drawn on the floor using a wheelchair in three different scenarios. The test evaluates the performance of the user navigation using: first a conventional wheelchair, secondly a standard electric-powered wheelchair manually controlled, and then

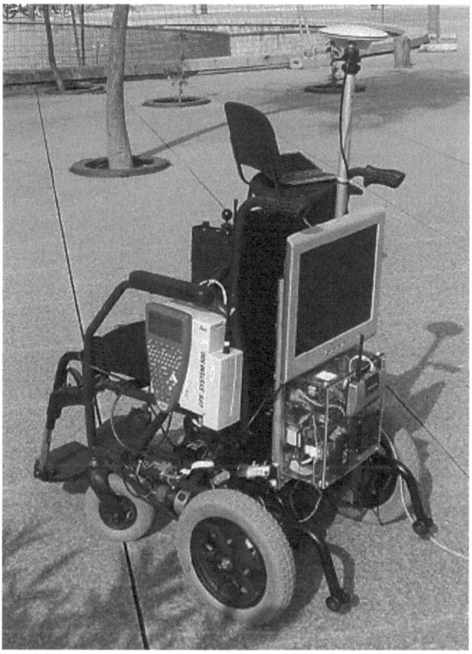

Fig. 7. The autonomous wheelchair prototype

an autonomous wheelchair prototype with shared control [72]. These tests were all designed to measure the interactions among physical and cognitive capabilities to perform this simple task with more or less assistance.

In our experiments, the wheelchairs have been tested by a group of 24 neurological and orthopedic inpatients who needed a daily use of wheelchair – 10 males (41.7%) and 14 females (58.3%); mean age 67.7 years – during a 4-week period. Exclusion criteria were patients bedridden, patients walking autonomously, presence of global aphasia, and blindness. Each subject underwent a structured clinical evaluation and assessment of cognitive, emotional, and functional abilities. This entire procedure was performed by a trained physician.

Of all the 24 persons involved in the experiment, 14 finished correctly the first test, while only 12 were able to finish the second. The third experiment, though, was successfully completed by all 24 persons.

In the first experiment, the ability to finish the test was not correlated with cognitive disabilities, as there was no significant difference at cognitive level between people reaching the end of the line and those not succeeding. The main differences between them were their functional status and their emotional state, as expected. People lacking strength or motivation failed to complete the experiment.

In the second scenario, subjects were provided with standard electric-powered wheelchair to perform the same task in another part of the garden to avoid the learning effect. In this case they had a joystick to steer the wheelchair. This experiment showed revealing facts as in this case the cognitive abilities proved to be a necessary factor to complete the task. Subjects physically able to operate a wheelchair with diminished cognitive abilities were unable to drive the wheelchair from A to B. It is interesting to note that some people who could finish the line in experiment 1 could not accomplish experiment 2, mainly those presenting cognitive disabilities. In fact, the percentage of failure amazingly increased in this second test.

In the third scenario, the agent-based electric-powered wheelchair was given to the subjects to perform the same task. This time the system performed a shared control, correcting trajectories when the users moved away from the line. Therefore all the users were able to finish the experiment without further problems. The system was able to give support subjects with cognitive or physical disabilities or suffering both. It is, however, interesting to note that when the wheelchair took control, sometimes the users tended to overcompensate motion with the joystick. This is an important factor to take into account to develop more reliable shared control strategies.

6 Conclusions

Mobility assistance is going to be of key importance in developed countries given the increasing age of the population. Research has focused on robotics-based wheelchairs, yielding sensors to assist their users. Most wheelchairs are equipped with range sensors and odometers to receive input and also with different interfaces depending on the users' condition. The control architectures of the chair tend to be hybrid: goals are calculated in a deliberative way whereas all safety mechanisms are implemented in a reactive, behavior-based way. Shared control, the most popular user/machine interaction choice, is mostly implemented in two ways: either the user chooses one or several behaviors from a predefined set (crossdoor, follow corridor, etc.) or the wheelchair takes control when a dangerous situation is detected. Some wheelchairs provide total control for users that cannot effectively drive them but can request a simple set goals via, for example, a voice recognition system. These wheelchairs work very much like an autonomous robot.

Real world experiments – real environment and real users – to probe the validity and appropriateness of assistive technologies mark a new step forward in its deploying. The use of agent technology in this field is opening new ways of interaction and creating new solutions. The ultimate goal of the interaction between robotics, agent systems, and the user is to enhance autonomy and up-grade the quality and complexity of services offered. Nevertheless, some important topics as safeness and security have to be redefined in the future in order to broaden the applicability of this approach [54, 70].

An open topic is the acceptability of this technology. Senior citizens facing some disabilities need to find easy to learn this technology as well as be confident with its usage in their preferred environment. This implies an effort to provide the appropriate infrastructure elsewhere. Also, it should be *easy* to adapt these technological solutions to different environments.

Acknowledgments

This work has been partially supported by the Spanish Ministerio de Educación y Ciencia (MEC), project No. TIN2004-07741. Case studies have been developed thanks to IRCCS Santa Lucia (Rome).

References

1. Building a society for all ages, United Nations Department of Public Information. DPI/2264, 2002
2. Ciole R. and Trusko, B. 1999. HealthCare 2020: Challenges for the Millenium, Health Management Technology: 34–38
3. L.J. Burton. A shoulder to lean on: assisted living in the US. *American Demographics*, 19: 45–51, 1997
4. E. Prassler, J. Scholz, and P. Fiorini. A robotic wheelchair for crowded public environments. *IEEE Robotics and Automation Magazine*, 8: 38–45, 2001
5. I. Volosyak, O. Kouzmitcheva, D. Ristic, and A. Gräser. Improvement of visual perceptual capabilities by feedback structures for robotic system FRIEND. *IEEE Transactions on Systems, Man and Cybernetics. Part C: Applications and Reviews*, 35(1): 66–74, 2005
6. S.D. Ivanoff and U. Sonn. Changes in the use of assistive devices among 90-year-old persons. *Aging Clinical and Experimental Research*; 17(3): 246–251, 2005
7. H. Yu, M. Spenko, and S. Dubowsky. An adaptive shared control system for an intelligent mobility aid for the elderly. *Autonomous Robots*, 15(1): 53–66, 2003
8. G. Wasson, J. Gunderson, S. Graves, and R. Felder. An assistive robotic agent for pedestrian mobility. *Proceedings of International Conference on Autonomous Agents*, 2001, pp 169–173
9. I. Shklovski, Y. Chung, and R. Adams. Robotic walker interface: designing for the elderly. *Extended Abstracts of the 2004 Conference on Human Factors and Computing Systems, Vienna, Austria*, 2004, pp 24–29
10. D.A. Norman. Design rules based on analyses of human error. *Communications of the ACM*, 26: 254–258, 1983
11. E.L. Weiner. *Human Factors of Advanced Technology (Glass Cockpit) Transport Aircraft*, NASA TR 177528, Moffett Field, CA: NASA Ames Research Center, 1989
12. World Health Organization. Fifty-fourth World Health Assembly for international use on 22 May 2001 – resolution WHA54.21
13. J.M. Guralnik and E.M. Simonsick. Physical disability in older Americans. *Journals of Gerontology*, 48: 3–10, 1993

14. G.V. Ostir, S. Volpato, J.D. Kasper, L. Ferrucci, and J.M. Guralnik. Summarizing amount of difficulty in ADLs: a refined characterization of disability. Results from the women's health and aging study. *Aging (Milano)*, 13: 465–72, 2001
15. A.R. Feinstein, B.R. Josephy, and C.K. Wells. Scientific and clinical problems in indexes of functional disability. *Annals of Internal Medicine*, 105: 413–420, 1986
16. S. Katz, A.B. Ford, R.W. Moskowitz, B.A. Jackson, and M.W. Jaffe. Studies of illness in the aged. The index of ADL: a standardized measure of biological and psychosocial function. *Journal of the American Medical Association*, 185: 914–919, 1963
17. M.P. Lawton and E.M. Brody. Assessment of older people: self-maintaining and instrumental activities of daily living. *Gerontologist*, 9: 179–186, 1969
18. T. Uhlig, A. Finset, and T.K. Kvien. Effectiveness and cost effectiveness of comprehensive rehabilitation programs. *Current Opinion in Rheumatology*, 15(2): 134–140, 2003
19. R. Baker, S. Bell, E. Baker, S. Gibson, V. Holloway, R. Pearce, Z. Dowling, P. Thomas, V. Assey, and L.A. Wareing, "A randomized controlled trial of the effects of multi-sensory stimulation for people with dementia, Br. j. clin. psychol. ISSN 0144-6657, 2001, 40(1)81–96
20. J.M. Guralnik. The evolution of research on disability in old age. *Aging Clinical and Experimental Research*, 17(3): 165–167, 2005
21. D.E. Crews. Artificial environments and an aging population: designing for age-related functional loss. *Journal of Physiological Anthropology and Applied Human Science*; 24: 103–109, 2005
22. G. Bourhis, K. Moumen, P. Pino, S. Rohmer, and A. Pruski, "Assisted navigation for a powered wheelchair. Systems Engineering in the service of humans: Proc. of the IEEE Int. Conf. on Systems, Man and Cybernetics, 1993, 17–20; 553–558
23. G. Bourhis and Y. Agostini. The VAHM robotized wheelchair: system architecture and human–machine interaction. *Journal of Intelligent Robotic Systems*, 22(1): 39–50, 1998
24. H.A. Yanco. Wheelesley: a robotic wheelchair system: indoor navigation and user interface, assistive technology and artificial intelligence. *Applications in Robotics, User Interfaces and Natural Language Processing*, Berlin Heidelberg New York: Springer, 1998, pp 256–268
25. A. Lankenau and T. Röfer. The role of shared control in service robots – the Bremen autonomous wheelchair as an example. In: T. Röfer, A. Lankenau, and R. Moratz (eds.), *Service Robotics –Applications and Safety Issues in an Emerging Market*, Workshop Notes, 2000, pp 27–31
26. A. Fattouh, M. Sahnoun, and G. Bourhis. Force feedback joystick control of a powered wheelchair: preliminary study. *Systems, Man and Cybernetics, IEEE International Conference*, 3: 2640–2645, 2004
27. J.M. Detriche and B. Lesigne. Robotic system MASTER. *Proceedings of European Conference on the Advancement of Rehabilitation Technology, Stockholm, Sweden*, 1990, pp 12–15
28. B. Shire. Microcomputer-based scanning interface for powered wheelchair. *RESNA 10th Annual Conference, San Jose, CA*, 1987, pp 541–543
29. J.L. Jaffe. A case study: the ultrasonic head controlled wheelchair and interface. *Center: Technology Transfer News*, 1(2), 1990

30. R. Simpson and S.P. Levine. NavChair: an assistive wheelchair navigation system with automatic adaptation. In: Mittal, et al. (eds.), *Assistive Technology and AI*, LNAI 1458, Berlin Heidelberg New York: Springer, 1998, pp 235–255
31. R.C. Simpson and S.P. Levine. Voice control of a powered wheelchair. *IEEE Transactions on Neural Systems and Rehabilitation Engineering*, 10(2): 122–125, 2002
32. P. Pino, P. Amoud, and E. Brangier. A more efficient man machine interface: fusion of the interacting Telethesis and smart wheelchair projects. *Proceedings of 2nd International Conference on Knowledge-Based Intelligent Electronic System*, 1998, pp 21–23
33. H.A. Yanco. Integrating robotic research: a survey of robotic wheelchair development. *AAAI Spring Symposium on Integrating Robotic Research, Stanford, CA*, 1998
34. H.P. Moravec and A.E. Elfes. High resolution maps from wide angle sonar. *Proceedings of EEE International Conference on Robotics & Automation (ICRA)*, 1985, pp 116–121
35. C. Mandel, K. Huebner, and T. Vierhuff, 2005, "Towards an autonomous wheelchair: cognitive aspects in service robotics." Proc. of TAROS 2005, pp 165–172
36. S. Diaz, C. Amaya Rodriguez, F. Diaz Del Rio, A. Civit Balcells, and D. Cagigas Muniz. TetraNauta: a intelligent wheelchair for users with very severe mobility restrictions. *Proceedings of the 2002 International Conference on Control Applications*, 2: 778–783, 2002
37. H. Wang, C.-U. Kang, T. Ishimatsu, and T. Ochiai. Auto navigation on the wheel chair. *Proceedings of Artificial Life and Robotics (AROB '96), Beppu, Japan*, 1996
38. C. Mandel, K. Huebner, and T. Vierhuff. Towards an autonomous wheelchair: cognitive aspects in service robotics. *Proceedings of Towards Autonomous Robotic Systems (TAROS 2005)*, 2005, pp 165–172
39. E. Fabrizi, G. Oriolo, S. Panzieri, and G. Ulivi. Enhanced uncertainty modeling for robot localization. In: M. Jamshidi, F. Pierrot, and M. Kamel (eds.), *Robotic and Manufacturing Systems*, Vol. 7, *Proceedings of 7th International Symposium on Robotics with Application (ISORA'98), Anchorage, AL*, USA: TSI, 1998, pp 313–320
40. J.H. Connell and P. Viola. Cooperative control of a semi-autonomous mobile robot. *Proceedings of the IEEE Conference on Robotics and Automation, Cincinnati, OH*, 1990, pp 1118–1121
41. D. Miller. Assistive robotics: an overview. In: V. Mittal, et al. (eds.), *Assistive Technology and AI*, LNAI-1458, Berlin Heidelberg New York: Springer, 1998, pp 126–136
42. R.S. Rao, K. Conn, S.H. Jung, J. Katupitiya, T. Kientz, V. Kumar, J. Ostrowski, S. Patel, and C.J. Taylor. Human robot interaction: applications to smart wheelchairs. *Proceedings of IEEE International Conference on Robotics and Automation, Washington, DC*, 2002
43. J. Borenstein and Y. Koren. The vector field histogram: a fast obstacle-avoidance for mobile robots. *IEEE Journal of Robotics and Automation*, 7(3): 278–288, 1991
44. N.L. Katevas, N.M. Sgouros, S.G. Tzafestas, G. Papakonstantinou, P. Beattie, J.M. Bishop, P. Tsanakas, and D. Koutsouris. The autonomous mobile robot SENARIO: a sensor-aided intelligent navigation system for powered wheelchairs. *IEEE Robotics and Automation Magazine*, 4(4): 60–70, 1997

45. R. Simpson and S. Levine. Development and evaluation of voice control for a smart wheelchair. *Proceedings of Annual RESNA Conference, Washington, DC*, RESNA, 1997, pp 417–419
46. J. Crisman and M. Cleary. Progress on the deictic controlled wheel-chair. In: V. Mittal, H. Yanco, J. Aronis, and R. Simpson (eds.), *Assistive Technology and Artificial Intelligence*, Berlin Heidelberg New York: Springer, 1998, pp 137–149
47. P. Nisbet, J. Craig, P. Odor, and S. Aitken. 'Smart' wheelchairs for mobility training. *Technology and Disability*, 5: 49–62, 1995
48. T. Gomi and A. Griffith. Developing intelligent wheelchairs for the handicapped. In: Mittal et al. (eds.), *Assistive Technology and AI*, LNAI 1458, Berlin Heidelberg New York: Springer, 1998, pp 150–178
49. W. Gribble, R. Browning, M. Hewett, E. Remolina, and B. Kuipers. Integrating vision and spatial reasoning for assistive navigation. *Proceedings of AAAI Workshop on Integrating Artificial Intelligence and Assistive Technology, Madison, WI*, 1998
50. B. Kuipers. The spatial semantic hierarchy. *Artificial Intelligence*, 119: 191–233, 2000
51. D. Fox, W. Burgard, and S. Thrun. The dynamic window approach to collision avoidance. *IEEE Robotics and Automation Magazine*, 4(1): 23–33, 1997
52. H. Choset and J. Burdick. Sensor-based exploration: the hierarchical generalized voronoi graph. *The International Journal of Robotics Research*, 19(2): 96–125, 2000
53. J. Fox, M. Beveridge, and D. Glasspool. Understanding intelligent agents: analysis and synthesis. *AI Communications*, 16: 139–152, 2003
54. J. Fox and S. Das. *Safe and Sound: Artificial Intelligence in Hazardous Applications*, Menlo Park/Cambridge: AAAI/MIT, 2000
55. V. Shankararaman, V. Ambrosiadou, T. Panchal, and B. Robinson. Agents in health care. In: V. Shankararaman (ed.), *Workshop on Autonomous Agents in Health Care*, New York: ACM-AAAI, ACM, 2000, pp 1–11
56. J. Vazquez-Salceda, J.A. Padget, U. Cortes, A. Lopez-Navidad, and F. Caballero. Formalizing an electronic institution for the distribution of human tissues. *Artificial Intelligence in Medicine*, 27(3): 233–258, 2003
57. L. Godo, J. Puyol-Gruart, J. Sabater, V. Torra, P. Barrufet, X. Fabregas. A multi-agent system approach for monitoring the prescription of restricted use antibiotics. *Artificial Intelligence in Medicine*, 27(3): 259–282, 2003
58. R.M. Vicari, C.D. Flores, A.M. Silvestre, L.J. Seixas, M. Ladeira, and H. Coelho. A multi-agent intelligent environment for medical knowledge. *Artificial Intelligence in Medicine*, 27(3): 335–366, 2003
59. Y. Xu, D. Sauquet, P. Degoulet, and M.C. Jaulent. Component-based mediation services for the integration of medical applications. *Artificial Intelligence in Medicine*, 27(3): 283–304, 2003
60. M.D. Beer, T. Bench-Capon, and A. Sixsmith. Using agents to deliver effective integrated community care. In: V. Shankararaman (ed.), *Workshop on Autonomous Agents in Health Care*, Barcelona: ACM Press, 2000, pp 35–45
61. DEFIE. Open architecture for a flexible and integrated environment for disabled and elderly people (http://www.rigel.li.it/rigel/progetti/DEFIE/)
62. S. Franklin and A. Graesser. Is it and agent, or just a program?: a taxonomy for autonomous agents. In: J.P. Muller, M.J. Wooldridge, and N.R. Jennings (eds.), *Intelligent Agents III – Agent Theories, Architectures, and Languages*, N. LNAI 1193, Berlin Heidelberg New York: Springer, 1996

63. S. Russell and P. Norvig. *Artificial Intelligence – A Modern Approach.* Upper Saddle River, NJ/San Jose, CA: Prentice Hall/AAAI, 1995
64. L. Steels. When are robots intelligent autonomous agents? *Journal of Robotics and Autonomous Systems*, 15: 3–9, 1995
65. G. Beavers and H. Hexmoor. Types and limits of agent autonomy. *Proceedings of International Workshop on Computational Autonomy – Potential, Risks and Solutions AAMAS03, Melbourne, Australia*, 2003, pp 1–9
66. C. Castelfranchi. Founding agent's autonomy on dependence theory. *Proceedings of ECAI'01, Berlin*, 2001, pp 353–357
67. D. Vanhooydonck, E. Demeester, M. Nuttin, and H. Van Brussel. Shared control for intelligent wheelchairs: an implicit estimation of the user intention. *Proceedings of the 1st International Workshop on Advances in Service Robotics, Bardolino, Italy*, 2003, pp 176–182
68. A. Lankenau and T. Röfer. Smart wheelchairs – state of the art in an emerging market. *Künstliche Intelligenz*, 14(4): 37–39, 2000
69. H. Hexmoor. A cognitive model of situated autonomy. In: Kowalczk, Wai Loke, Reed, and William (eds.), *Advances in Artificial Intelligence*, LNAI2112, Berlin Heidelberg New York: Springer, 2001, pp 325–334
70. U. Cortès, R. Annicchiarico, J. Vázquez-Salceda, C. Urdiales, L. Cañamero, M. López, M. Sànchez-Marrè, C. Caltagirone. Assistive technologies for the disabled and for the new generation of senior citizens: the e-Tools architecture. *AI Communications*, 16: 193–207, 2003
71. A.B. Martínez, J. Escoda, T. Benedico, U. Cortés, R. Annicchiarico, C. Barrué, and C. Caltagirone. Patient driven mobile platform to enhance conventional wheelchair, with multiagent system supervisory control. *Multi-Agent Systems and Applications IV: 4th International Central and Eastern European Conference on Multi-Agent Systems, CEEMAS 2005, Budapest, Hungary*, LNAI 3690, 2005, p. 92
72. C. Barrué, U. Cortés, R. Annicchiarico, J. Escoda, A.B. Martínez, S. Willmott, and C. Caltagirone. Testing e-Tools: real users with shared control. *Artificial Intelligence and Medicine*, 2006 (in press)

Modeling Treatment Processes Using Information Extraction*

Katharina Kaiser and Silvia Miksch

Summary. Clinical Practice Guidelines (CPGs) are important means to improve the quality of care by supporting medical staff. Modeling CPGs in a computer-interpretable form is a prerequisite for various computer applications to support their application. However, transforming guidelines in a formal guideline representation is a difficult task. Existing methods and tools demand detailed medical knowledge, knowledge about the formal representations, and a manual modeling.

In this chapter we introduce methods and tools for formalizing CPGs and we propose a methodology to reduce the human effort needed in the translation from original textual guidelines to formalized processable knowledge bases.

The idea of our methodology is to use Information Extraction methods to help in the semiautomation of guideline content formalization of treatment processes. Thereby, the human modeler will be supported by both automating parts of the modeling process and making the modeling process traceable and comprehensible.

Our methodology, called LASSIE, represents a novel method applying a stepwise procedure. The general idea is to use this method to formalize guidelines in any guideline representation language by applying both general steps (i.e., language-independent) and language-specific steps.

In order to evaluate both the methodology and the Information Extraction system, a framework was implemented and applied to several guidelines from the medical subject of otolaryngology. The framework has been applied to formalize the guidelines in the formal Asbru plan representation. Findings in the evaluation indicate that using semiautomatic, stepwise Information Extraction methods are a valuable instrument to formalize CPGs.

1 Introduction

Errors in healthcare are a leading cause of death and injury. Kohn et al. [1] mention that, for example, preventable adverse events are a leading cause of death in the United States. In their studies they state that at least 44,000 and

* This work is supported by the *Fonds zur Förderung der wissenschaftlichen Forschung – FWF* (Austrian Science Fund), grants P15467-INF and L290-N04.

K. Kaiser and S. Miksch: *Modeling Treatment Processes Using Information Extraction*, Studies in Computational Intelligence (SCI) **48**, 189–224 (2007)
www.springerlink.com

perhaps as many as 98,000 Americans die in hospitals each year as a result of medical errors.

Thus, clinical practice guidelines (CPGs) were introduced to increase the quality of care. CPGs are "systematically developed statements to assist practitioners and patient decisions about appropriate healthcare for specific circumstances" [2]. They typically address a specific health condition and provide recommendations to the physician about issues such as who and how to investigate for the problem and how to treat it.

In spite of a substantial level of interest, CPGs have failed to influence clinician behavior significantly. One main reason for this is that guidelines are initially published as textual documents, which require the clinicians to interrupt their workflow to locate, read, and process. If CPGs are embedded within clinical decision support systems (DSSs) integrated within the workflow of clinicians work habits and patient management, they may modify clinicians practices. Thus, to make physicians follow the guidelines, they have to be presented in a structured format that can be used by clinical DSSs.

Therefore, many researchers have proposed frameworks for modeling CPGs in a computer-interpretable and -executable format. Asbru, EON, GLIF, Guide, Prodigy, and PROforma are described by [3] and have been compared by [4]. These frameworks are tailored for specific classes of guidelines, specific users, and specific organizations. Each of these frameworks provides specific guideline representation languages. Most of these language are sufficiently complex that the manual formalization of CPGs is a challenging, but burdensome and time-consuming task. Existing methods and tools to support this task demand detailed medical knowledge, knowledge about the formal representations, and a manual modeling. Furthermore, formalized guideline documents mostly fall far short in terms of readability and understandability for the human domain modeler.

In Sect. 2 we describe tools and methods to model computer-interpretable CPGs. In Sect. 3 we propose our novel methodology to semiautomatically transform process information into a formal representation by a stepwise procedure. We demonstrate the applicability by transforming CPGs into the Asbru representation.

2 Modeling Computer-Interpretable Clinical Practice Guidelines

To support the formalization of CPGs into a guideline representation language various methods and tools exist, ranging from simple editors to sophisticated graphical applications as well as methods that support a step-wise modeling.

2.1 Markup-Based Tools

2.1.1 Stepper

Stepper[1] [5] is a mark-up tool for narrative guidelines. The goals of the Stepper project are to develop both a stepwise method for formalization (in this context, XML transformation) of text documents of clinical guidelines and an XML editor enhanced with features to support this method.

Stepper has been designed as a document-centric tool, which takes a guideline text as its starting point and splits the formalization process into multiple user-definable steps, each of which corresponds to an interactive XML transformation. The result of each step is an increasingly formalized version of the source document. An embedded XSLT processor carries out noninteractive transformation. Both the mark-up and the iterative transformation process are carried out by rules expressed in a new transformation language based on XML, the so-called XKBT (XML Knowledge Block Transformation). Stepper's transformation process consists of six steps:

1. *Input text format.* The format of the original guideline text is XHTML, the XML version of HTML.
2. *Coarse-grained semantic mark-up.* Basic blocks of the text are marked (e.g., headings, sentences) and parts without operation semantics are removed.
3. *Fine-grained semantic mark-up.* Complex sentences are rearranged into simpler ones and background knowledge is added. In addition, a data dictionary is created, which describes the clinical parameters involved.
4. *Universal knowledge base.* The original document is transformed into a universal knowledge base. This involves changing the structure of the document to achieve modularity, which is assumed to involve medical experts in part.
5. *Export-specific knowledge base.* The representation is adapted to ease the export to the target representation. Therefore, an export-specific knowledge base is produced from the universal one.
6. *Target computational representation.* The ultimate format is produced by the knowledge engineer. This step is assumed to be performed fully automatically using XSL style sheets.

By using the Stepper method and tool it is possible to transform CPGs into fragments of operational code (e.g., Java) or into parts of a guideline representation language (e.g., Asbru).

Stepper's main advantage is the documentation of all activities, which allows to easily review the transformation process. Stepper also provides an interface showing the interconnection between the source text and the model.

[1] http://euromise.vse.cz/stepper-en/aplikace_stepper/index.php (Accessed: Sep. 17, 2005).

2.1.2 GEM Cutter

The *GEM Cutter* [6] is a tool with the aim to facilitate the transformation of CPGs into the Guideline Elements Model (GEM) format [7], an XML-based guideline document model. The model encodes considerable information about guideline recommendations in addition to the recommendations themselves, including the reason for each recommendation, the quality of evidence that supports it, and the recommendation strength assigned by the developers.

The authoring process for GEM guidelines takes place in three steps:

1. The GEM document, which has an XML-based syntax, is created based on the original guideline using the GEM Cutter (see Fig. 1). The elements of the GEM document are then stored in a relational design database.
2. *Knowledge Customization.* meta-information is added, the guideline can be locally adapted, and abstract concepts of the guideline can be implemented. This step is guided by the *knowledge customization wizard.*
3. *Knowledge Integration* into the clinical workflow depending on local circumstances.

The GEM Cutter shows the original guideline document together with the corresponding GEM document and makes it possible to copy text from the

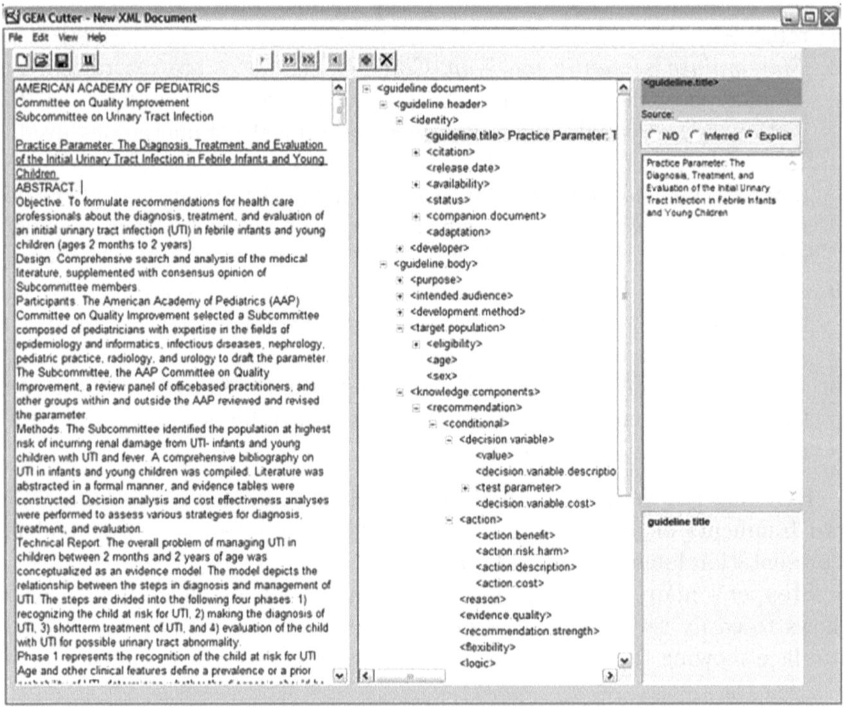

Fig. 1. GEM Cutter [8]. The left pane shows the guideline text, the middle pane shows the GEM tree segment and the right pane shows the Element Segment

guideline to the GEM document. The GEM document is displayed in tree structure format. Each item on the tree represents a GEM element, which can contain text and can be edited.

2.1.3 Document Exploration and Linking Tool/Addons (DELT/A)

DELT/A [9] provides a relatively easy way to translate free text into various (semi-)formal, XML-based representations. It achieves this by displaying both the original text and the translation, and showing the user which parts of the formal code correspond to which elements of the original text. This not only makes it easier to author plans, but also to understand the resulting constructs in terms of the original guideline.

DELT/A[2] provides two main features (1) linking between a textual guideline and its formal representation, and (2) applying design patterns in the form of macros.

DELT/A allows the definition of links between the original guideline and the target representation, which gives the user the possibility to find out where a certain value in the XML-language notation comes from. If someone wants to know the origin of a specific value in the XML file DELT/A can be used to jump to the correlating point in the text file where the value is defined and the other way round. The second feature is the usage of macros. A macro combines several XML elements, which are usually used together. Thus, using macros allows creating and extending specific XML files more easily through the usage of common design patterns.

DELT/A (see Fig. 2 for its user interface) supports the following tasks:

Authoring and augmenting guidelines. The user wants to be able to take a new guideline in plain text and create an (XML-based) representation of it, and to add links to the corresponding parts of a guideline to an already existing XML file.

Understanding the (semi-)formal representation of guidelines. For a guideline in a (semi-)formal representation, the user wants to be able to see where values in the different parts of the representation's code come from, and how parts of the original text were translated into it. This is important not just for knowledge engineers, but also for physicians, who want to get an understanding of the language.

Structuring the syntax of the (semi-)formal representation. DELT/A provides a structured list of elements of the target language – the macros – that need to be done in a way that best supports the authoring of plans. This list will also provide a good starting point for teaching material and possible subsets of the language for special purposes.

By means of these features the original text parts need not be stored as part of the target representation elements. The links clearly show the source

[2] http://ieg.ifs.tuwien.ac.at/projects/delta/ (Accessed: Sep. 9, 2005).

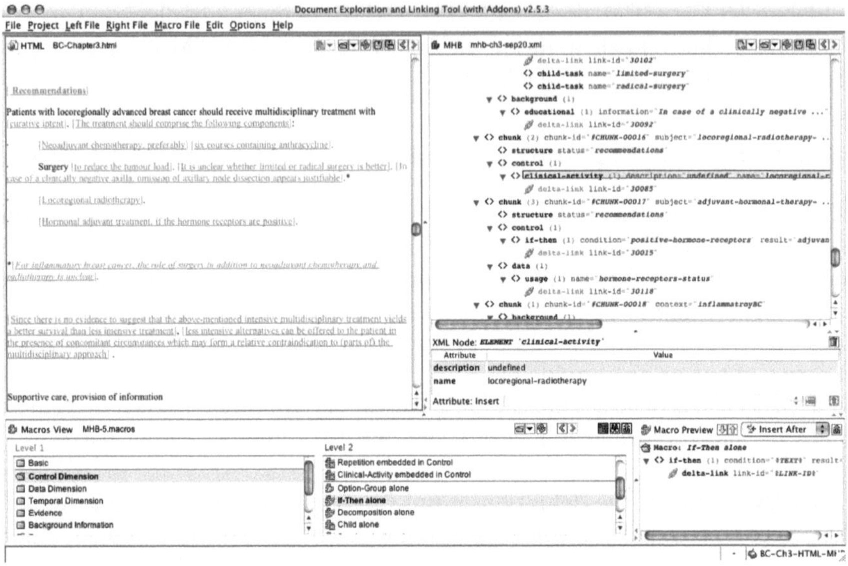

Fig. 2. Document Exploration and Linking Tool/Addons. The left pane shows a guideline document in textual format. The right pane shows a formal representation of the document. The bottom pane shows the Macros that can be used to support the formalization task by templates of several models

of each element in the target representation. Additionally, there is no need to produce a guideline in natural language from the target representation since the original text remains unaltered.

2.1.4 Uruz/Degel – Digital Electronic Guideline Library

Degel[3] [10] is a generic framework with tools to support guideline classification, semantic markup, context-sensitive search, browsing, run-time application, and retrospective quality assessment. It is applicable for any XML-based guideline representation, currently supporting Asbru and GLIF [3]. It supports the gradual migration of free text guidelines to formal representations.

Semantic markup is performed using the Uruz Web-based guideline markup-tool. It can also be used to create a guideline document de-novo (i.e., without using any source) by directly writing into the knowledge roles of a selected target ontology. The editor can modify the contents or add new content. This enables implicit knowledge to become more explicit, further facilitating the task of the knowledge engineer who fully formalizes the guideline.

[3] http://medinfo.ise.bgu.ac.il/medlab/ResearchProjects/RP_DeGeLhtm.htm (Accessed: Aug. 25, 2005).

Several features are especially tailored to Asbru, such as the plan-body wizard (PBW), which is used for defining the guideline's control structure. The PBW enables a user to decompose the actions embodied in the guideline into atomic actions and other sub-guidelines, and to define the control structure relating to them (e.g., sequential, parallel, repeated application). The PBW, used by medical experts, significantly facilitates the final formal specification by the knowledge engineer.

To be truly sharable, guidelines need to be represented in a standardized fashion. Thus, Uruz enables the user to embed in the guideline document terms originating from standard vocabularies, such as ICD-9-CM (International Classification of Diseases) for diagnosis codes, CPT-4 (Current Procedural Terminology) for procedure codes, and LOINC-3 (Logical Observation Identifiers, Names and Codes) for observations and laboratory tests.

2.2 Graphical Tools

2.2.1 AsbruView

Within the Asgaard/Asbru project a graphical user interface to Asbru [3] was developed, which supports the development of guidelines and protocols, called AsbruView[4] [11].

Asbru is a complex language, which cannot be fully understood by physicians, who have no or hardly any training in formal methods. AsbruView is a tool to make Asbru accessible to physicians, and to give any user an overview of a plan hierarchy. AsbruView is based on visual metaphors to make the underlying concepts easier to grasp. This was done because not only is the notation foreign to physicians, but also the underlying concepts. AsbruView provides four views: topological view (see Fig. 3a), temporal view (see Fig. 3b), SOPOView, and XML View.

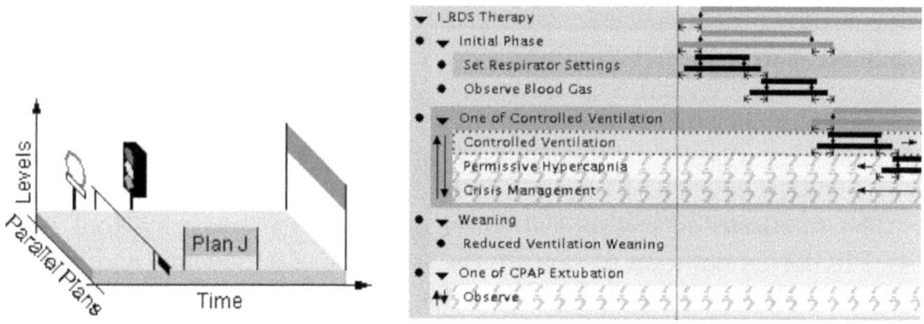

(a) Topological View **(b)** Temporal View

Fig. 3. AsbruView, (**a**) topological view, (**b**) temporal view

4 http://www.asgaard.tuwien.ac.at/tools/asbruview.html (Accessed: June 12, 2005).

The metaphors and graphical representation of AsbruView have proved to be useful in communicating Asbru's concepts to physicians. Users get a better overview of the therapy steps than from tables, while at the same time being able to see the precise temporal constraints of plans (which is not the case with flowcharts).

2.2.2 Protégé

Protégé[5] is an open source ontology development and knowledge acquisition environment [12]. It is a Java tool, which provides an extensible architecture for the creation of customized knowledge-based tools and assists users in the construction of large electronic knowledge bases. Protégé has an intuitive user interface that enables developers to create and edit domain ontologies and supports customized user-interface extensions, incorporates the Open Knowledge Base Connectivity (OKBC) knowledge model, and interacts with standard storage formats such as relational databases, XML, and RDF.

Protégé is a "meta-tool" that helps users construct domain-specific knowledge acquisition systems that application experts can use to enter and browse the content knowledge of electronic knowledge bases. It is also a knowledge-base editing tool, which supports the construction of a domain ontology, the design of customized knowledge-acquisition forms, and entering domain knowledge. Furthermore, it serves as a platform, which can be extended with graphical widgets for tables, diagrams, and animation components to access other knowledge-based systems embedded applications. Protégé is a library, which other applications can use to access and display knowledge bases.

Protégé is also used to author guidelines in various models (e.g., EON, GLIF, Prodigy, PROforma). Thereby, a part of the modeling can be accomplished using predefined graphical symbols. These symbols are arranged in a diagram and linked by graphs. See Fig. 4 for an example. The underlying data is entered by Web masks.

2.2.3 Arezzo

The first implementation of software to create, visualize, and enact PROforma [13] guidelines was *Arezzo*. It consists of three main modules (1) the Composer, (2) the Tester, and (3) the Performer (see Fig. 5).

The *Composer* is a graphical editor or knowledge authoring tool, which uses PROforma notation to capture the structure of a guideline and generate an executable specification (see Fig. 6 for an overview). The building blocks used to construct a guideline of any level of complexity are the four PROforma task types. Data items and their properties to be collected during protocol enactment are also defined using the Composer.

The *Tester* is used to test the guideline logic before deployment.

[5] http://protege.stanford.edu (Accessed: June 15, 2005).

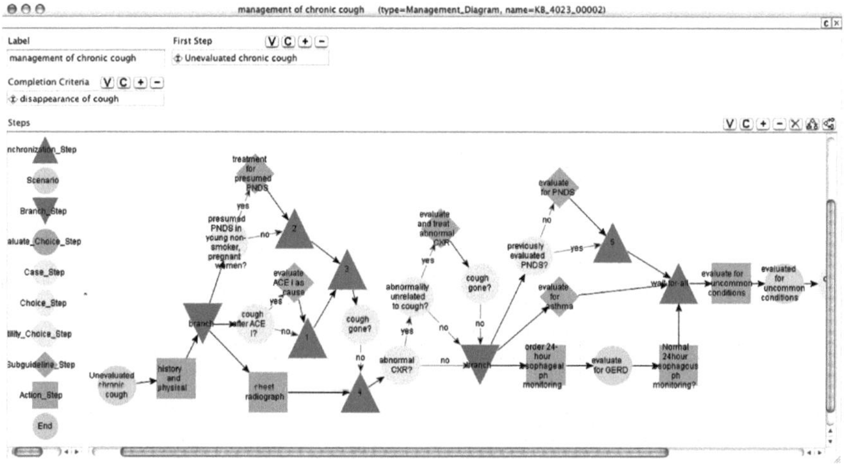

Fig. 4. View of Protégé being used to author a guideline for managing chronic cough. The guideline model being used in this application is Dharma, part of the EON framework

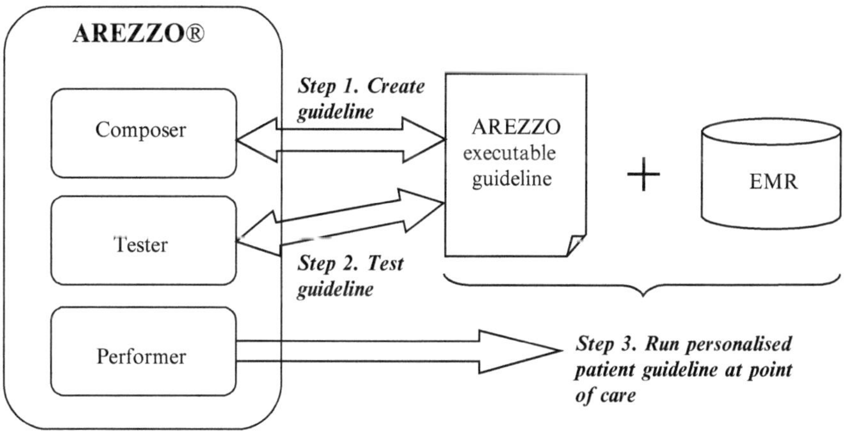

Fig. 5. Overview of the Arezzo application [14]

The *Performer* executes guidelines defined in the PROforma language. It interprets the guideline specification and during guideline enactment it prompts the user to perform actions, collect data, carry out procedures, and make decisions as required.

2.2.4 Tallis

Tallis [16] is a new Java implementation of PROforma-based authoring and execution tools developed by Cancer Research UK. It is based on a later version of the PROforma language model and consists of a Composer (to support

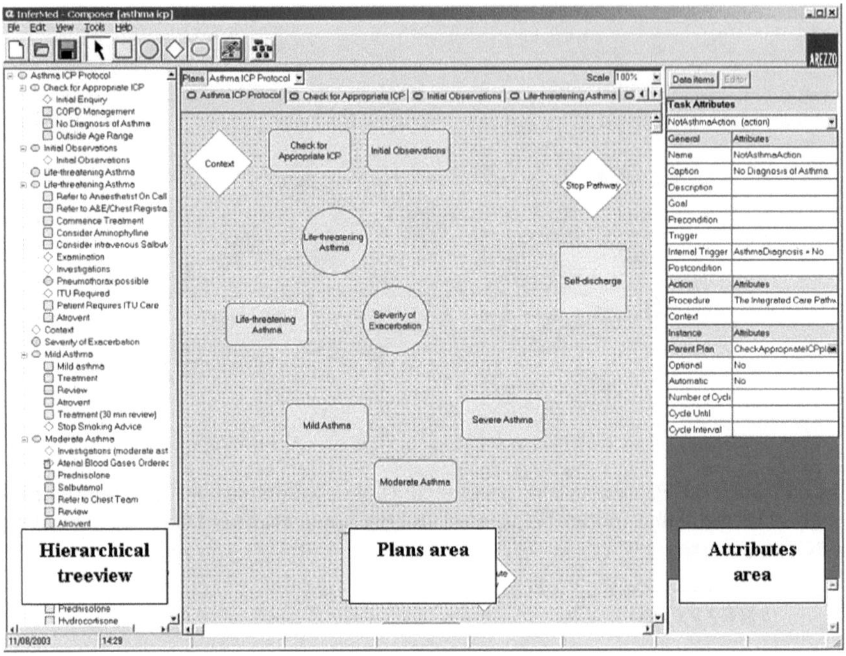

Fig. 6. AREZZO Composer [15]. The three-panel screen, with a hierarchical tree view of the guideline tasks in the left pane, task-authoring tool in the middle pane, and the attributes-authoring tool in the right pane

creation, editing, and graphical visualization of guidelines), Tester, and Engine (to enact guidelines and allow them to be manipulated by other applications). Tallis is also designed for delivering Web-based services; applications will run on any platform and integrate with other components, including third party applications. The Tallis Publisher forms part of the Tallis software suite. It has been built to allow guidelines to be published and enacted over the WWW.

2.3 Multistep Methodologies

In the course of time most of the guideline representation languages have produced a very extensive syntax. Due to this complexity the modeling process of a CPG into such a language is a very challenging task. Nowadays, researchers know the requirements to such a language and the resulting complexity. Often, they develop both a particular guideline representation language and methodologies to model guidelines together. Many of these methodologies result in a multistep approach, as a one-step or even a two-step modeling process was shown to be not sufficient to the modeler [17,18].

Some tools have already been developed to support multistep methods, such as *Stepper* [5] or the *GEM Cutter* [6]. But there are also other methodologies that were developed either together with the representation language (e.g., SAGE [19]) or afterward when it was obvious that the modeling process needed systematically structuring and adaptation for the various groups of modelers, such as knowledge engineers and physicians (e.g., MHB [18,20]).

2.3.1 SAGE – The Standards-Based Shareable Active Guideline Environment

The Standards-based Shareable Active Guideline Environment (SAGE) [19] uses standardized components that allow interoperability of guideline execution elements with standard services provided within vendor clinical information systems. It includes organization knowledge to capture workflow information and resources needed to provide decision-support in enterprise setting. It synthesizes prior guideline modeling work for encoding guideline knowledge needed to provide situation-specific decision support and to maintain linked explanatory resource information for the end-user.

The SAGE methodology for developing a guideline knowledge base consists of six main steps (cp. Fig. 7).

1. Clinicians must create clinical scenarios that are detailed enough to support integration of executable guideline content into real clinical workflow.
2. Clinicians extract the knowledge and logic needed to generate these recommendations from guideline texts, medical literature, and clinical expertise. The extraction process requires clinicians to select, interpret, augment, and operationalize guideline statements to disambiguate concepts.
3. Clinical concepts used in the extracted guideline logic are identified.
4. Concepts identified as part of the required guideline logic are instantiated as detailed data models that correspond to constraints on classes of "virtual medical record" (vMR). The vMR supports a structured data

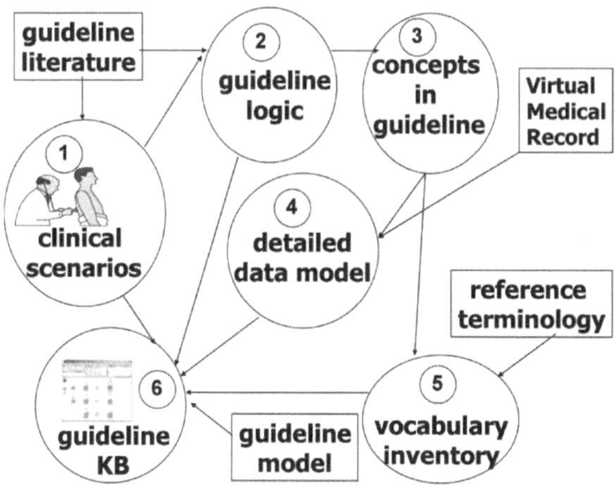

Fig. 7. Steps in modeling clinical practice guidelines for integrating into workflow. The arrows represent information flow [21]

model for representing information related to individual patients, domains for values of attributes in the data model, and queries through which guideline DSS can test the various patient states.
5. Guideline concepts in terms of standard terminologies are specified. To implement a computerized guideline in a particular institution, terms used in a guideline knowledge base to describe patient states must be mapped to terms in that institutions electronic patient record. Standard terminologies, such as SNOMED CT2[6] (the Systematized Nomenclature of Medicine Clinical Terms) and LOINC-3[7], provide the necessary shared semantics for such mappings.
6. Clinical scenarios and guideline logic are translated into a computer–interpretable model of guidelines. The SAGE methodology calls for explicit modeling of guideline usage as part of the executable guideline specification. As such, it assumes that a guideline does not dictate the workflow in a clinic, but the guideline knowledge base specifies how a DSS reacts to events in the care process.

When encoding a guideline for SAGE, clinical experts must interpret the guideline statements and create one ore more plans that will support the guideline goals in the specific work environment of their healthcare organization.

2.3.2 MHB – A Many-Headed Bridge between Guideline Formats

Transforming the original guideline text into a formal guideline representation is a difficult task requiring both the skill of a computer scientist and medical knowledge. To bridge this gap, an intermediate representation called MHB [18,20] has been designed. It is called a *Many-Headed Bridge* between informal representations such as free text and tables and more formal representations such as Asbru, GLIF, or PROforma [3].

The overall structure of an MHB file is a series of *chunks* corresponding to a certain bit of information in the natural language guideline text (i.e., a sentence, part of a sentence, more than one sentence). The information in a chunk is structured in various dimensions. MHB provides eight different dimensions:

1. *Control flow dimension.* It is used to define when to do what. Therefore, two means are offered to express this (1) *decisions* in the form of "if-then" statements and (2) *decomposition*, where a task and its subtasks are named.
2. *Data flow dimension.* It consists of the description of the data processing involved in diagnosis and treatment. It is composed of the "definition" and the "usage" of the data item.

---

[6] http://www.snomed.org (Accessed: Sept. 17, 2005).
[7] http://www.regenstrief.org/loinc/ (Accessed: Oct. 4, 2005).

3. *Temporal aspects dimension.* MHB covers the complexity of Asbru in modeling temporal aspects and is extended by more standard concepts such as average or precise duration. That means that for each start, end, and duration, the minimum, maximum, estimate, and precise value can be given.
4. *Evidence dimension.* Thereby, a "grade" is given to show the overall strength of the evidence supporting a scientific conclusion and a "level" is given for every single literature reference that this statement is built on. The level depends on the quality and the design of the study.
5. *Background information dimension.* Information about intentions, effects, relations, and so on can be stated.
6. *Resources.* The resources consumed by an action are described, such as *personal* resources, *devices*, and *financial* costs.
7. *Patient related aspects dimension.* These are other issues which see treatment from the patient perspective, such as *risk*, *patient discomfort*, and *health prospective.*
8. *Structure dimension.* Thereby, the position of the chunk within the guideline document can be stated (i.e., introduction, definition, recommendations, etc.).

MHB not only provides constructs to express the essential knowledge, but also allows for a modeling with the degree of detail necessary for further modeling purposes. When translating an MHB guideline to a guideline representation format such as Asbru, together with the original guideline text, it forms a better basis for guideline formalization than the original guideline text alone.

Experiences [18] have shown that MHB is easier to understand than, for instance, Asbru for those without computer background, although a significant effort in training was necessary. Furthermore, it is easier to create an MHB model than an Asbru model from the original guideline text and it is easier to create an Asbru model based on MHB than based on the original guideline.

3 LASSIE: Semiautomatic Modeling Using Information Extraction

In Sect. 2 we have shown various tools and methodologies to create a guideline model in a formal guideline representation language. The major drawback for all those tools and methods is that they demand for a burdensome and time-consuming manual modeling. Furthermore, they mostly lack readability/understandability once the guideline document is formalized in the representation language. If the modeling process is carried out in multiple steps, often the traceability of each step is not possible. Some languages provide no or only rudimental support to select the appropriate syntax for modeling a particular part of a guideline. Thus, we propose a new methodology that accomplishes parts of the modeling automatically and provides traceability for each modeling process step.

3.1 Our Approach

Inspired by multistep modeling methodologies, such as Stepper, SAGE, or GEM, we defined a stepwise approach, which should be applicable for various representation languages (see Fig. 8) [22]. It facilitates the formalization process by using various intermediate representations (IRs) that are obtained by stepwise procedures. The IRs are specific templates that can present the desired information. The transformation from one representation to another is applied using Information Extraction (IE) methods (see [23,24] for surveys).

IRs cover the representation of a particular piece of information (i.e., actions, processes, sequences, parameter definitions, etc.) [22]. They are XML-based documents and are constructed by refining the preceding representation. The stepwise procedure also enables the user to interact, to alter and to improve the output of each step in order to enhance the output of subsequent steps. This is necessary as the whole process of computerization, and especially the first steps of formalization, cannot be fully automated due to the content of original textual guidelines, which might be ambiguous, vague, and incomplete. Guidelines for intended users of medical personnel do not explicitly describe common knowledge required to accomplish their daily work (e.g., what is "fever" and at which blood temperature do we define "high fever"?). If guidelines have to be executed in a computer-supported way it is necessary to model this implicit information. Due to the lack of this knowledge in an explicit form, it is not possible to model this information automatically. In our

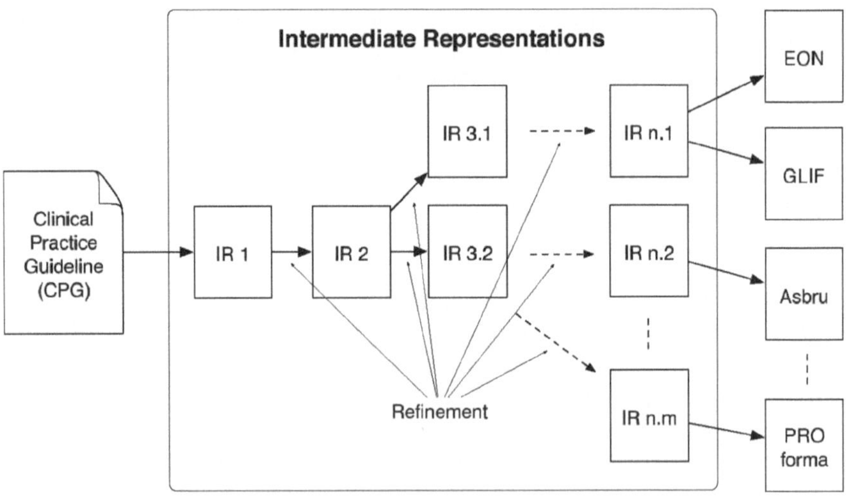

Fig. 8. Idea of the modeling approach. Starting from the guideline document at the left side the stepwise approach using IRs obtains a formalized guideline in a guideline representation language on the right side

system we are restricted to the processing of explicitly described information in the guidelines. If additional knowledge is required it has to be added by a domain expert.

To process as large a class as possible of documents and information we need specific heuristics. These are applied to a specific form of information, for instance:

Different kinds of information. Each kind of information (e.g., processes, parameters) needs specific methods for processing. By presenting only one kind of information the application of the associated method is simpler and easier to trace.

Different representations of information. We have to take into account various ways in which the information might be represented (i.e., structured, semistructured, or free text).

Different kinds of guidelines. CPGs exist for various diseases, various user groups, various purposes, various organizations, and so on, and have been developed by various guideline developers' organizations. Therefore, we can speak about different classes of CPGs that may contain similar guidelines.

Hereby, we want to emphasize that is not our intention to develop new representations for clinical guidelines. The IRs are only means in our approach to semiautomatically generate a formal representation in any guideline representation language.

3.2 The Methodology

CPGs present effective treatment processes. One challenge when authoring CPGs is the detection of individual processes and their relations and dependencies. We will demonstrate that it is possible to formalize processes using IE and present a framework for modeling guidelines in Asbru [3] as proof of concept (see Fig. 9).

Our multistep transformation methodology, called *LASSIE*[8], facilitates the formalization process by using various IRs that are obtained by stepwise procedures. LASSIE is intended to be a semiautomatic approach. This enables the user not only to correct the transformations, but also to augment them by implicit knowledge necessary for a subsequent execution.

In the remainder of this section we present the steps that extract process information from clinical guidelines using heuristic algorithms. These algorithms are based on extraction patterns whose derivation is described in this section. The output of this method is a unified format, which can be transformed into the final representation, but which is independent of the final guideline representation language. In order to create the guideline in the Asbru format we describe how the IR can be transformed into Asbru.

[8] modeLing treAtment proceSSes using Information Extraction.

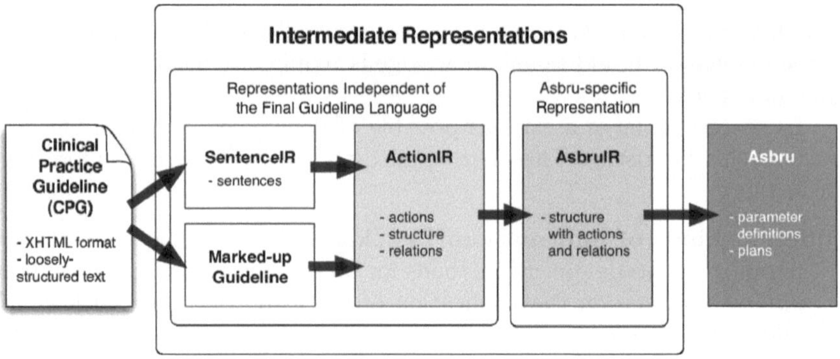

Fig. 9. Steps to (semi-)automatically gain an Asbru representation of CPGs. To gain process information from a CPG the first two steps are accomplished in order to have a representation independent of the final guideline language

3.2.1 Developing Extraction Rules

Information Extraction (IE) is an emerging Natural Language Processing (NLP) technology whose function is to process unstructured, natural language text, to locate specific pieces of information, or facts in the text, and to use these facts to fill a database [25]. Similar to IE systems are *wrappers* which aim to locate relevant information in semistructured data [26] and often do not need to apply NLP techniques due to a less grammatical structure of the information resources.

Approaches for developing IE systems. For developing both IE and wrapper systems two approaches can be applied (1) the Knowledge Engineering approach and (2) the automatic learning approach.

The former is customized manually to a given task (e.g., [27–29]). But manually generating extraction rules is a cumbersome and time-consuming task. Thus, research has been directed toward automating this task. The automatic approach takes a set of documents and outputs a set of extraction patterns by using Machine Learning techniques. Automatic learning systems can be categorized in three groups:

1. *Supervised learning systems*, where a large set of training data is required to learn the rules using Machine Learning techniques (e.g., [30–32])
2. *Semisupervised learning systems* (e.g., [33, 34])
3. *Unsupervised learning systems*, where rules are learned by a small set of seed rules and an annotated corpus using bootstrapping methods (e.g., [35, 36])

To cope with the problems of "wrapper generation" and "wrapper maintenance" rule-based methods have been especially popular in recent years. Some techniques for generating rules in the realm of text extraction are called "wrapper induction" methods. These techniques have proved to be rather successful for IE tasks in their intended domains, which are collections of documents such as Web pages generated from a template script [37–39]. However, wrapper induction methods do only extend well to documents specific to the induced rules.

In *semiautomatic* wrapper generation Machine Learning approaches are applied. Tools may support the design of the wrapper. Some approaches offer a declarative interface where the user shows the system what information to extract (e.g., [38, 39]). *Automatic* wrapper generation tools use unsupervised learning techniques. Therefore, no training sets are necessary, just a post-generation tuning (e.g., [40, 41]).

When developing an IE system one has to incorporate numerous criteria to decide which approach to apply [23]. These are the availability of training data, which counts for an automatic learning approach, or the availability of linguistic resources and knowledge engineers, where the Knowledge Engineering approach may be favored. Also the level of performance required and the stability of the final specifications are important factors which may be better fostered by the Knowledge Engineering approach.

Required extraction rules. Rules for IE are developed from a training set of documents – in our case clinical practice guidelines. For our system, we defined patterns on three levels, whereas patterns at a certain level serve as concept classes in the preceding levels (1) phrase level patterns, (2) sentence level patterns, and (3) discourse level patterns. Pattern rules were designed using the atomic approach [23]. Thereby, a domain module is built that recognizes the arguments to an event and combines them into template structures strictly on the basis of intelligent guesses rather than syntactic relationships. In doing so domain-relevant events are assumed for any recognized entities, leading to high recall, but much overgeneration, and thus low precision. Further development would result improving filters and heuristics for combining the atomic elements, improving precision.

Medical terms (i.e., drug agents, surgical procedures, and diagnostic terms) are based on a subset of the Medical Subject Headings (MeSH)[9] of the United States National Library of Medicine. We adapted them according for missing terms, different wordings, acronyms, and varying categorization.

Phrase level patterns. They are used for identifying basic entities, such as *time*, *dosage*, *iteration*, and *condition* expressions, which build the attributes of actions. They are defined by regular expressions.

Sentence level patterns. They use phrase level patterns, medical terms, and trigger words for the medical terms to identify medical actions and their attributes. The trigger words are mainly verbs and indicate the application of a therapy (e.g., the administration of a drug agent or the implementation of a surgical procedure) or the avoidance of a therapy. Sentence level

[9] http://www.nlm.nih.gov/mesh/ (Accessed: Dec. 12, 2004).

patterns are delimiter-based and use syntactic constraints. We can categorize the patterns in two groups (1) patterns for free text and (2) patterns for telegraphic text.

The former are applied to free text, which has a grammatical structure and is usually identified in paragraphs, but also in list elements. These patterns indicate that therapy instruments (i.e., agent terms and surgical procedures) combined with trigger terms (e.g., "activate," "indicate," "perform," "prescribe") appearing in the same clause identify relevant sentences. The particular clauses must not be condition clauses. Phrase level patterns, such as <`dosage`>, <`duration`>, <`condition`>, and so on can be arbitrarily combined with <`therapy instrument`> <`trigger`> pairs. But information concerning a treatment recommendation can be distributed in several sentences. These sentences including additional information (e.g., "The standard dose is 40–45 mg/kg/day.") neither contain a therapy instrument nor a trigger term, but also have to be identified by sentence patterns.

Telegraphic text patterns are applicable in list elements. In these elements often ungrammatical text is formulated. Often, only a therapy instrument indicates the relevancy of an element. Other patterns exist for list elements indicating that these elements are relevant if within their context or in the paragraph preceding the list special terms appear. These terms (i.e., "remedy," "remedies," "measure," "measures," "medication," "medications") are important, because they specify actions that may not contain therapy instruments in the form of agent terms or surgical procedures (e.g., "Maintain adequate hydration (drink 6–10 glasses of liquid a day to thin mucus)").

Discourse level patterns. They are based on *sentence level patterns*, but are augmented to consider the structure and the layout of the documents. They are used to categorize sentences, merge them to actions, and find relationships between actions to structure them. To accomplish the latter task we analyzed treatment processes contained in the guidelines and detected the following processes, whereas some of them are identified by discourse level patterns:

- Processes without temporal dependencies
- Sequential processes
- Processes containing subprocesses
- Selections of processes
- Recurring processes

3.2.2 Gaining Process Information

To extract processes from CPGs we proceed in several steps which serve as filter segments of text containing treatment instructions from the documents and to generate processes. We propose a two-step approach to gain a representation that is independent of the subsequent guideline representation language (cp. Fig. 9). The first step is to extract relevant sentences containing treatment recommendations by marking-up the original guideline document. The subsequent step is to combine several sentences to one action and to structure the actions and detect relations among them. These two steps provide a basis for the subsequent transformation of the process information into any guideline representation language.

Extracting relevant sentences. This task is a first step toward our final guideline representation. We will achieve it by two modules (1) the segmentation and filtering module and (2) the template generation module (see Fig. 10 for an overview).

This first intermediate step is especially important as not the entire content of a guideline contains processes, which are to be modeled. Although health care consists of the three stages observation, diagnosis, and therapy [42] we only want to model the control flow regarding the therapy. Only about 20% of sentences of a guideline are of interest for modeling processes. On this account it is important to select the relevant sentences for modeling.

Thus, this task performs an automatic mark-up of sentences that are utilized to process the subsequent steps.

Segmentation and filtering. Detecting relevant sentences is a challenging task, which we undertake in two steps (1) detecting irrelevant text parts to exclude them from further processing and (2) detecting relevant sentences. Irrelevant text parts (i.e., sections, paragraphs) are associated with diagnosis, symptoms, or etiology, relevant sentences describe actions of a treatment process.

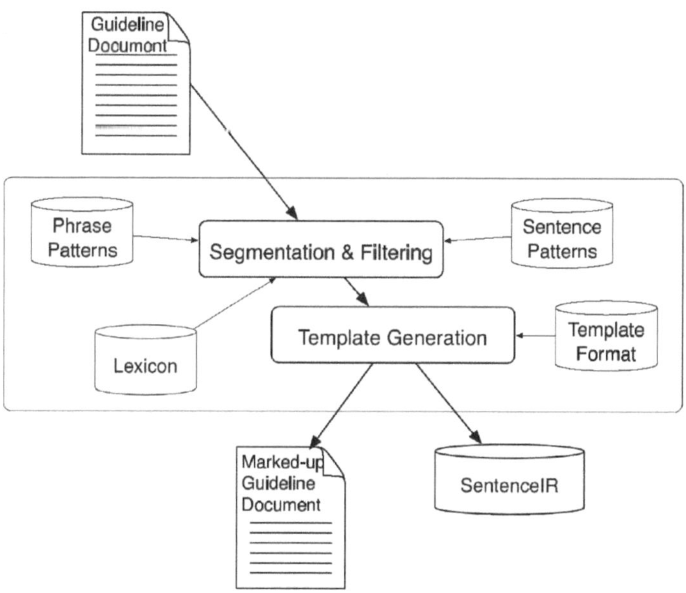

Fig. 10. Detecting relevant sentences. We split this task into two modules (1) segmentation and filtering module and (2) template generation module

The first filtering occurs at the section level. Sections in the document with captions indicating diagnosis or symptom declarations will be omitted in further processing. We can identify these captions by keywords such as "history," "diagnosis," "symptom," "clinical assessment," "risk factor," and so on.

Detecting relevant sentences is not a trivial task. First, we parse the entire document and split it into sentences. Then we process every sentence with regard to its context within the document and its group affiliation. Thereby, the context is obtained by captions (e.g., "Acute Pharyngitis Algorithm Annotations | Treatment | Recommendations:") and a group contains sentences from the same paragraph or the same list, if there are no sublists. Each sentence is then checked for relevance by applying *sentence level patterns*.

Template generation. After having collected the relevant sentences from the guideline, we can proceed with generating the IR *SentenceIR*. We generate two files: one file listing all relevant sentences and the marked-up guideline document (Listing 1.1 shows a part of a marked-up guideline document). Both are linked by applying the same id to the same sentences in order to give the user the possibility to see the *SentenceIR* representation and its corresponding textual representation using the DELT/A tool (cp. Fig. 11). The presentation of the template file and the guideline document are as simple as possible in order to support the user by detecting all relevant sentences.

Extracting required information and finding processes. The information contained in *SentenceIR* and the marked-up guideline document are the input for the next task (see Fig. 12 for an overview). Its goal is to structure

Listing 1.1. Excerpt of a source listing of the marked-up guideline document "Evidence-based clinical practice guideline for children with acute bacterial sinusitis in children 1–18 years of age" [43]. Relevant sentences are enclosed by HTML-like "a" tags

```
<li>
   <a id="delta:8">In children with risk factors for Streptococcus
      pneumoniae, it is recommended that Amoxicillin, high dose (80
      to 90 mg/kg/day) or Augmentin (with high dose amoxicillin
      component) be utilized as first-line therapy.
   </a>
   <ul type="disc">
      <li>
         <a id="delta:9">Note: Failure with amoxicillin is likely to
            be due to resistant Streptococcus pneumoniae, Haemophilus
             influenzae, or Moraxella catarrhalis.
         </a>
         <a id="delta:10">High dose amoxicillin will overcome
            Streptococcus pneumoniae resistance (changes in
            penicillin-binding proteins).
         </a>
         The clavulanic acid component of Augmentin is active
         against resistant Haemophilus influenzae and Moraxella
         catarrhalis (B-lactamase enzyme).
      </li>
   </ul>
</li>
```

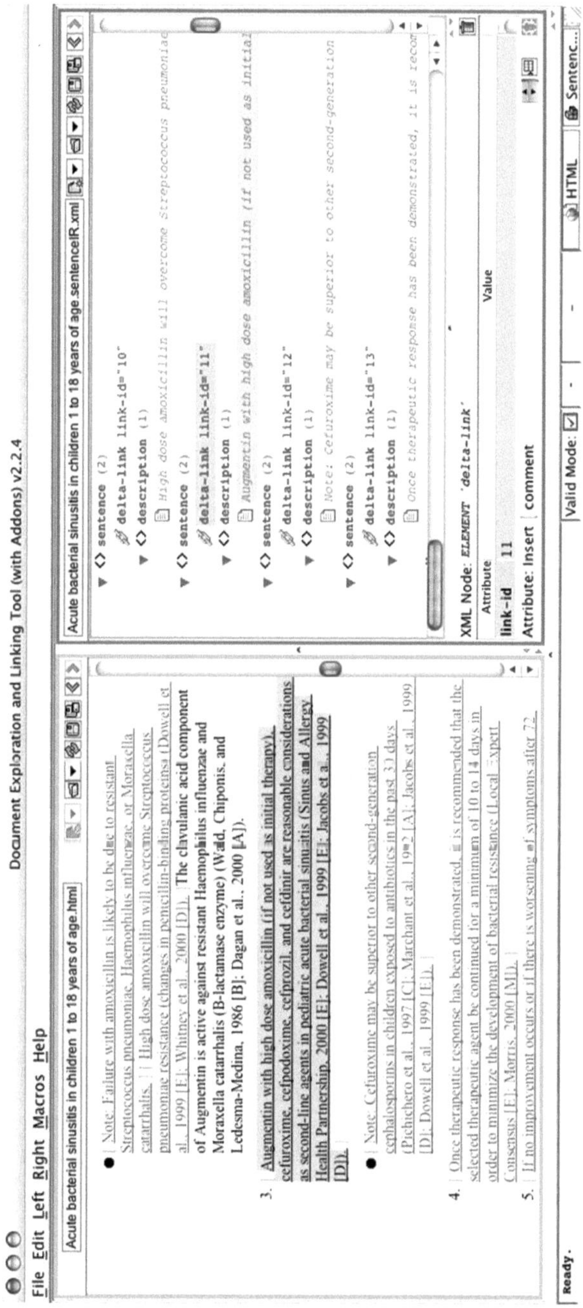

Fig. 11. The DELT/A tool showing the marked-up guideline on the left side and the *SentenceIR* file containing a list of all extracted sentences on the right side

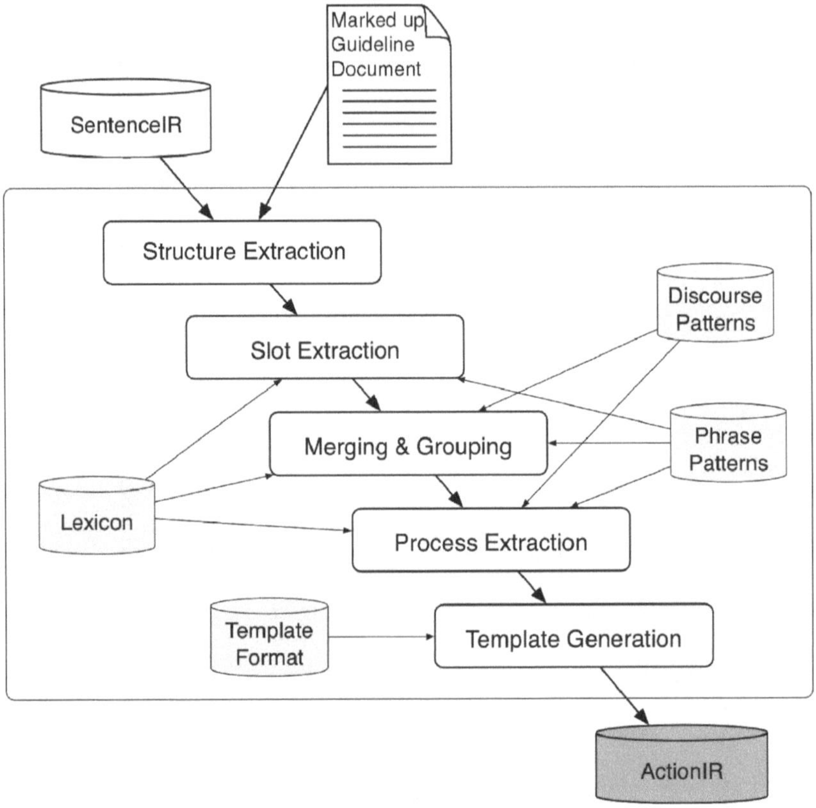

Fig. 12. Finding processes and extracting required information. We split this task into five modules (i.e., the structure extraction module, the slot extraction module, the merging and grouping module, the process extraction module, and the template generation module)

relevant sentences and find relationships between sentences. Again, the output of this task should be represented in a format that is independent of any desired guideline representation format.

Structure extraction. In this task we obtain the context of each sentence by means of hierarchical groups which is necessary for other subtasks, especially the merging and grouping and the process extraction. Every action is assigned to one group. The context of a sentence defines the affiliation to a group and is defined by the sentence's position in the hierarchical structure. We use the superior headings that establish several context items.

Slot extraction. This module is used to extract therapy instruments (i.e., agent terms and surgical procedures), dosage information in case of a drug administration, the duration of the therapy action, the iteration information of the action, as well as conditions which have to be fulfilled to perform an action. It uses both the lexicon and the *phrase level patterns.*

Merging and grouping. In this module we categorize sentences in actions or negative actions and annotations. Annotations always belong to at least one action (or negative action). They cannot exist alone. This module extensively applies *discourse level patterns.*

First, we check whether a sentence describes an action or a negative action. Negative actions are instructions that an action should not be performed, often under specific conditions (e.g., "Do not use aspirin with children and teenagers because it may increase the risk of Reyes syndrome."). Most guideline representation languages will handle such actions by inverting the condition. Languages may exist which will handle these in other ways. Therefore, we provide a representation for such actions that can be used in a general way.

Furthermore, we identify annotations and assign them to their corresponding actions or negative actions using *name-alias coreferencing* and *definite description coreferencing* based on therapy instruments and their hypernyms. We do not apply pronoun-antecedent coreference.

Process extraction. To group actions and to detect relationships between actions we use *discourse level patterns.* We will describe those used by this module later.

The default relationship among processes is that there is no synchronization in their execution. To group actions to a *selection* they must fulfill the following requirements (1) the actions have to belong to the same group, and (2) agents or surgical procedures must have the same superordinate. For instance, processes describing the administration of *Erythromycin*, *Cephalexin*, and *Clindamycin* within one group are combined in a *selection*, as all these agents are antibiotics. If actions are grouped in a selection, one of these actions has to be selected to be executed.

Furthermore, we try to detect relations between actions that are explicitly mentioned within the text as well as relations that are implicitly given by the document structure. The former is very difficult to detect, as we often cannot detect the reference of the relation within the text (e.g., "After 10–14 days of failure of first line antibiotic ..."). Nevertheless, we found heuristics that arrange actions or action groups if the reference is unambiguously extractable out of the text. These heuristics can be grouped in two categories (1) detecting sentences describing relations between actions, and (2) detecting actions that are described in the preceding heuristic. A relation is mainly identifiable by a relation term (e.g., "before," "after," "during," "while"). If such a term appears, we are searching for therapy instruments, as these describe most of our actions. After we have detected these terms, we search for actions containing the particular instruments. If we have found both the source action and the destination action we can create a new relation.

We use patterns of the document structure (e.g., "Further Treatment" appears `after` "Treatment" or "Treatment" appears `before` "Follow-Up") to detect implicitly given relations. These patterns are part of discourse level patterns to determine relations between several groups.

Template generation. The template of this IR has to contain actions as well as their relations. It has to be simple and concise and it has to illustrate from which original data the current information was built. We split the new *ActionIR* template in three parts (1) an area for actions, (2) an area for relations, and (3) an area for the structure illustrating the hierarchy and nesting of groups.

An *action* contains the action sentence, the assigned annotation sentences, treatment instruments and their MeSH ids, information about the dosage, duration, or iteration of a drug administration, and conditions. If the action is part of a selection, it is stated by the selection id. DELT/A links are inherited from the *SentenceIR* representation in order to provide the traceability of the process from both the original guideline document and the *SentenceIR* document. Listing 1.2 shows an example instance.

Relations are stated by their type (e.g., succeeding, preceding, overlapping) and the concerned actions by their DELT/A ids.

Listing 1.2. Action instance of an *ActionIR* template for the guideline "Evidence-based clinical practice guideline for children with acute bacterial sinusitis in children 1–18 years of age" [43]

```
<action id="8" parent="5" group="18" selection="0">
   <delta-link link-id="8"/>
   <description>In the child with no risk factors for
        penicillin-resistant Streptococcus pneumoniae standard dose
        amoxicillin or Augmentin (with standard dose Amoxicillin
        component) may be considered as initial therapy.
   </description>
   <agents>
      <agent MeSH="D000658" name="amoxicillin"/>
      <agent MeSH="D019980" name="Augmentin"/>
   </agents>
   <condition>
      <item>In the child with no risk factors for penicillin-resistant
           Streptococcus pneumoniae
      </item>
   </condition>
   <annotations>
      <annotation>Note: Forty-six percent of isolates at Children's
           Hospital Medical Center of Cincinnati, Ohio have
           intermediate or high Penicillin-resistant Streptococcus
           pneumoniae and local data supports that 15% of children
           locally may fail initial therapy with standard dose
           amoxicillin.
         <delta-link link-id="9"/>
      </annotation>
   </annotations>
   <context>
      <item>Antibiotic Treatment</item>
   </context>
</action>
```

3.2.3 Modeling Plans in *Asbru*

Now we wanted to verify whether the information obtained by the process extraction task is in a format that can be utilized to transform it into a computer-interpretable guideline representation. We have chosen the language Asbru [3] which was developed to embody CPGs as time-oriented skeletal plans. We process the representation *AsbruIR* to subsequently generate an *Asbru* guideline.

A step toward Asbru

In the next step we extract Asbru-specific information and integrate it in an other IR. This new format contains several actions and their temporal specifications to generate both atomic and cyclical plans in Asbru. The IR *AsbruIR* contains the following refined Asbru-specific data:

- Temporal information of durations and iterations are refined and calculated if necessary
- Conditions are refined and classified in categories (e.g., "diagnosis," "patient," "allergy") if possible
- Interval relations are modeled
- Actions and structure are merged
- Auxiliary actions are inserted

Figure 13 gives an overview of the steps required to obtain the new representation.

Slot Refinement. A lot of the information we have extracted so far is not in an Asbru-interpretable format. For instance, phrases, such as *every 4–6 weeks*, describe an iteration, but to use it in Asbru it has to be itemized in values and units. Therefore, we use phrase patterns with an Asbru-specific emphasis. In case of an iteration we also define its type (e.g., iterations defined by the frequency or by the period between two recurrences). Similarly we proceed with "duration" instances.

To better cope with various conditions we classify them into patient-, disease-, and allergy-specific conditions. Furthermore, in case of a negative action we mark each condition.

Interval relations are integrated in the particular actions by using temporal conditions. Asbru is able to cope with both incomplete and uncertain temporal information and provides a powerful means to represent intervals: the *time annotation* (see Fig. 14). Reference [44] shows in detail which possibilities are available to model such interval relations.

Action Generation. This module addresses the merging of the action section and the structure section as well as the generation of auxiliary actions.

The *structure* section of the *ActionIR* representation contains the hierarchy of the guideline document and is now filled with the particular actions.

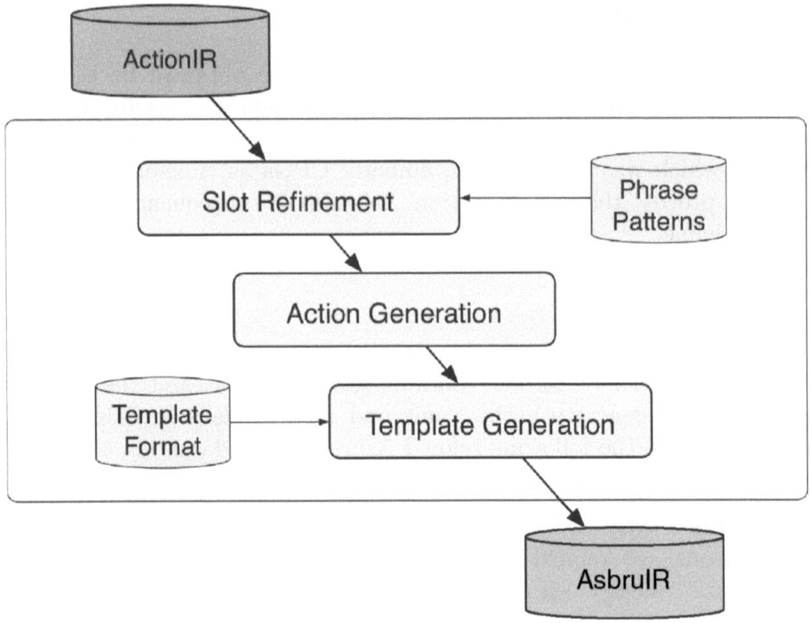

Fig. 13. Refining process information and generating auxiliary actions. We split this task into three modules (i.e., slot refinement module, action generation module, and template generation module)

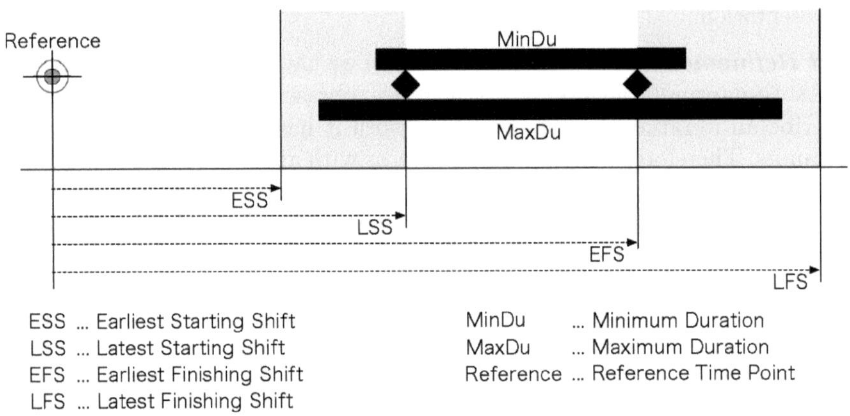

Fig. 14. Time interval in Asbru. The grey areas indicate periods when the action has to start and accordingly finish

For *select-one-of* actions we have to generate a special action which controls the choice of the particular actions. Although this kind of plan often appears in guidelines Asbru does not provide a separate modeling concept. Thus, the modeling is elaborate and we will support it in this IR. *Select-one-of* actions must have a parent action able to invoke each single action including a constraint that the parent action has to complete after the finishing of the selected action. Listing 1.3 shows an example.

Listing 1.3. Example of a parent action constituting a *select-one-of* relation for actions with plan ids "6" and "7"

```
<action id="SELECT_0" parent="5" group="16">
   <condition>
      <item type="complete-condition" plan="6" state="completed"/>
      <item type="complete-condition" plan="7" state="completed"/>
   </condition>
</action>
```

Further auxiliary actions are generated in order to represent the entire guideline hierarchy.

Template Generation. For this representation we focus on automatic processing to generate an Asbru protocol. For the human user it is difficult to get an overall outline of the guideline as actions are displayed in their hierarchical structure. Due to the refined itemization the information is not so easily readable (in the sense of understandable). Therefore, we additionally state it as string information. Listing 1.4 shows an example of an *AsbruIR* instance.

Listing 1.4. Instance of an *AsbruIR* template

```
<action id="25" parent="SELECT_1" group="18" selection="1">
   <delta-link link-id="25" />
   <description>For those allergic to amoxicillin:
        Trimethoprim-sulfamethoxazole (TMP/SMX): one double strength
        tab BID 10 days
   </description>
   <agents>
      <agent MeSH="D015662" name="Trimethoprim-sulfamethoxazole">
         <iteration term="BID" specification="CYCLICAL">
            <frequency value="12" unit="h" />
            <minimum value="2"  unit="h" />
            <maximum value="10" unit="h" />
         </iteration>
         <duration term="10 days">
            <minimum value="10" unit="d" />
            <maximum value="10" unit="d" />
         </duration>
      </agent>
   </agents>
   <condition>
      <item allergy="amoxicillin">For those allergic to amoxicillin</
           item>
   </condition>
   <annotations>
      <annotation>Trimethoprim-sulfamethoxazole (TMP/SMX) is a
           potential first-line antibiotic.
         <delta-link link-id="28" />
      </annotation>
      <annotation>Studies have shown effectiveness with 3 to 14 days.
         <delta-link link-id="32" />
      </annotation>
   </annotations>
</action>
```

Obtaining Asbru

The final step in our approach is the generation of an Asbru guideline. We accomplish this task using XSLT[10].

We therefore built several XSLT templates to transform the required Asbru segments. If these segments are combined they might represent an Asbru guideline. Starting from the IR *AsbruIR* the templates have to map the following concepts: plans and parameter definitions. For more information about the Asbru language and its modeling requirements for processes refer to [44].

Plans. They are the basic building blocks of Asbru guidelines. Our XSLT templates have to constitute several kinds of plans which arise from *AsbruIR*:

1. *Atomic plans.* This plan cannot be refined. Example: user-performed plans.
2. *Cyclical plans.* This plan iteratively calls another plan. The modeling depends on whether the iteration is frequency-based or period-based.
3. *Plans containing subplans.* Plans can be nested. Due to the hierarchical structure of guidelines this is a very frequent concept. Asbru provides the possibility to model various kinds of synchronization among the subplans. Plans contain several optional child elements. For our modeling we only use "conditions" and "plan-body."

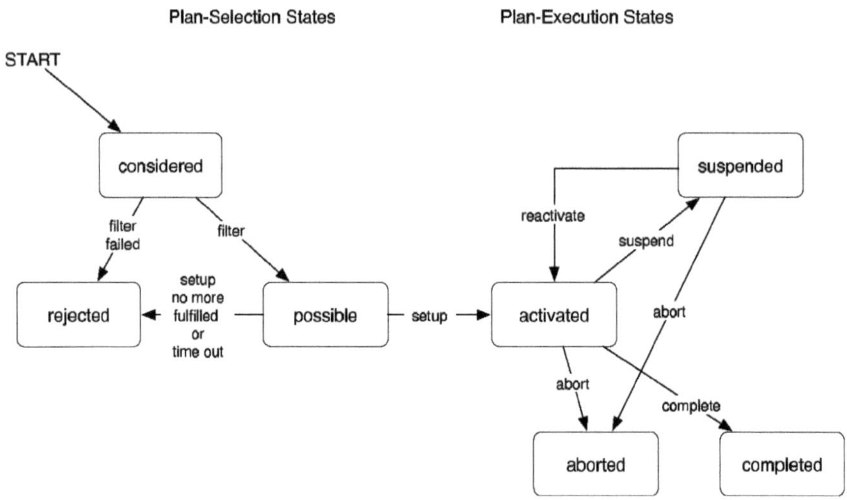

Fig. 15. Plan states and conditions in Asbru. The arrows specify the type of condition that must apply to switch from one state to another

[10] XSLT is an acronym for eXtensible Stylesheet Language (XSL) Transformation. It is an XML-based language used for the transformation of XML documents.

4. *Conditions.* They control the execution of a plan by enabling plan instances to receive a certain plan state. Figure 15 describes the conditions that must apply to switch from one state to an other. Conditions can only map temporal constraints. The concept of "conditions" as appearing in *ActionIR* is not equal to Asbru's "conditions" concept and thus has to be modeled by other concepts which appear in the "plan-body" element.
5. *Plan-body.* It contains the information about the events when executing the plan. There are several possibilities, which are all described in [45]. For our modeling we only use:
   - *Subplans.* A set of plan steps performed in parallel or sequentially.
   - *Cyclical-plan.* A plan repeated several times.
   - *Single-step.* A single step of plan execution; for instance, a plan activation.
   - *User-performed.* This plan is executed through some action by the user, which is not further modeled in the system.

Parameter definitions. In Asbru variables are referred to as parameters. Parameters may have quantitative as well as qualitative character and are defined in the "domain-defs" section. In many cases the definition of parameters has to be done manually as they often reflect implicit or tacit knowledge.

We use parameters in many condition statements. Listing 1.5 shows an example of parameter definitions for a guideline.

Listing 1.5. Parameter definitions for an Asbru guideline

```
<domain-defs>
   <domain name="Acute_pharyngitis">
      <parameter-group title="Diagnosis parameters">
         <parameter-def name="for_treatment_of_culture_
             positive_cases_of_GABS_pharyngitis" required="no" type="
             any">
            <raw-data-def mode="manual" use-as-context="no" user-text="
                Diagnosis is GABS pharyngitis?"/>
         </parameter-def>
         <parameter-def name="for_streptococcal_pharyngitis" required="
             no" type="any">
            <raw-data-def mode="manual" use-as-context="no" user-text="
                Diagnosis is streptococcal pharyngitis?"/>
         </parameter-def>
         <parameter-def name="for_strep_pharyngitis" required="no" type
             ="any">
            <raw-data-def mode="manual" use-as-context="no" user-text="
                Diagnosis is strep pharyngitis?"/>
         </parameter-def>
         <parameter-def name="for_treatment_of_ GABS_pharyngitis"
             required="no" type="any">
            <raw-data-def mode="manual" use-as-context="no" user-text="
                Diagnosis is GABS pharyngitis?"/>
         </parameter-def>
      </parameter-group>
      <parameter-group title="Allergy parameters">
         <parameter-def name="In_PCN-allergic_patients" required="no"
             type="any">
            <raw-data-def mode="manual" use-as-context="no" user-text="
                Patient is allergic to PCN?"/>
```

```
        </parameter-def>
        <parameter-def name="In_PCN-_and_erythromycin-
            allergic_patients" required="no" type="any">
          <raw-data-def mode="manual" use-as-context="no" user-text="
              Patient is allergic to PCN and erythromycin?"/>
        </parameter-def>
      </parameter-group>
    </domain>
</domain-defs>
```

Using different templates we are able to generate Asbru plans with various levels of detail. For instance, we can create plans at a very low level where an action in an *AsbruIR* representation corresponds to exactly one Asbru plan – no matter if the action contains iterative instructions or a bundle of treatment instructions. The highest level in Asbru modeling would be the itemization of iterative instructions and further subplans.

AsbruIR is a mixture between single- and multislot templates. It consists of actions, whereas one action might consist of several sentences (i.e., action sentence and several annotation sentences). But this action may consist of several (alternative) sub-actions, which is shown in the "agents" section of the template: each agent is separately presented and can therefore form a separate plan in Asbru.

Furthermore, nontemporal conditions (e.g., *In case of penicillin allergy: oral cephalexin* 750 mg x 2 *or cefadroxil* 1 g x 1.) have to be modeled by "if-then-else" statements containing subplans that are activated depending on the condition's result (see Listing 1.6).

Listing 1.6. Asbru: Plan for an **if-then-else** statement. The plan contains a subplan including an **ask** statement, where the parameter value is queried, and an **if-then-else** statement, where the value is compared to a constant. In case of match the **then-branch** gets executed

```
<plan name="PLAN_7" title="In case of penicillin allergy: oral
     cephalexin 750 mg x 2 or cefadroxil 1 g x 1 (Deeter et al., 1992;
     DARE-953519, 1999) [A].">
   <delta-link link-id="7"/>
   <plan-body>
      <subplans retry-aborted-subplans="no" type="any-order"
          wait-for-optional-subplans="no">
         <wait-for>
            <all/>
         </wait-for>
         <ask>
            <parameter-ref name="In_case_of_penicillin_allergy"/>
            <time-out>
               <now/>
            </time-out>
         </ask>
         <if-then-else>
            <simple-condition>
               <comparison type="equal">
                  <left-hand-side>
                     <parameter-ref name="In_case_of_penicillin_allergy
                         "/>
                  </left-hand-side>
                  <right-hand-side>
                     <qualitative-constant value="yes"/>
                  </right-hand-side>
```

```
                </comparison>
            </simple-condition>
            <then-branch>
                <plan-activation>
                    <plan-schema name="SELECT_PLAN_7">
                        <delta-link link-id="7"/>
                    </plan-schema>
                </plan-activation>
            </then-branch>
        </if-then-else>
      </subplans>
   </plan-body>
</plan>
```

Modeling Asbru is very tedious. But based on well structured and extensive data it is possible to create the necessary Asbru statements using sophisticated XSLT templates. Due to their size and complex syntax Asbru guidelines are not comprehensible for a human user, but they can be executed in a computer-supported way.

3.3 Results

In order to evaluate our methodology we applied a framework for translating otolaryngology guidelines into Asbru. We therefore chose evidence-based guidelines for treatment and management featuring temporal aspects of flows and divided the set of documents into a training set of six guidelines and a test set of 12 guidelines. The training set was used to adapt the extraction rules according to special characteristics of the clinical specialty. The test set was then used to evaluate both the IE part and our proposed methodology. Two persons participating the evaluation generated key target templates for the tasks for each guideline which were compared to the automatically generated output templates of LASSIE. The input data for the second and every subsequent step were the key target templates of the particular previous step. Based on this data we compiled the number of total possible correct responses (POS), the number or correct values (COR), and the number of values generated by the system (ACT). Using these values we generated the recall and precision scores, which are used to measure IE systems [46].

$$\text{recall} = \frac{\text{COR}}{\text{POS}}, \tag{1}$$

$$\text{precision} = \frac{\text{COR}}{\text{ACT}}. \tag{2}$$

Recall measures the ratio of correct information extracted from the texts against all the available information present in the text. That means, it specifies how well the system finds what you want. Precision measures the ratio of correct information that was extracted against all the information that was extracted. That means, it specifies how well the system filters what you do not want.

It is hardly possible to develop a system which delivers only correct results. Systems are often optimized with respect to one score.

Thus, we have to consider two cases for the *mark-up task*:

1. The system should detect almost all relevant sentences and probably will spuriously detect some irrelevant sentences, too.
2. The system should hardly detect irrelevant sentences as relevant and probably will ignore some relevant sentences.

Systems with an emphasis on the first case will gain a higher recall, but may concurrently derive a decreased precision. Systems with an emphasis on the second case will gain a higher precision at the expense of a decreased recall. To optimize the benefit of this task it is more important to provide almost all relevant sentences rather than reading the remaining ones, about 80%, of the guideline to detect the lacking relevant sentences. After continuous improvement we gained a recall score of 90.8% and a precision score of 94.9% which constitutes a benefit even if the recall score is less than 100%.

For the *process extraction task* overall recall and precision are 84.0% and 86.8%, respectively. Apart from the evaluation of the overall task we also analyzed the *slot extraction* and *sentence categorization and assignment* subtasks. Thereby, the optimization regarding recall and precision has to be done individually for each of the subtasks and slots, respectively. For detailed evaluation results see [44].

Furthermore, we also wanted to constitute the benefit of the process steps by the users. We measured the benefit on the basis of the effort manually modeling of adjusting the processes using the DELT/A tool. In [44] we have shown that users benefit from automating the last two transformation steps (i.e., obtaining the *AsbruIR* and *Asbru* representations) and that based on the correct representation in *ActionIR* an almost errorless transformation into *Asbru* is possible.

4 Conclusion

Modeling CPGs is a complex task which has to be assisted by both physicians and knowledge engineers. Bearing those two user groups in mind a method is demanded supporting them in their particular fields of functions: the physicians have to be less overcharged by the formal specifications and the knowledge engineers have to be fostered by providing medical knowledge. Based on this conceptual formulation and already existing methods and tools we developed a stepwise procedure for modeling treatment processes using IE – the LASSIE methodology.

Findings in our evaluation discussed in [44] indicate that using semi-automatic, step-wise IE methods are a valuable instrument to formalize CPGs. We have developed several IE and transformation rules, which we integrated in a framework and applied them to several guidelines of the specialty of otolaryngology. Thereby, we firstly generate a simple representation of treatment instructions (i.e., actions), which are independent from the final guideline representation language. Based from this independent representation we can secondly transform the information in further steps into the guideline representation languages. To proof our methodology we applied the framework to formalize guidelines in the formal *Asbru* plan representation.

Nevertheless, some problems and shortcomings of guideline modeling with LASSIE are not solved so far. Although the review of the modeling process using DELT/A is a great support, its representation and usage is unfamiliar for physicians. They have difficulties using DELT/A as most of them are not familiar with XML, the concept of macros, and any representation format that is not pure natural language text.

Anyhow, LASSIE offers distinct benefits, in particular:

- Automating of the modeling process
- Disburdening of the physicians in the modeling process by providing a medical knowledge base
- Structuring of the guideline information
- Decomposition of guidelines into parts containing various kinds of information
- Making the modeling process traceable and comprehensible
- The applicability for many guideline representation languages
- Supporting the guideline development process in order to better structure guidelines, identifying ambiguities, inconsistencies, and incompleteness

Furthermore, the methodology may also influence the application of the concept of "living guidelines," an approach to update guidelines on a more continuous basis than the usual practice of revision every two to five years. Scientific and pragmatic knowledge is growing faster every year and therefore a guideline is a static document, which cannot be modified easily. To become flexible, adaptable documents the aim is to develop guidelines, which present up-to-date and state-of-the-art knowledge to practitioners. To make this possible, guidelines have to be modular in structure, so that only part of a guideline must be adjusted and not the whole document needs revision.

References

1. Kohn L.T., Corrigan J.M., and Donaldson M.S., editors. *To Err Is Human: Building a Safer Health System.* National Academy Press, Washington, DC, 2000
2. Field M.J. and Lohr K.N., editors. *Clinical Practice Guidelines: Directions for a New Program.* National Academies Press, Institute of Medicine, Washington DC, 1990
3. de Clercq P.A., Blom J.A., Korsten H.H.M., and Hasman A. Approaches for creating computer-interpretable guidelines that facilitate decision support. *Artificial Intelligence in Medicine*, 31(1):1–27, 2004

4. Peleg M., Tu S.W., Bury J., Ciccarese P., Fox J., Greenes R.A., Hall R., Johnson P.D., Jones N., Kumar A., Miksch S., Quaglini S., Seyfang A., Shortliffe E.H., and Stefanelli M. Comparing Computer-Interpretable Guideline Models: A Case-Study Approach. *Journal of the American Medical Informatics Association (JAMIA)*, 10(1):52–68, 2003
5. Svátek V. and Růžička M. Step-by-step mark-up of medical guideline documents. *International Journal of Medical Informatics*, 70(2–3):319–335, 2003
6. Polvani K.-A., Agrawal A., Karras B., Deshpande A., and Shiffman R. *GEM Cutter Manual.* Yale Center for Medical Informatics, 2000
7. Shiffman R.N., Karras B.T., Agrawal A., Chen R., Marenco L., and Nath S. GEM: a proposal for a more comprehensive guideline document model using XML. *Journal of the American Medical Informatics Association (JAMIA)*, 7(5):488–498, 2000
8. Gem cutter: Screenshot. http://gem.med.yale.edu/GEM_Cutter/gem_cutter.htm, 2005. [retrieved: Oct. 20, 2005]
9. Votruba P., Miksch S., and Kosara R. Facilitating knowledge maintenance of clinical guidelines and protocols. In Fieschi M., Coiera E., and Li Y.-C.J., editors, *Proceedings from the Medinfo 2004 World Congress on Medical Informatics*, pp. 57–61. IOS Press, 2004
10. Shahar Y., Young O., Shalom E., Mayaffit A., Moskovitch R., Hessing A., and Galperin M. DEGEL: A hybrid, multiple-ontology framework for specification and retrieval of clinical guidelines. In Dojat M., Keravnou E., and Barahona P., editors, *Proceedings of the 9th Conference on Artificial Intelligence in Medicine in Europe, AIME 2003*, volume 2780 of *LNAI*, pp. 122–131, Protaras, Cyprus, Springer, Berlin Heidelberg New York, 2003
11. Kosara R. and Miksch S. Metaphors of movement: a visualization and user interface for time-oriented, skeletal plans. *Artificial Intelligence in Medicine, Special Issue: Information Visualization in Medicine*, 22(2):111–131, 2001
12. Gennari J.H., Musen M.A., Fergerson R.W., Grosso W.E., Crubézy M., Eriksson H., Noy N.F., and Tu S.W. The evolution of protégé: an environment for knowledge-based systems development. *International Journal of Human Computer Studies*, 58(1):89–123, 2003
13. Sutton D.R. and Fox J. The syntax and semantics of the PRO*forma* guideline modeling language. *Journal of the American Medical Informatics Association (JAMIA)*, 10(5):433–443, 2003
14. Arezzo overview. http://www.infermed.com/arezzo/arezzo-components/, 2006. [retrieved: March 22, 2006]
15. Arezzo composer. http://www.infermed.com/arezzo/arezzo-create-guideline/, 2006. [retrieved: March 22, 2006]
16. R. Steele and Fox J. Tallis PROforma primer – introduction to PROforma language and software with worked examples. Technical report, Advanced Computation Laboratory, Cancer Research, London, UK, 2002
17. Balser M., Coltell O., van Croonenborg J., Duelli C., van Harmelen F., Jovell A., Lucas P., Marcos M., Miksch S., Reif W., Rosenbrand K., Seyfang A., and ten Teije A. Protocure: Integrating formal methods in the development process of medical guidelines and protocols. In Kaiser K., Mikschc S., and Tu S.W., editors, *Computer-based Support for Clinical Guidelines and Protocols. Proceedings of the Symposium on Computerized Guidelines and Protocols (CGP 2004)*, volume 101 of *Studies in Health Technology and Informatics*, pp. 103–107, Prague, Czech Republic, IOS Press, 2004

18. Seyfang A., Miksch S., Polo-Conde C., Wittenberg J., Marcos M., and Rosenbrand K. MHB - a many-headed bridge between informal and formal guideline representations. In *Proceedings of the 10th Conference on Artificial Intelligence in Medicine in Europe, AIME 2005*, volume 3581 of *LNAI*, pp. 146–150, Aberdeen, UK, Springer, Berlin Heidelberg New York, 2005
19. Campbell J.R., Tu S.W., Mansfield J.G., Boyer J.I., McClay J., Parker C., Ram P., Scheitel S.M., and McDonald K. The SAGE guideline model: A knowledge representation framework for encoding interoperable clinical practice guidelines. In *Proceedings of the AMIA Annual Symposium*, November 2003
20. Seyfang A., Miksch S., Marcos M., Wittenberg J., Polo-Conde C., and Rosenbrand K. Bridging the gap between informal and formal guideline representations. In *European Conference on Artificial Intelligence (ECAI-2006)*, 2006, forthcoming
21. Tu S.W., Musen M.A., Shankar R., Campbell J., Hrabak K., McClay J., Huff S.M., McClure R., Parker C., Rocha R., Abarbanel R., Beard N., Glasgow J., Mansfield G., Ram P., Ye Q., Mays E., Weida T., Chute C.G., McDonald K., Mohr D., Nyman M.A., Scheital S., Solbrig H., Zill D.A., and Goldstein M.K. Modeling guidelines for integration into clinical workflow. In Fieschi M., Coiera E., and Li Y.-C.J., editors, *Proceedings from the Medinfo 2004 World Congress on Medical Informatics*, pp. 174–178. IOS Press, 2004
22. Kaiser K., Akkaya C., and Miksch S. How can information extraction ease formalizing treatment processes in clinical practice guidelines? A method and its evaluation. *Artificial Intelligence in Medicine*, 2006 doi:10.1016/j.artmed.2006.07.011
23. Appelt D.E. Introduction to information extraction. *AI Communications*, 12:161–172, 1999
24. Cowie J. and Lehnert W. Information extraction. *Communications of the ACM*, 39(1):80–91, 1996
25. Yangarber R. *Scenario Customization for Information Extraction*. PhD thesis, New York University, New York, January 2001
26. Kushmerick N., Weld D.S., and Doorenbos R.B. Wrapper induction for information extraction. In *International Joint Conference on Artificial Intelligence*, Nagoya, 1997
27. Hobbs J.R., Appelt D., Tyson M., Bear J., and Islael D. SRI international: description of the FASTUS system used for MUC-4. In *Proceedings of the 4th Message Understanding Conference (MUC-4)*, pp. 268–275, 1992
28. Ayuso D., Boisen S., Fox H., Gish H., Ingria R., and Weischedel R. BBN: Description of the PLUM system as used for MUC-4. In *Proceedings of the Fourth Message Understanding Conference (MUC-4)*, pp. 169–176, 1992
29. Yangarber R. and Grishman R. NYU: Description of the Proteus/PET system as used for MUC-7 ST. In *Proceedings of the 7th Message Understanding Conference: MUC-7*, Washington, DC, 1998
30. Riloff E. Automatically constructing a dictionary for information extraction tasks. In *Proceedings of the National Conference on Artificial Intelligence (AAAI)*, pp. 811–816, 1993
31. Soderland S. Learning information extraction rules for semi-structured and free text. *Machine Learning*, 34(1–3):233–272, 1999
32. Cunningham H., Maynard D., Bontcheva K., and Tablan V. GATE: A framework and graphical development environment for robust NLP tools and

applications. In *Proceedings of the 40th Anniversary Meeting of the Association for Computational Linguistics (ACL'02)*, Philadelphia, July 2002
33. Riloff E. and Jones R. Learning dictionaries for information extraction by multi-level bootstrapping. In *Proceedings of the National Conference on Artificial Intelligence (AAAI)*, pp. 474–479. AAAI/MIT, 1999
34. Agichtein E. and Gravano L. Snowball: extracting relations from large plaintext collections. In *Proceedings of the 5th ACM International Conference on Digital Libraries*, 2000
35. Riloff E. An empirical study of automated dictionary construction for information extraction in three domains. *Artificial Intelligence*, 85(1–2):101–134, 1996
36. Yangarber R., Grishman R., Tapanainen P., and Huttunen S. Automatic acquisition of domain knowledge for information extraction. In *Proceedings of the 18th International Conference on Computational Linguistics (COLING 2000)*, Saarbrücken, Germany, August 2000
37. Muslea I., Minton S., and Knoblock C. A hierarchical approach to wrapper induction. In Etzioni O., Müller J.P., and Bradshaw J.M., editors, *Proceedings of the International Conference on Autonomous Agents*, pp. 190–197, Seattle, WA, USA, ACM, 1999
38. Kushmerick N. Wrapper induction: efficiency and expressiveness. *Artificial Intelligence*, 118(1–2):15–68, 2000
39. Baumgartner R., Flesca S., and Gottlob G. Visual Web information extraction with lixto. In *Proceedings of the Conference on Very Large Databases (VLDB)*, 2001
40. Doorenbos R.B., Etzioni O., and Weld D.S. A scalable comparison-shopping agent for the world-wide web. In Johnson W.L. and Hayes-Roth B., editors, *Proceedings of the International Conference on Autonomous Agents*, pp. 39–48, Marina del Rey, CA, USA, ACM, 1997
41. Crescenzi V., Mecca G., and Merialdo P. Roadrunner: towards automatic data extraction from large web sites. In *Proceedings of the Conference on Very Large Databases (VLDB)*, pp. 109–118, 2001
42. Van Bemmel J.H. and Musen M.A., editors. *Handbook of Medical Informatics*. Springer, Berlin Heidelberg New York, 1997
43. Cincinnati Children's Hospital Medical Center. Evidence based clinical practice guideline for children with acute bacterial sinusitis in children 1 to 18 years of age. Cincinnati Children's Hospital Medical Center, Cincinnati, OH, 2001
44. Kaiser K. *LASSIE – Modeling Treatment Processes Using Information Extraction*. PhD thesis, Institute of Software Technology & Interactive Systems, Vienna University of Technology, 2005
45. Seyfang A., Kosara R., and Miksch S. Asbru 7.3 Reference Manual. Technical Report Asgaard-TR-2002-1, Institute of Software Technology & Interactive Systems, Vienna University of Technology, Vienna, Austria, Europe, 2002
46. Lehnert W., Cardie C., Fisher D., McCarthy J., Riloff E., and Soderland S. Evaluating an information extraction system. *Journal of Integrated Computer-Aided Engineering*, 1(6), 1994

Introduction to Neonatal Facial Pain Detection Using Common and Advanced Face Classification Techniques

Sheryl Brahnam, Loris Nanni, and Randall Sexton

Summary. Assessing pain in neonates is a challenging problem. Neonates cannot describe their pain experiences but must rely exclusively on the judgments of others. Studies demonstrate, however, that proper diagnosis of pain is impeded by observer bias. It has therefore been recommended that neonatal pain assessment instruments include evaluations that have bypassed an observer. In this article, we describe the Infant COPE project and our work using face classification to detect pain in a neonate's facial displays. We begin by providing an introduction to face classification that includes an outline of some common and advanced algorithms. We then describe a small database we designed specifically to investigate classifier performance in this problem domain. This is followed by a summary of the experiments we have performed to date, including some preliminary results of current work. We believe these results indicate that the application of face classification to the problem of neonatal pain assessment is a promising area of investigation.

1 Introduction

Pain is an important indicator of medical conditions. It is also the source of suffering. Health professionals are responsible for diagnosing pain, determining when pain intervention is necessary, and developing treatment plans [1]. To accomplish these tasks, health professionals employ a variety of assessment tools for evaluating patient self-reports. In the case of preverbal children, methods have been devised to help them communicate their pain experiences. These children can indicate their pain levels, for example, by pointing to drawings of faces that express increasing levels of discomfort [2]. Neonatal pain assessment, in contrast, depends exclusively on the judgment of others. A growing body of evidence suggests that failing to diagnose and alleviate pain in newborns can have devastating and long-term effects [3]. Developing accurate pain assessment instruments for neonates is thus inherently problematical and yet most crucial.

S. Brahnam et al.: *Introduction to Neonatal Facial Pain Detection Using Common and Advanced Face Classification Techniques*, Studies in Computational Intelligence (SCI) **48**, 225–253 (2007)
www.springerlink.com

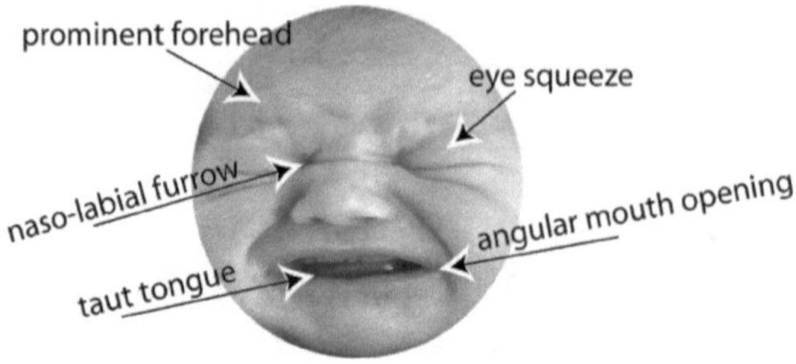

Fig. 1. Characteristics of neonatal facial displays of pain

To diagnose pain in neonates, health professionals draw on physiological and behavioral information. Among the many physiological indicators of pain are changes in heart and respiratory rates, blood pressure, vagal tone, and palmar sweating [4]. Inferring neonatal states from physiological measures is difficult, however. The physiological parameters associated with pain are often indistinguishable from those produced by other stressful events [5], and physiological responses can vary widely from newborn to newborn [6].

Significant behavioral indicators of pain include gross body movement, crying, and facial expressions [6]. The gold standard in infant pain assessment is the face. Facial responses to pain are more specific and consistent than other known behavioral and physiological responses [7]. For this reason, the majority of pain assessment instruments developed for newborns incorporate observations of facial activity. Figure 1 illustrates some of the patterns – prominent forehead, eye squeeze, naso-labial furrow, taut tongue, and an angular opening of the mouth – that characterize neonatal pain displays [8].

Even though facial activity is easier to decipher then physiological measures and other behavioral indicators such as crying, instruments that have relied on facial information have proven unsatisfactory primarily because of problems with observer bias [9]. Bias is defined as the tendency for a person to alter responses to a stimulus over time and when the parameters of the situation change [10]. Several factors influence an observer's propensity toward bias. Some of these include the personality of the observer, perception of the measure, the context, and desensitization due to repeated exposure to patient suffering [1,11].

One way to reduce bias is to incorporate evaluations that have not been made by an observer. Several researchers have begun investigating machine assessment of common pain indicators. Lindh et al. [12], for instance, have reported some success detecting pain as it relates to heart rate variability, and Petroni et al. [13] have trained neural networks to discriminate differences in neonatal cries, including a cry in response to pain. Developing classification systems using these pain indicators, however, has limited practicality. Given the robust population of most neonatal units, implementing systems that distinguish different types of cries for individual neonates would be difficult to accomplish, and monitoring physiological measures would probably require tethering neonates to ungainly sensors. A more practical approach is to utilize the gold standard and develop machine vision systems that unobtrusively scan a neonate's face for signals of pain.

This article describes the Infant COPE (Classification Of Pain Expressions) project [14, 15]. A short-term goal of this project is to investigate the feasibility of using holistic face recognition techniques to detect pain signals in newborn facial displays. The long-term goal is to develop working systems that can be implemented in neonatal units.

Face recognition is a vital area of research in computer vision, neuroscience, and psychology. Development has been fueled by government security interests, algorithmic developments, and the availability of large databases of faces for comparative studies [16]. Application areas where face recognition technology has been successfully employed include biometrics, information security, law enforcement, surveillance, and access control.

Most of these application areas involve the identification of people. However, since gender, age, and race are closely tied to identification, these facial characteristics have been the focus of many investigations [17–19]. Another area of research, especially relevant to the neonatal pain detection problem, is face expression classification. This has important uses in human computer interaction and security.

Applying face classification to a medical task is a new area of research. Golomb and Sejnowski [20] have noted a number of areas where it could be beneficial. However, aside from our own research, we are aware of only one other study that has applied face classification to an actual medical problem, and that is the work of Gunaratne and Sato [21]. They successfully used a mesh-based approach to estimate asymmetries in facial actions to determine the presence of facial motion dysfunction for patients with Bell's palsy.

In most application areas, holistic algorithms are preferred because they are easy to implement and have been shown to outperform other methods [22]. In addition, they allow the classifier to determine the best set of features to use. However, holistic algorithms suffer from what is commonly referred to as the *curse of dimensionality*. The pixel values of image files contain a very small number relevant to the classification problem. Processing large numbers of insignificant values greatly increases computational complexity and degrades classification performance. For this reason, most holistic classification systems apply various methods to reduce dimensionality. In Sect. 2, we describe several common and advanced holistic face recognition algorithms as well as several feature reduction techniques.

We spend the remainder of the article discussing our work. In Sect. 3, we describe the first Infant COPE database and study design. This database contains 204 images of 26 neonates between the ages of 18 h and 3 days. The neonates were photographed while experiencing a variety of stress-inducing stimuli, including the pain of a heel lance. Special care was taken in the design of the database to produce a set of images that would be challenging to classify.

In Sect. 4, we present a description of the methods used in our classification experiments, including the development of two evaluation protocols, designated A and B. In protocol A, we assume sample facial displays of new subjects are available for classifier relearning. Protocol B, which is more rigorous, assumes the classifier must work out-of-the-box on a set of unknown infants.

In Sect. 4, we review the classification experiments we have performed thus far using the Infant COPE database. This section includes a few unpublished reports of current work as well as a survey of published work. In our experiments, we have obtained classification scores of 100% accuracy using protocol A and 95.38% accuracy using protocol B. We believe these results indicate that the application of face classification to the problem of neonatal pain assessment is a promising area of investigation.

We conclude the article in Sect. 6 by discussing plans for future work on the Infant COPE project. We also mention extending our face classification research to include other patients who have difficulty articulating their pain experiences.

2 Holistic Face Classification

> *As the language of the face is universal, so it is very comprehensive. It is the shorthand of the mind, and crowds a great deal in a little room.*
>
> Jeremy Collier

The face, as the English bishop Jeremy Collier (1650–1726) noted, does indeed crowd a great deal of information into a very small space. A face can reveal the age, sex, emotional state, current focus of attention, and, to some degree, the medical condition of a person. It forms impressions, whether grounded in fact or not, regarding a person's character, and these may significantly influence the behavior of others. It is the center of oral communication, is highly plastic and expressive, and plays a vital role in the development of human relations and the self. That the face is able to convey such a wealth of information is all the more astonishing given the remarkable similarity between faces. Much of the visual information contained within a face is highly redundant. What varies is but a small set of relationships between features and slight differences in textures, complexions, and shapes.

Given this high redundancy, it is no wonder that isolating the *essential features* that provide the keys to understanding faces within a particular problem domain has proven a difficult task. One method of representing faces is to measure the relative distances between important facial key points: eye corners, mouth corners, nose tip, and chin edge. Although this approach has the advantage of drastically reducing the number of features to be considered, a major drawback has been the difficulty in determining a priori the best set of key points to measure [23, 24].

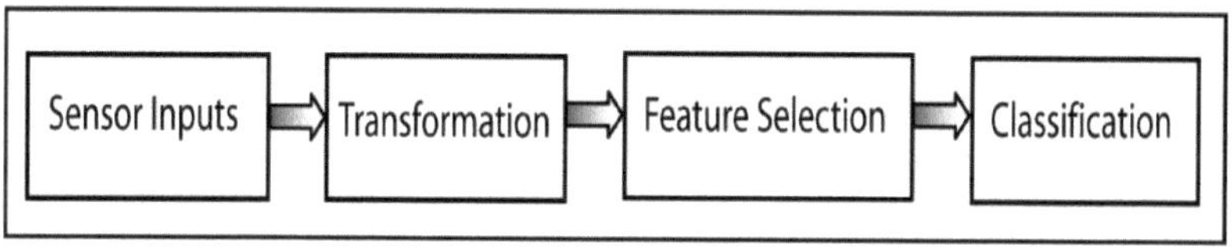

Fig. 2. General schematic of holistic face classification systems

An alternative approach is to process faces holistically [25]. Holistic techniques discover the relevant features a posteriori from raw sensor inputs (image pixels, for example) and have been shown to outperform classification systems that rely on facial key points [22]. In holistic systems, face images are represented as single points in a high dimensional vector space. Processing vectors in such a space is usually computationally complex. To contend with the curse of dimensionality, the original feature space, as shown in Fig. 2, is generally transformed and relevant variables selected.

Transformation can occur within the spatial domain using statistical methods such as principal component analysis (PCA) and linear discriminant analysis (LDA) or within the frequency domain using such methods as the discrete Fourier transform, Gabor wavelet transform, and discrete cosine transform (DCT). The basic principle of a transform is to take N sensor inputs and arrive at another set of N rotated values. Although the two sets of values carry the same amount of energy and information, the transforms tend to decorrelate the features and redistribute most of the energy contained in the raw input into a smaller number of components, thus allowing for *feature extraction.*

To reduce the feature set further, feature subsets can be constructed using a search strategy and a *feature selection* function (e.g., the minimum error of the classifier). As an exhaustive search is usually computationally infeasible, other heuristic techniques have been developed to circumvent this problem. These include branch and bound [26] and suboptimal search methods such as sequential forward selection (SFS) [27] and sequential forward floating selection (SFFS) [28]. The advantages of selecting a subset of salient features include decreasing processing time, reducing noise, and increasing classifier generalization and accuracy [29–31]. For an overview of feature selection methods, see [32, 33].

In the classification stage, numerous methods, most significantly nearest neighbor, neural networks, and support vector machines (SVMs), have been applied to a number of face classification problems. A naive nearest neighbor classifier is usually employed in all techniques that adopt dimensionality reduction as a method for classification, as with, for instance, PCA and LDA. Classification in this case involves projecting an unknown face vector onto the transformed face space and measuring its distance from representative face classes within the same space. PCA seeks a projection that best represents the data, and LDA seeks a projection that best separates the data. PCA and

LDA have successfully been used to classify faces according to identity [34–36], gender [19, 37, 38], age [24], race [18, 39], and facial expression [40–42].

Neural networks have been employed in many face classification problems: gender classification [43], face recognition [44], and classification of facial expressions [42]. Kohonen [45] was one of the first to use a linear autoassociative neural network to store and recall face images. Autoassociative neural networks associate input patterns with themselves [46]. It is interesting to note that a linear autoassociative neural network is equivalent to PCA [47].

Early surveys of neural network face classification techniques can be found in [48] and [24]. Two of the most promising are the probabilistic decision-based neural network (PDBNN) [49] and the neural network simultaneous optimization algorithm (NNSOA) [50]. PDBNN is a classification neural network with a hierarchical modular structure. The network consists of one subnet representing the face class. Training is performed with DBNN learning rules, where the teacher provides the network with the correctness of the classification but with no exact target values, and locally unsupervised globally supervised (LUGS) learning is applied. The subnet is trained with an unsupervised training algorithm. The global training is performed to fine-tune decision boundaries by employing reinforced or antireinforced learning when a pattern in the training set is misclassified.

NNSOA uses a modified genetic algorithm to search for a parsimonious network and for a global solution in a supervised multilayer feedforward neural network [50]. This algorithm has been shown to be successful in finding solutions that generalized well for real-world examples [50–52]. In terms of face classification, NNSOA has only been applied to the neonatal pain display detection problem [53]. However, it has successfully tackled a number of medical classification tasks, including diagnosing breast lumps, diabetes and predicting heart disease [54].

SVM is a powerful binary classifier. It determines a decision boundary in the feature space by constructing the optimal separating hyperplane (OSH) that distinguishes the classes. Using SVMs to classify faces is a recent development [55–57], yet SVMs have already established a proven track record [16, 48, 57]. They typically outperform PCA and LDA [55, 56, 58] and provide performance comparable to neural networks. Of particular interest to this study are the experiments of [56], where SVMs outperformed human test subjects given the same face classification task.

Readers wanting a more comprehensive survey of face classification techniques should refer to [16]. DCT is described below in Sect. 2.1. The feature selection algorithms SFS and SFFS are outlined in Sect. 2.2. PCA, LDA, SVM, and NNSOA, the four classifiers we have experimented with using the initial Infant COPE database, are described in detail in Sects. 2.3–2.6. We conclude this introduction to face classification in Sect. 2.7 by listing software that implements many of the algorithms discussed in this section.

2.1 Discrete Cosine Transform

The DCT, developed by Ahmed et al. [59], is closely related to the discrete Fourier transform in that it transforms signals, or images, from the spatial domain to the frequency domain by means of sinusoidal basis functions, with the difference that DCT adopts only real sinusoidal functions. It is a linear separable transformation. The two-dimensional DCT transform is equivalent to a one-dimensional DCT performed along a single dimension followed by a one-dimensional DCT in the other dimension.

Compared to other input independent transforms, DCT has the advantage of packing the most useful information into the fewest coefficients, introducing only a small error in the reconstructed images. In addition, DCT algorithms are usually more efficient than other transforms. In particular, the DCT transform offers numerous advantages over PCA, including producing good quality images at suitable compression ratios and the ability to perform in real time situations due to its computational efficiency. Also, in contrast to the PCA transform, which determines the most representative eigenvectors dependently on the set of images (see Sect. 2.3), the DCT basis is independent of the set of images.

DCT compresses the representation of the data by discarding redundant information. As most DCT components from real-world images are typically very small in magnitude, most of the salient information exists in the coefficients with low frequencies. Given an ensemble of images, the most informative DCT coefficients can be chosen for that ensemble by determining which coefficients have the greatest variance. This was the approach adopted in [60], where the DCT components were sorted according to their variance over the images in the training set. Since components in different locations have different orders of magnitude, the components were normalized in the interval $[-1, 1]$. In other methods of feature extraction, DCT is not applied on the entire image, but is taken from square-sampling windows, see [61] for an example. In Fig. 3, we show an example of a neonatal face image and its DCT coefficients.

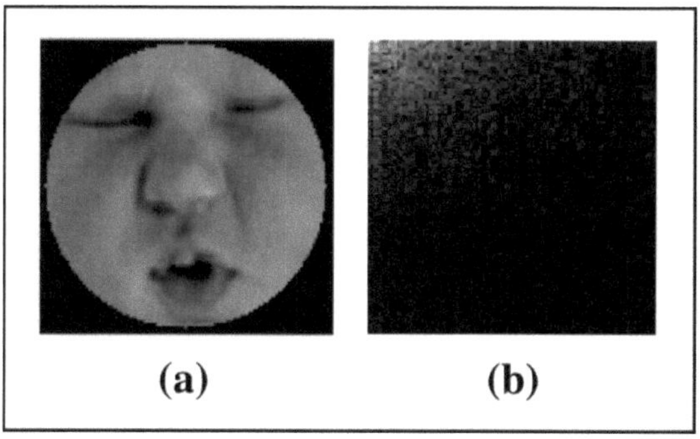

Fig. 3. Gray value image (**a**) and its DCT coefficients (**b**)

Because DCT transform provides a good compromise between information packing ability and computational complexity, it has been adopted in the image compression standard of the joint photographic experts group (JPEG).

2.2 Sequential Forward Selection and Sequential Forward Floating Selection

SFS and SFFS are top–down searches that successively delete features from a set of original candidate features to obtain a smaller optimal set of features. As the number of subsets to be considered grows exponentially with the number of original features, these algorithms provide a heuristic for determining the best order to transverse the feature subset space.

With SFS, first used in [27], the best feature subset, S_k of size k, is constructed by adding a single feature to the subset, S_{k-1}, with $k-1$ initially equal to 0, which gives the best performance for the new subset. In other words, a desirable set of k features are selected incrementally, beginning with the evaluation of each feature using a criterion function. The feature with the best value is added to the empty set S. All possible two-dimensional vectors containing the single feature in S are then evaluated using the criterion function. The winning vector replaces the elements in S. All possible three-dimensional vectors containing the two-dimensional vector in S are then evaluated, with the winner again replacing S. This process is repeated k times.

SFS is superior to an exhaustive search in that only $n(n + 1)/2$ subsets need be examined. However, it is generally suboptimal since, once the features are selected, they cannot be reevaluated and discarded.

SFFS, developed by Pudil et al. [28], improves SFS by backtracking after the inclusion of a new feature. At this point, each feature in S_k is excluded, and each new set S'_{k-1} is compared with S_{k-1}. If S'_{k-1} outperforms S_{k-1}, then it replaces S_{k-1}.

SFFS has proven superior to SFS in many comparison studies [28,31,33]. SFFS is more complex than SFS, and the search takes longer, but it evaluates more subsets than SFS and appears to obtain better feature subsets.

2.3 Principal Component Analysis

The central idea behind PCA is to find an orthonormal set of axes pointing in the direction of maximum covariance in the data. In terms of facial images, the idea is to find the orthonormal basis vectors, or the eigenvectors, of the covariance matrix of a set of images, with each image treated as a single point in a high dimensional space. It is assumed that facial images form a connected subregion in the image space. The eigenvectors map the most significant variations between faces and are preferred over other correlation techniques that assume every pixel in an image is of equal importance, (see, for instance, [62]). Since each image contributes to each of the eigenvectors, the

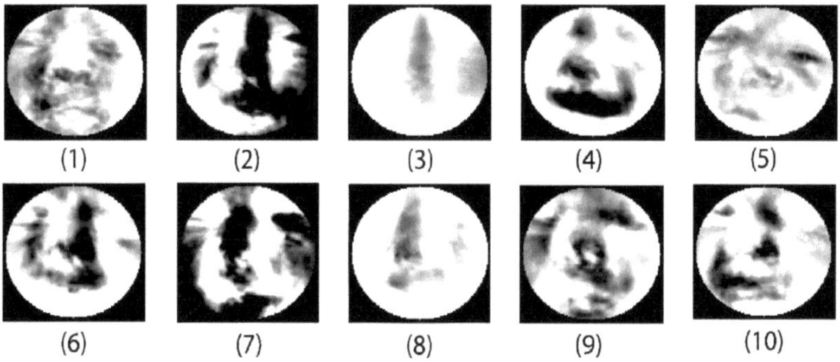

Fig. 4. The first ten eigenfaces of the 204 neonatal images, with the eigenfaces ordered by magnitude of the corresponding eigenvalue

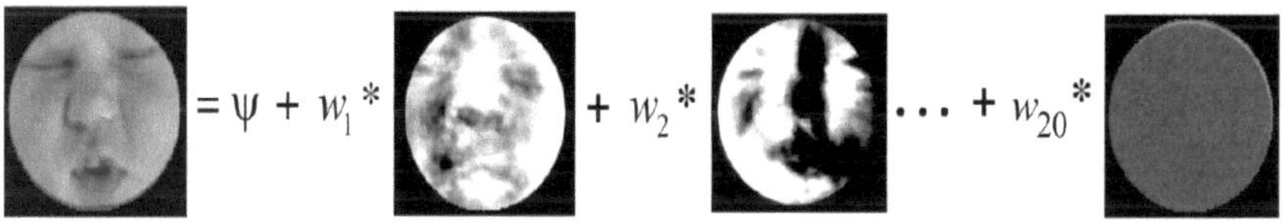

Fig. 5. Illustration of the linear combination of eigenfaces. The face to the left can be represented as a weighted combination of eigenfaces plus ψ, the average face (see number 2 in Fig. 4)

eigenvectors resemble ghostlike faces when displayed. For this reason, they are often referred to in the literature as *holons* [44] or *eigenfaces* [35], and the new coordinate system is referred to as the *face space* [35]. Examples of eigenfaces are shown in Fig. 4. Individual images can be projected onto the face space and represented exactly as weighted combinations of the eigenface components (see Fig. 5).

The resulting vector of weights that describes each face can be used both in face classification and in data compression. Classification is performed by projecting a new image onto the face space and comparing the resulting weight vector to those of a given class [35]. Compression is achieved by reconstructing images using only those few eigenfaces that account for the most variability [63]. PCA classification and compression are discussed in more detail below.

2.3.1 PCA Classification

The principal components of a set of images can be derived directly as follows. Let $\mathbf{I}(x, y)$ be a two-dimensional array of intensity values of size $N \times N$. $\mathbf{I}(x, y)$ may also be represented as a single point, a one-dimensional vector $\mathbf{\Gamma}$ of size N^2. Let the set of face images be $\mathbf{\Gamma}_1, \mathbf{\Gamma}_2, \mathbf{\Gamma}_3, \ldots, \mathbf{\Gamma}_M$, and let

$$\mathbf{\Phi}_k = \mathbf{\Gamma}_k - \mathbf{\Psi} \tag{1}$$

represent the mean normalized column vector for a given face $\mathbf{\Gamma}_k$, where

$$\mathbf{\Psi} = \frac{1}{M}\sum_{k=1}^{M}\mathbf{\Gamma}_k \tag{2}$$

is the average face of the set.

PCA seeks the set of M orthonormal vectors, $\mathbf{u}_k$, and their associated eigenvalues, $\boldsymbol{\lambda}_k$, which best describes the distribution of the image points. The vectors $\mathbf{u}_k$ and scalars $\boldsymbol{\lambda}_k$ are the eigenvectors and eigenvalues, respectively, of the covariance matrix:

$$\mathbf{C} = \frac{1}{M}\sum_{k=1}^{M}\mathbf{\Phi}_k\mathbf{\Phi}_k^{\mathrm{T}} = \mathbf{A}\mathbf{A}^{\mathrm{T}} \tag{3}$$

where the matrix $\mathbf{A} = [\mathbf{\Phi}_1, \mathbf{\Phi}_2, \ldots, \mathbf{\Phi}_M]$ [35].

The size of $\mathbf{C}$ is $N^2 \times N^2$ which for typical image sizes is an intractable task [35]. However, since typically $M < N^2$, that is, the number of images is less than the dimension, there will only be $N - 1$ nonzero eigenvectors. Thus, the N^2 eigenvectors can be solved in this case by first solving for the eigenvectors of a $M \times M$ matrix, followed by taking the appropriate linear combinations of the data points $\mathbf{\Phi}$ [35].

PCA is closely associated with the singular value decomposition (SVD) of a data matrix. SVD can be defined as follows:

$$\mathbf{\Phi} = \mathbf{U}\mathbf{S}\mathbf{V}^{\mathrm{T}} \tag{4}$$

where $\mathbf{S}$ is a diagonal matrix whose diagonal elements are the singular values, or eigenvalues, of $\mathbf{\Phi}$, and $\mathbf{U}$ and $\mathbf{V}$ are unary matrices. The columns of $\mathbf{U}$ are the eigenvectors of $\mathbf{\Phi}\mathbf{\Phi}^{\mathrm{T}}$ and are referred to as *eigenfaces*. The columns of $\mathbf{V}$ are the eigenvectors $\mathbf{\Phi}^{\mathrm{T}}\mathbf{\Phi}$ and are not used in this analysis.

Faces can be classified by projecting a new face $\mathbf{\Gamma}$ onto the face space as follows:

$$\omega_k = \mathbf{u}_k^{\mathrm{T}}(\mathbf{\Gamma}_k - \mathbf{\Psi}) \tag{5}$$

for $k = 1, \ldots, M$ eigenvectors.

The weights form a vector $\mathbf{\Omega}_k^{\mathrm{T}} = [\omega_1, \omega_2, \ldots, \omega_{M'}]$, which contains the projections onto each eigenvector. Classification is performed by calculating the distance of $\mathbf{\Omega}_k$ from $\mathbf{\Omega}$, where $\mathbf{\Omega}$ represents the average weight vector defining some class [35].

Two commonly used distance measures are the sum of absolute differences, also known as the L_1 metric, and the Euclidean distance, also know as the L_2 metric. If we have two points, $A(x_1, y_1)$ and $B(x_2, y_2)$, the L_1 distance between A and B is $abs(x_1 - x_2) + abs(y_1 - y_2)$. The L_2 metric is $\sqrt{(x_1 - x_2)^2 + (y_1 - y_2)^2}$.

2.3.2 PCA Data Compression

Since the eigenfaces are ordered, with each one accounting for a different amount of variation among the faces, images can be reconstructed using only those few eigenfaces, $M' \ll M$ in (4), that account for the most variability [63]. As noted above, PCA results in a dramatic reduction of dimensionality and maps the most significant variations in a dataset. For this reason, it is often used to transform and reduce features when performing other classification procedures.

2.3.3 Outline of PCA Face Classification

The basic steps necessary to perform PCA training and testing using face images are outlined in Table 1. These steps follow from the presentation given above.

2.4 Linear Discriminant Analysis

While PCA is optimal for reconstructing images from a low dimensional space, it is not optimal for discrimination. PCA yields projection directions that maximize the total scatter across all classes. LDA, or Fisher's linear discriminants, in contrast, is a supervised learning procedure that projects the images onto a subspace that maximizes the between-class scatter and minimizes the within-class scatter of the projected data. A classical technique in pattern recognition, LDA is an example of a *class specific method* in that it shapes the scatter in order to make it more reliable for classification [64]. There has

Table 1. Outline of PCA training and testing steps

PCA training	PCA testing
Using a set of training feature vectors: 1. Compute the average feature vector, $\mathbf{\Psi}$ 2. Subtract $\mathbf{\Psi}$ from the feature vectors to obtain $\mathbf{\Gamma}$, the mean adjusted dataset 3. Derive eigenfaces for $\mathbf{\Gamma}$ using SVD 4. Obtain the weight vectors, or eigenvalues, for each $\mathbf{\Gamma}_k$ by projecting it onto the resulting face space 5. Reduce dimensionality by retaining only the most significant eigenvalues 6. Obtain the class vectors, $\mathbf{\Omega}$, by averaging the eigenvalues of each $\mathbf{\Gamma}_k$ belonging to each class	Using a set of testing feature vectors: 1. Subtract $\mathbf{\Psi}$ from the feature vectors to obtain $\mathbf{\Gamma}$ 2. Obtain the weight vectors, or the eigenvalues, for each $\mathbf{\Gamma}_k$ by projecting $\mathbf{\Gamma}_k$ onto the face space derived using the training set 3. Reduce dimensionality as was done with the training set 4. Classify each $\mathbf{\Gamma}_k$ based on its distance from $\mathbf{\Omega}$, using a distance metric

been a tendency to prefer LDA to PCA because LDA deals directly with discrimination between classes, whereas PCA aims at faithfully representing the data. It has been shown that LDA outperforms PCA only when large and representative training datasets are given [65].

2.5 Support Vector Machines

SVMs, introduced in [66], belong to the class of maximum margin classifiers. They perform pattern recognition between two classes by finding a decision surface that has maximum distance to the closest points in the training set. The data points that define the maximum margin are called support vectors.

SVMs are designed to solve two-class problems and are thus ideally suited to the neonatal pain detection task. SVMs produce the pattern classifier (1) by applying a variety of kernel functions (linear, polynomial, radial basis function, and so on) as the possible sets of approximating functions, (2) by optimizing the dual quadratic programming problem, and (3) by using structural risk minimization as the inductive principle, as opposed to classical statistical algorithms that maximize the absolute value of an error or of an error squared.

Different types of SVM classifiers are used depending upon the type of input patterns: a linear maximal margin classifier is used for linearly separable data, a linear soft margin classifier is used for linearly nonseparable, or overlapping, classes, and a nonlinear classifier is used for classes that are overlapped as well as separated by nonlinear hyperplanes. Each of these cases is outlined below. Readers interested in using SVM should consult [67].

2.5.1 Outline of SVM

Suppose, there is a set of training data, $\mathbf{x}_1$, $\mathbf{x}_2$, ..., $\mathbf{x}_k$. where $\mathbf{x}_i \in \mathbf{R}^n$ and $i = 1, 2, \ldots, k$. Each $\mathbf{x}_i$, belonging as it does to one of two classes, has a corresponding value y_i, where $y_i \in \{1, 1\}$.

Linear maximal margin classifier. The goal is to build the hyperplane that maximizes the minimum distance between the two classes. This hyperplane is called the OSH and has the form:

$$f(\mathbf{x}) = \sum_{i=1}^{k} \alpha_i y_i \mathbf{x}_i \cdot \mathbf{x} + b \tag{6}$$

where α and b are the solutions of a quadratic programming problem.

Unknown test data $\mathbf{x}_t$ can be classified by simply computing (7).

$$f(x) = \text{sign}(w_0 \cdot x_t + b_0) \tag{7}$$

Examining (7), it can be seen that the hyperplane is determined by all the training data, $\mathbf{x}_i$, that have the corresponding attributes of $\alpha_i > 0$. We call this kind of training data *support vectors*. Thus, the OSH is not determined by the training data per se but rather by the support vectors.

Linear soft margin classifier. The objective in this case is to separate the two classes of training data with a minimal number of errors. To accomplish this, some non-negative slack variables, $\xi_{i,i} = 1, 2, \ldots, k$, are introduced into the system. The penalty, or regularization parameter, C, is also introduced to control the cost of errors. The computation of the linear soft margin classifier is the same as the linear maximal margin classifier. Thus, we can obtain OSH using (6) and (7).

Nonlinear classifier. In this case, kernel functions such as the polynomial or RBF are used to transform the input space to a feature space of higher dimensionality. In the feature space, a linear separating hyperplane is sought that separates the input vectors into two classes. In this case, the hyperplane and decision rule for the nonlinear training pattern is (8).

$$f(x) = \text{sign}\left(\sum_{i=1}^{K} \alpha_i y_i\right) K(\mathbf{x}_t, \mathbf{x}) + b) \tag{8}$$

Where, α_i and b are the solutions of a quadratic programming problem and $K(\mathbf{x}_t, \mathbf{x})$ is a kernel function.

2.6 Neural Network Simultaneous Optimization Algorithm

NNSOA is a global search procedure that searches from one population of NN solutions to another, focusing on the area that provides the current best solution, while continuously sampling the total parameter space. NNSOA is a slight modification of a genetic algorithm (GA) used in previous NN studies (see [51]). NNSOA takes advantage of the GA's ability to search multiple points (or solutions) at one time, unlike gradient search techniques, such as backpropagation, that are able to search for only one solution at a time. As explained below, what makes NNSOA unique is the addition of a penalty in the objective function. This penalty enables NNSOA to eliminate unneeded weights in the NN architecture. Thus, NNSOA is able to produce solutions that generalize better than those found using gradient search techniques.

Because NNSOA uses a genetic algorithm for the search procedure, it is not limited to differentiable functions, as is the case with gradient search techniques. Thus, NNSOA can have objective functions that add a penalty for the number of nonzero weights in a solution. NNSOA is able to eliminate unneeded weights in a solution by intermittently exchanging solution weights with hard zeros and then evaluating whether that substitution helped or hindered the network's ability to predict using normal GA operations.

Backpropagation does not have the ability to zero out weights in a solution. Therefore, in a backpropagation network, or in any gradient search technique used for searching for optimal weights in a NN solution, the search must find a solution that has values for these unneeded weights that will, in effect, zero each other out when producing estimates. This works well for training data but is likely to introduced additional errors in the estimates when these solutions are applied to out-of-sample data. A solution found by the NNSOA completely eliminates this possibility of additional error because the unneeded weights are set to a hard zero. This ability to zero out weights in a solution provides additional feature reduction as those inputs that are of no value to a solution are basically removed from the solution. In addition, those inputs that offer the most value can easily be isolated by examining the weights of the NN solution.

Another advantage of NNSOA is that it finds the appropriate NN architectures by searching for the correct number of hidden nodes in a solution. This is done by starting a network with only one hidden node. After a user specified number of generations (MAXHID), the best solution out of the population of solutions is saved, and an additional hidden node is added to the architecture and trained for another MAXHID generation. The previous best solution is included in this additional training by replacing one of the randomly initialized solutions with the best solution found in the previous architecture. Since adding an additional node to the architecture increases the number of weights in the solutions equal to the number of inputs plus one, the additional weights for this best solution are set to hard zeros. The process of adding an additional hidden node after every MAXHID generation continues until the current best solution is worse than the previous architecture's best solution. At this point, the number of hidden nodes is set to the number of hidden nodes in the previous architecture, and the NN continues with the training process for a user defined number of generations. Once the MAXGEN number of generations has been reached, training is complete.

2.6.1 Outline of NNSOA

NNSOA classification is performed as follows:

Initialization. A population of 12 solutions is created by drawing random real values from a uniform distribution $[-1, 1]$ for input weights. The output weights are determined by ordinary least squares (OLS).

Evaluation. Each member of the current population is evaluated by an objective function based on its sum of squared error (SSE) value in order to assign each solution a probability for being redrawn in the next generation. To search for a parsimonious solution, a penalty value is added to the SSE for each nonzero weight (or active connection). The penalty for keeping an additional weight varies during the search and is equal to the current value of the root-mean-squared error (RMSE). This means that the penalty for keeping additional weights is high at the beginning of the training process when errors are high. As the optimization process gets closer to the final solution, errors decrease and the penalty value becomes smaller. Based on the objective function, each of the 12 solutions in the population is evaluated. The probability of being drawn in the next generation is calculated by dividing the distance of the current solution's objective value from the worst objective value in the generation by the sum of all distances in the current generation.

Reproduction. A mating pool of 12 solutions is created by selecting solutions from the current population based on their assigned probability. This is done by selecting a random number in the range of 0–1 and comparing it to the cumulative probability of the current solution. When it is found that the random value is less than the current solution's cumulative probability, the current string is drawn for the next generation. This is repeated until the entire new generation is drawn. It should be noted that a given solution can be drawn more than once or not at all, depending on its assigned probability.

Crossover. Once reproduction occurs, providing a combination of solutions from the previous generation, the 12 solutions are then randomly paired so that six pairs are produced. A point is randomly selected for each pair. New solutions are produced by switching the weights above the randomly generated point. In this fashion, 12 new solutions are generated for the next generation.

Mutation. For each weight in a population of solutions, a random number is drawn; if the random value is less than 0.05, the weight is replaced by a value randomly drawn from the entire weight space. By doing this, the entire weight space is globally searched, thus enhancing the algorithm's ability to find global solutions.

Mutation 2. For each weight in the population of solutions, a random number is drawn; if the random value is less than 0.05, the weight is replaced by a hard zero. As a result of doing this, unneeded weights are identified as the search continues for the optimum solution. After this operator is performed, this new generation of 12 solutions begins again with evaluation, and the cycle continues until it reaches 70% of the maximum set of generations.

Convergence enhancement. Once 70% of the maximum set of generations has been completed, the best solution replaces all the strings in the current generation. The weights of these 12 identical solutions are then modified by adding a small random value to each weight. These random values decrease to an arbitrarily small number as the number of generations increases to its set maximum number.

Termination. The algorithm terminates on a user specified number of generations.

2.7 Face Recognition Software Tools

Because of its excellent visualization tools and platform independence, MATLAB [68] by MathWorks is commonly used for experimenting with face recognition algorithms and problems. Numerous toolboxes have been developed that provide MATLAB users with routines for handling images and statistical pattern recognition tasks. MathWorks, for instance, offers an excellent image processing toolbox that includes a DCT transform function. MathWorks also produces a neural network toolbox for designing and visualizing neural network algorithms, with built-in support for many common neural network algorithms.

An excellent MATLAB toolbox for experimenting with statistical pattern recognition is PRTools [69]. It is free for academic research. PRTools provides over 200 routines, including PCA, LDA, SVM, and several feature selection algorithms. The SVM implementation in PRTools, however, is limited. For a more comprehensive package, the OSU SVM MATLAB toolbox developed by Ohio State University is an excellent choice. It is available at sourceforge.net. Links to additional software and resources are available at www.face-rec.org.

3 Infant COPE Database and Study Design

Of critical importance in developing the preliminary Infant COPE database was the selection of stimuli used to provoke facial displays in the neonates. The objective was to obtain a representative and challenging set of images for evaluating face classification systems of pain.

In early neonatal pain studies that explored facial activity, infants were typically exposed to two categories of noxious stimuli, a pain-inducing event (pin prick or puncture of a lancet) and a noninvasive tactile experience, such as rubbing the leg or foot with cotton and alcohol. Swabbing with cotton triggers a high degree of facial activity, affording researchers the opportunity of isolating the facial behaviors specific to pain experiences [70]. Contemporary studies typically introduce additional stimuli, such as exposure to bright light [11] or a diaper change [71]. These stimuli are calculated to produce facial behaviors that are similar to those produced in reaction to pain. Diaper change, for instance, often provokes a crying expression, and exposure to bright light triggers eye squeeze.

For the initial Infant COPE study, four noxious stimuli were selected: (1) the puncture of a heel lance, (2) friction, produced by swabbing on the external lateral surface of the heel, (3) an air stimulus on the nose, and (4) transport from one crib to another. Since classifiers easily discriminate changes in lighting, an air stimulus, rather than exposure to bright light, was selected to elicit eye squeeze. The fourth stressor, bodily transportation, was a logistic necessity. The infants had to be moved to a special crib to obtain an unobstructed view of the neonate's face. Like diaper change, moving an infant to another crib is a major bodily disturbance that often provokes crying. Instead of waiting for a period of time to calm the infant after being moved, we replaced diaper change with the transportation event.

3.1 Subjects

This study complied with the protocols and ethical directives for research involving human subjects at Missouri State University and St John's Health

System, Inc. Informed consent was obtained from a parent, usually the mother in consultation with the father. Most parents were recruited in the neonatal unit of a St John's Hospital sometime after delivery. Only mothers who had experienced uncomplicated deliveries were approached.

A total of 204 color photographs were taken of 26 Caucasian neonates (13 boys and 13 girls) ranging in age from 18 h to 3 days. Six males had been circumcised the day before the photographs were taken, and the last feeding time before the photography session ranged from 45 min to 5 h. All infants were in good health.

3.2 Apparatus

All photographs were taken using a Nikon D100 digital camera under ambient lighting conditions in a room separated from other newborns.

3.3 Procedure

The facial expressions of the newborns were photographed in one session. All stimuli were administered by an attending nurse. Following the requirements of standard medical procedures, photographs of the four stimuli were taken in the following sequence:

1. Transport from one crib to another (Rest/Cry): after being transported from one crib to another, the neonate was swaddled and a series of photographs was taken over the course of 1 min. The state of the neonate was noted as either crying or resting for each photograph taken in the series.
2. Air Stimulus: after resting for at least one additional minute, the neonate's nose was exposed to a puff of air emitted from a squeezable plastic camera lens cleaner. A series of pictures of the neonate's face was taken immediately after the air puff contacted the infant's face.
3. Friction: after resting for at least 1 min, the neonate received friction on the external lateral surface of the heel with cotton wool soaked in 70% alcohol for 10–15 s. The face of the neonate was repeatedly photographed during the friction rubbings.
4. Pain: after resting for at least 1 min, the external lateral surface of the heel was punctured for blood collection. Several continuous photographs of the neonate's face were taken, starting immediately after introduction of the lancet and while the skin of the heel was squeezed for blood samples.

3.4 Expression Categories

We divided the facial expressions that resulted from the four stimuli into five facial expression categories: rest, cry, air stimulus, friction, and pain. Of the 204 photographs taken, 67 are rest, 18 are cry, 23 are air stimulus, 36 are friction, and 60 are pain.

The five facial expressions for two subjects are illustrated in Fig. 6. The rest category includes yawns, alert expressions, and the faces of sleeping neonates. The pain category includes images of neonates crying as well as other facial behaviors elicited by the pain stimulus. Figure 7 provides example images in the pain category and demonstrates the diverse expressiveness found in this category. The cry category includes all images of crying infants except those provoked by the pain stimulus. Figure 7 provides samples from the cry category for comparison with the pain images. The challenge the initial Infant COPE database offers classifier systems is especially apparent by comparing the middle pain/cry image in Fig. 7 to the middle nonpain/cry image in Fig. 8.

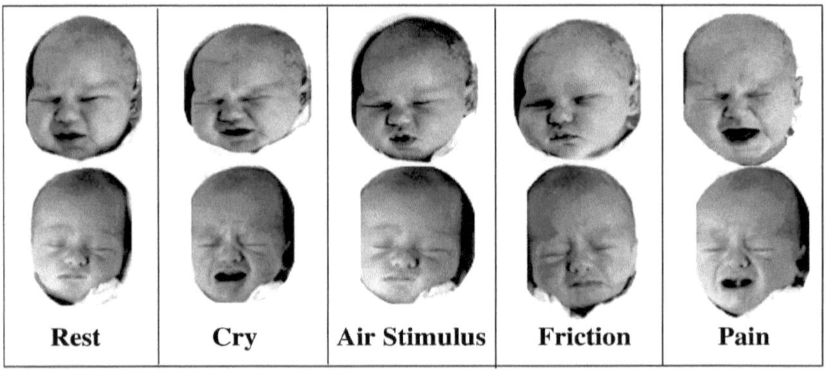

Fig. 6. Examples of the five facial expressions in the infant COPE database

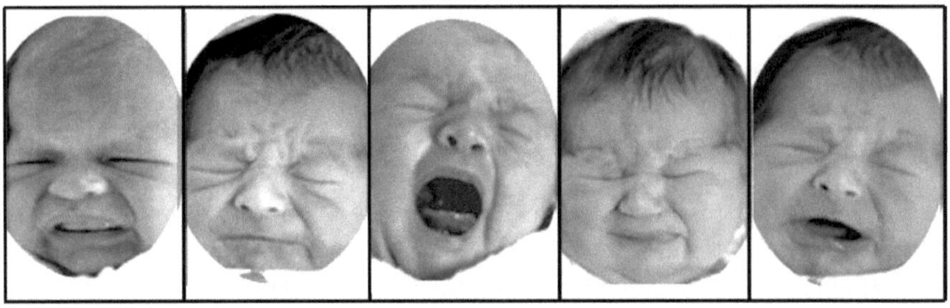

Fig. 7. Examples of pain expressions

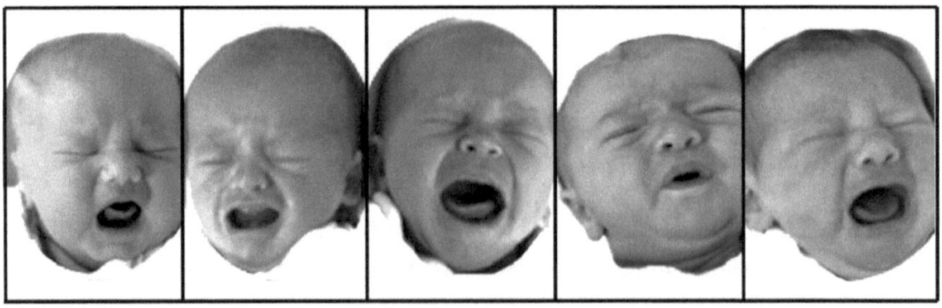

Fig. 8. Examples of cry expressions not elicited by the pain stimulus

4 Method

In this section, we outline the method used in the classification experiments performed thus far using the initial Infant COPE database. In Sect. 4.1, we present details regarding the division of the five expression categories discussed above into the binary classification classes of pain and nonpain. In Sect. 4.2, we describe two evaluation protocols that are targeted for two situations – one where sample facial displays are available for new infants and another where no samples are available for new infants. We also discuss the rationale behind the development of these two protocols. In Sect. 4.3, we provide a general outline and description of the procedures used in the classification experiments surveyed in Sect.5.

4.1 Classification Classes

Since the main objective of the Infant COPE project is to develop neonatal pain detection systems, most classification experiments performed to date have focused on distinguishing pain responses from other expressions. For this purpose, the 204 color photographs were divided into two classes: pain and nonpain. All the rest, cry, air stimulus, and friction photographs formed the nonpain class for a total of 140 images. The remaining 60 images formed the pain class.

4.2 Evaluation Protocols

Two evaluations protocols, designated protocol A and protocol B, have been developed for evaluating classification systems using the Infant COPE database.

Protocol A. Used in the classification experiments reported in [15, 53], this protocol presents the best-case scenario by assuming that samples of individual subjects will be available to personalize the classifier, as is the case with most commercial speech recognition software. Multiple but different samples of neonatal pain and nonpain facial expressions from all subjects are used in the testing and training sets.

As expected, personalizing classifiers in this way greatly enhances classifier performance (see Sect. 5), but this classification task is not easy. In Sect. 3.4, we pointed out the diversity in expressiveness in the Infant COPE database, especially in the category of pain. As evident in Fig. 9, care was taken that all images of a given subject within a particular expression category contained clearly discernable differences in either facial orientation or configuration.

Protocol B. Used in the classification experiments reported in [14], this protocol presents the worst case scenario by assuming that the classifier will be trained on one set of subjects and then applied out of the box to an unknown set of future newborns. In this evaluation protocol, images are divided by subject, and the testing set contains images of subjects that are not used in

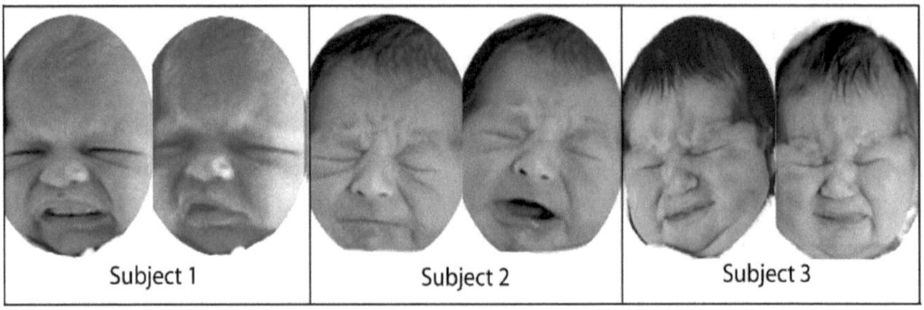

Fig. 9. Example of face configuration and orientation differences in pain images within three subject classes

the training set. Protocol B is more realistic since the hospital stay for most newborns is only between 3 and 4 days. This protocol is also the most difficult to classify.

4.3 Outline of Experimental Procedures

Outlined in Fig. 10 are the general experimental procedures used in the classification experiments reviewed in Sect. 5. The experimental procedures can be divided into the following stages: image preprocessing, feature extraction, and classification.

In the image preprocessing stage, the input images were normalized and rotated so that faces were upright and the eyes intersected the same horizontal axis. The original images, size $3,008 \times 2,000$ pixels, were also reduced to 100×120 pixels and cropped.

In the feature extraction stage, color information was discarded and the facial features centered within an ellipse. The rows within the ellipse were concatenated to form an input vector of dimension 8,583 with entries ranging in value between 0 and 255. The raw input vectors were then transformed using PCA or DCT, and the dimensionality reduced further using one of the feature selection functions described in Sect. 3.

Finally, in the classification stage, PCA, LDA, SVMs, and NNSOA classifiers were trained and tested following evaluation protocols A or B.

5 Experiments

This section surveys the classification experiments we have performed to date using the Infant COPE database. SVM and NNSOA, the most advanced classifiers explored thus far, have consistently performed well. NNSOA, for instance, classified the facial expressions into the classes of pain and nonpain with 100% accuracy using protocol A and 95.38% using protocol B. SVM has produced classification scores that compare well with NNSOA. In [14,15],

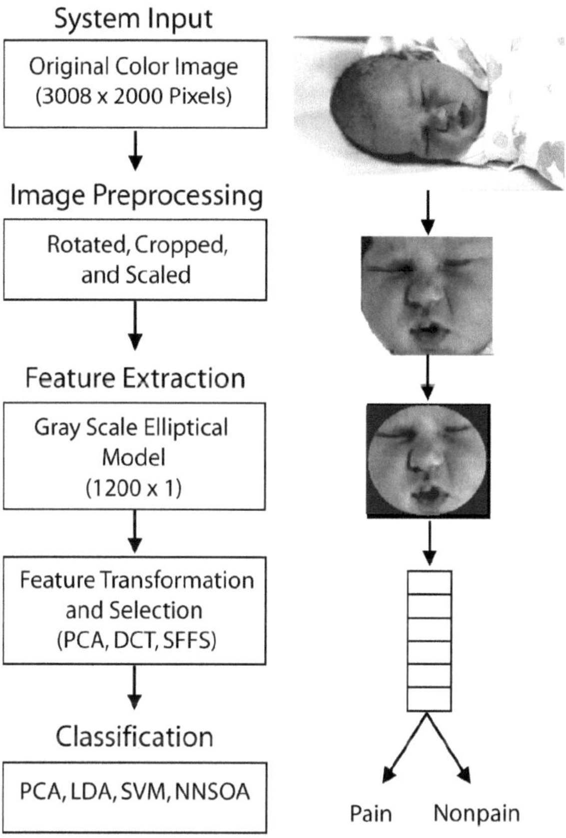

Fig. 10. Outline of experimental procedures

we performed comprehensive investigations of SVM using five kernels: linear, RBF, polynomial degree 2, polynomial degree 3, and polynomial degree 4. We found no statistical difference in performance between NNSOA and SVMs with the linear and polynomial kernels in our experiments using protocol B [14]. Because application of the RBF kernel resulted in poor performance, RBF kernel classification scores are not presented in what follows. The reader is referred to [14, 15] for those results. However, PCA and LDA classification scores using the L_1 metric are provided for baseline comparison.

For this discussion we divide the experiments according to the protocol used. In Sect. 5.1, we survey experimental results using protocol A, and in Sect. 5.2 we compare classifier performance using protocol B. We conclude the survey with a brief description of current work in Sect. 5.3.

5.1 Experimental Results Using Protocol A

Thus far we have performed two pain detection experiments using protocol A: an experiment reported in [15] that investigated PCA, LDA, and SVM classifier performance and another reported in [53] that examined NNSOA performance using protocol A. In these experiments, the PCA transform was used to reduce dimensionality of the elliptical model vectors (refer to Fig. 10). Feature reduction was accomplished by performing a series of linear SVM experiments. These determined that the top 70 PCA coefficients were optimal for the classification task.

In the PCA, LDA, and SVM experiments, we employed a simple cross-validation technique. The pain and nonpain classification classes were randomly divided into 10 segments, and 9 out of the 10 segments were used in the training session. The remaining segment was used in testing. An average classification score was then computed for the testing set of images in that segment. This process was repeated ten times, with the ten classification scores averaged for a final performance score. It is these final performance scores that are reported in Table 2 for PCA, LDA, SVM, and NNSOA.

The NNSOA experiments were more rigorous in that we applied the leave-one-out method of cross-validation. This method used all but one image for the training set. The remaining image formed the testing set. As a result, the number of NNSOA networks trained and tested equaled the number of images in the Infant COPE dataset. By applying the leave-one-out method rather than the cross-validation technique employed in the PCA, LDA, and SVM experiments, we were able to gain confidence in the ability of NNSOA to find consistently good solutions because we were assured that each observation had been tested.

Table 2 compares the average classification scores obtained using protocol A for PCA, LDA, Linear SVM, SVMs with polynomial degrees 2, 3, and 4, and NNSOA. For the SVM experiments, we set the regularization parameter, C, to 1. Other values for C were tried, but they did not significantly affect performance.

Referring to Table 2, we see that NNSOA classified the images with 100% accuracy. SVM with polynomial kernels of degree 2 (86.50%), degree 3 (88.00%), and degree 4 (82.17%) did not perform as well. There was no

Table 2. Summary of PCA, LDA, SVM, and NNSOA experiments using protocol A, as reported in [15,53]

Classifier	Transform	Features selected	Recognition rate (%)
PCA with L_1 distance	PCA	70	80.33
LDA with L_1 distance	PCA	70	83.67
Linear SVM	PCA	70	83.67
Polynomial SVM degree = 2	PCA	70	86.50
Polynomial SVM degree = 3	PCA	70	88.00
Polynomial SVM degree = 4	PCA	70	82.17
NNSOA	PCA	40	100.00

difference in performance between LDA and a linear SVM, both of which performed marginally better than PCA.

As noted in Table 2, NNSOA classified the images using only 24 PCA components. Recall from Sect. 2.6 that NNSOA eliminates unneeded weights, resulting in a parsimonious architecture. An added advantage of eliminating these weights is the identification of relevant features.

5.2 Experimental Results Using Protocol B

Protocol B is more difficult, as none of the subjects in the testing set were used in the training set (see Sect. 4.2). Following the requirements of Protocol B, we performed a total of 26 experiments for each classifier. For each of the 26 subjects, the set of facial images for that subject became the testing set while the facial images of the remaining 25 subjects became the training set. The classification rates of the 26 experiments were then averaged for a final classification score.

In [14], we report a series of experiments using protocol B that applied the PCA transform. As in the experiments using protocol A, dimensionality was reduced by selecting the top 70 components.

Table 3 compares the average classification scores reported in [14] for PCA, LDA, NNSOA, linear SVM, and SVMs with polynomial degrees 2, 3, and 4. Referring to Table 3, we see that NNSOA had the highest classification rate with 90.20% accuracy, followed by an SVM with a linear kernel (82.35%). However, a statistical analysis showed that there was no significant difference in performance between the various SVM methods and NNSOA.

As with the experiments using protocol A, the SVM regularization parameter, C, was set to 1 for all SVM experiments. In Table 3 we also report the average number of PCA components (24) that were used by NNSOA across the 26 networks.

Table 3. Summary of PCA, LDA, SVM, and NNSOA experiments using protocol B as reported in [14]

Classifier	Transform	Features selected	Recognition rate (%)
PCA with L_1 distance	PCA	70	80.39
LDA with L_1 distance	PCA	70	76.96
Linear SVM	PCA	70	82.39
Polynomial SVM degree = 2	PCA	70	79.90
Polynomial SVM degree = 3	PCA	70	80.39
Polynomial SVM degree = 4	PCA	70	72.06
NNSOA	PCA	24	90.20

5.3 Current Work

Our current work is centered on protocol B, as it is the most realistic and challenging protocol developed so far. At present we are conducting experiments using the DCT transform and two methods of feature reduction: sorting by variance and SFFS. Application of the first method involved sorting the DCT coefficients by variance, as in [60]. We then performed a series of linear SVM experiments that determined that the top 80 coefficients were optimal for the classification task. In the second method, we applied SFFS [28], as described in Sect. 2, to select a feature set of only 15 DCT coefficients. The SFFS selection criterion function was the minimum error of linear SVM classification. In the discussion that follows, we label the first method DCT + VAR and the second DCT + SFFS.

In Table 4 we present preliminary results for SVM with a linear kernel and NNSOA. We have not yet completed experiments using SVM with the polynomial kernels. Examining Table 4, we discover an unexpected result: a slightly lower classification score for NNSOA + SFFS (93.14%) compared with NNSOA + VAR (95.38%). In the DCT + VAR experiment, NNSOA reduced the number of coefficients needed for optimum NNSOA classification to an average of 27. NNSOA found all 15 coefficients selected by SFFS relevant for classification. It is probably the case that SFFS selects a better subset of features than NNSOA, but the problem for NNSOA + SFFS is that the features selected were overfitted for the NNSOA objective function. Although in both experiments (DCT + VAR and DCT + SFFS) SVM with a linear kernel produced lower scores than NNSOA, a statistical analysis has discovered no significant difference in performance between the two classifiers.

Our preliminary investigation also shows no statistical difference in performance between linear SVM using DCT + VAR and linear SVM using the top 70 PCA components reported in [14] (see Sect. 5.2). However, NNSOA classification performance with DCT + VAR coefficients is statistically superior to NNSOA using the 70 PCA components.

To round off the SFFS studies, we are also currently investigating classifier performance using PCA + SFFS. It will be interesting to compare classifier performance using PCA + SFFS with DCT + SFFS.

Table 4. Summary of preliminary experiments using protocol B with DCT coefficients

Classifier	Transform and selection method	Features selected	Recognition rate (%)
Linear SVM	DCT + VAR	80	87.53
Linear SVM	DCT + SFFS	15	89.17
NNSOA	DCT + VAR	27	95.38
NNSOA	DCT + SFFS	15	93.14

6 The Future

We believe that the results reported here and in earlier studies indicate a high potential for developing machine detection systems that could be used in neonatal pain assessment. In terms of future work, we are currently designing experiments that will investigate NNSOA and SVM classifier ensembles, as it appears that the two algorithms provide complementary information about the patterns to be classified. In addition, we plan on adding fiduciary points to the input vectors. It is possible that shape information, along with the gray scale texture information provided in the pixel values, will improve our pain detection systems.

We are also working on developing another Infant COPE database using video images of approximately 500 neonates. Video will allow us to investigate the dynamic and multidimensional nature of neonatal facial displays. The database will also include facial expressions evoked by additional stimuli, for example, the temperature change of removing a heel warmer applied to increase blood flow and the repeated deep pain of the heel squeezes that follow heel lancing.

Finally, we should mention that the Infant COPE project is not the only COPE project under development. We are planning pain expression studies that include other patients, such the profoundly mentally disabled and people with Alzheimer's disease, as these patients are also incapable of articulating their pain experiences. For anyone interested in this work, we will continuously update our progress on these projects at www.copedata.org.

Acknowledgments

The authors wish gratefully to acknowledge the partial funding of this project by Missouri State University, faculty grant #1015-22-2181. We also wish to acknowledge Chao-Fa Chuang, Ph.D. candidate, and Frank Y. Shih, director of the Computer Vision Laboratory, at New Jersey Institute of Technology for their participation in two early Infant COPE studies (see [14, 15]).

References

1. Stevens B, Johnston C, Gibbins S (2000) Pain assessment in neonates. In: Anand KJS, Stevens BJ, McGrath PJ (eds) Pain in neonates: 2nd revised and enlarged edition. Elsevier, New York, pp 101–134
2. Wong D, Baker C (1988) Pain in children: Comparison of assessment scales. Pediatr Nurs 14(1): 9–17
3. Grunau RE (2000) Long-term consequences of pain in human neonates. In: Anand KJS, Stevens BJ, McGrath PJ (eds) Pain in neonates: 2nd revised and enlarged edition. Elsevier, New York, pp 55–76

4. Coffman S, Alvarez Y, Pyngolil M, Petit R, Hall C, Smyth M (1997) Nursing assessment and management of pain in critically ill children. Heart Lung 26(3): 221–228
5. Van Cleve L, Johnson L, Pothier P (1996) Pain responses of hospitalized infants and children to venipuncture and intravenous cannulation. J Pediatr Nurs 11(3): 161–168
6. McGrath PA (1989) Pain in children: Nature, assessment, and treatment. Guildford Press, New York
7. Craig KD (1998) The facial display of pain in infants and children. In: Finley GA, McGrath PJ (eds) Measurement of pain in infants and children. IASP Press, Seattle, pp 103–121
8. Grunau RE, Grunau RVE, Craig KD (1987) Pain expression in neonates: Facial action and cry. Pain 28(3): 395–410
9. Prkachin KM, Solomon P, Hwang T, Mercer SR (2001) Does experience influence judgments of pain behaviour? Evidence from relatives of pain patients and therapists. Pain Res Manag 6(2): 105–112
10. McDowell I, Newall C (1996) Measuring health: A guide to rating scales and questionnaires. Oxford University Press, Oxford
11. Xavier Balda R, Guinsburg R, de Almeida MFB, de Araujo CP, Miyoshi MH, Kopelman BI (2000) The recognition of facial expression of pain in full-term newborns by parents and health professionals. Arch Pediatr Adolesc Med 154(10): 1009–1016
12. Lindh V, Wiklund U, Håkansson S (1999) Heel lancing in term new-born infants: An evaluation of pain by frequency domain analysis of heart rate variability. Pain 80(1–2): 143–148
13. Petroni M, Malowany A, Johnston C, Stevens B (1995) Identification of pain from infant cry vocalizations using artificial neural networks (ANNS). Int Soc Opt Eng 2492: 729–738
14. Brahnam S, Chuang C-F, Sexton R, Shih FY, Slack MR (in press) Machine assessment of neonatal facial expressions of acute pain. Decis Support Syst
15. Brahnam S, Chuang C-F, Shih FY, Slack MR (2006) Machine recognition and representation of neonate facial displays of acute pain. Artif Intell Med 36(3): 211–222
16. Zhao W, Chellappa R, Phillips PJ, Rosenfeld A (2000) Face recognition: A literature survey. ACM Comput Surv 35(4): 399–458
17. Moghaddam B, Yang M-H (2002) Learning gender with support faces. IEEE Trans PAMI 24(5): 306–311
18. O'Toole AJ, Abdi H, Deffenbacher KA, Bartlett JC (1991) Classifying faces by race and sex using an autoassociative memory trained for recognition. In: 13th annual conference on cognitive science. Hillsdale, NJ, pp 847–851
19. O'Toole AJ, Deffenbacher KA (1997) The perception of face gender: The role of stimulus structure in recognition and classification. Mem Cog 26: 146–160
20. Ekman P, Huang TS, Sejnowski TJ, Hager JC, Golomb B (1992) Final report to NSF of the planning workshop on facial expression understanding. Available at http://face-and-emotion.com/dataface/nsfrept/references.html
21. Gunaratne P, Sato Y (2003) Estimation of asymmetry in facial actions for the analysis of motion dysfunction due to paralysis. Int J Image Graph 3(4): 639–652
22. Lanitis A, Taylor CJ, Cootes TF (1997) Automatic interpretation and coding of face images using flexible models. IEEE Trans PAMI 19(7): 743–756

23. Burton AM, Bruce V, Dench N (1993) What's the difference between men and women? Evidence from facial measurement. Perception 22(2): 153–176
24. Valentin D, Abdi H, O,Toole AJ, Cottrell GW (1994) Connectionist models of face processing: A survey. Pattern Recognit 27(9): 1209–1230
25. Brunelli R, Poggio T (1993) Face recognition: Features versus templates. IEEE Trans PAMI 15(10): 1042–1052
26. Narendra PM, Fukunaga K (1977) A branch and bound algorithm for feature subset selection. IEEE Trans Comput 26: 917–922
27. Whitney A (1971) A direct method of nonparametric measurement selection. IEEE Trans Comput 20: 1100–1103
28. Pudil P, Novovicova J, Kittler J (1994) Floating search methods in feature selection. Pattern Recognit Lett 5(11): 1119–1125
29. Egmont-Petersen M, Dassen WRM, Reiber JHC (1999) Sequential selection of discrete features for neural networks: A bayesian approach to building a cascade. Pattern Recognit Lett 20(11–13): 1439–1448
30. Guyon I, Elisseeff A (2003) An introduction to variable and feature selection. J Mach Learn Res 3: 1157–1182
31. Kudo M, Sklansky J (2000) Comparison of algorithms that select features for pattern classifiers. Pattern Recognit 33(1): 25–41
32. Devijver PA, Kittler J (1982) Pattern recognition: A statistical approach. Prentice Hall, Englewood Cliffs
33. Jain A, Zongker D (1997) Feature selection: Evaluation, application, and small sample performance. IEEE Trans PAMI 19(2): 153–158
34. Swets DL, Weng J (1996) Using discriminant eigenfeatures for image retrieval. IEEE Trans PAMI 18(8): 831–837
35. Turk MA, Pentland AP (1991) Eigenfaces for recognition. J Cogn Neurosci 3(1): 71–86
36. Turk MA, Pentland AP (1991) Face recognition using eigenfaces. In: IEEE Computer Society Conference on Computer Vision and Pattern Recognition. Silver Spring, MD, pp 586–591
37. Jain A, Huang J (2004) Integrating independent components and linear discriminant analysis for gender classification. In: The sixth IEEE international conference on automatic face and gesture recognition, pp 159–163
38. Valentin D, Abdi H, Edelman BE, O'Toole AJ (1997) Principal component and neural network analyses of face images: What can be generalized in gender classification? J Math Psychol 41(4): 398–413
39. Lu X, Jain AK (2004) Ethnicity identification from face images. In: SPIE: Biometric Technology for Human Identification, pp 114–123
40. Cottrell GW, Metcalfe J (1991) Empath: Face, emotion, and gender recognition using holons. In: Touretzky D (ed) Advances in neural information processing systems. Morgan & Kaufman, San Mateo, CA, pp 564–571
41. Martinez AM, Benavente R (1998) The AR face database. CVC technical report #24. Available at http://rvl1.ecn.purdue.edu/~aleix/aleix_face_DB.html
42. Padgett C, Cottrell GW (1998) A simple neural network models categorical perception of facial expressions. In: Proceedings of the 20th annual cognitive science conference. Madison, WI, pp 806–807
43. Edelman BE, Valentin D, Abdi H (1998) Sex classification of face areas: How well can a linear neural network predict human performance. J Biol Syst 6(3): 241–264

44. Cottrell GW, Fleming MK (1990) Face recognition using unsupervised feature extraction. In: International conference on neural networks, pp 322–325
45. Kohonen T (1977) Associative memory: A system theoretic approach. Springer, Berlin Heidelberg New York
46. Valentin D, Abdi H, O'Toole AJ (1994) Categorization and identification of human face images by neural networks: A review of the linear autoassociative and principal component approaches. J Biol Syst 2(3): 413–429
47. Oja E (1992) Principal components, minor components and linear neural networks. Neural Netw 5: 927–935
48. Chellappa R, Wilson CL, Sirohey S (1995) Human and machine recognition of faces: A survey. Proc IEEE 83: 705–740
49. Lin SH, Kung SY, Lin LJ (1997) Face recognition/detection by probabilistic decision based neural network. IEEE Trans Neural Netw 8(1): 114–132
50. Sexton R, Dorsey R, Sikander N (2004) Simultaneous optimization of neural network function and architecture algorithm. Decis Support Syst 36: 283–296
51. Sexton RS, Dorsey RE, Johnson JD (1998) Toward a global optimum for neural networks: A comparison of the genetic algorithm and backpropagation. Decis Support Syst 22: 171–185
52. Sexton RS, Sriram RS, Etheridge H (2003) Improving decision effectiveness of artificial neural networks – A modified genetic algorithm approach. Decis Sci 34(3): 421–442
53. Brahnam S, Sexton R, Slack MR (in review) Recognizing neonatial facial expressions of pain using a neural network simultaneous optimization algorithm
54. Sexton RS, Dorsey RE (2000) Reliable classification using neural networks: A genetic algorithm and backpropagation comparison. Decis Support Syst 30: 11–22
55. Heisele B, Ho P, Poggio T (2001) Face recognition with support vector machines: Global versus component-based approach. In: The eighth IEEE international conference on computer vision, Vancouver, pp 688–694
56. Moghaddam B, Yang M-H (2000) Gender classification with support vector machines. In: The sixth IEEE international conference on automatic face and gesture recognition, pp 306–311
57. Phillips PJ (1998) Support vector machines applied to face recognition. Adv Neural Inf Process Syst 11: 803–809
58. Guo G, Li SZ, Chan KL (2001) Support vector machines for face recognition. Image Vis Comput 19: 631–638
59. Ahmed N, Natarajan T, Rao KR (1972) On image processing and a discrete cosine transform. IEEE Trans Comp 23(1): 90–93
60. Pan Z, Rust A, Bolouri H (2000) Image redundancy reduction for neural network classification using discrete cosine transforms. In: International joint conference on neural networks. Como, Italy, pp 149–154
61. Kohir VV, Desai UB (2000) Face recognition. IEEE Int Symp Circ Syst 5: 305–308
62. Kosugi M (1995) Human-face search and location in a scene by multi-pyramid architecture for personal identification. Syst Comput Jpn 26(6): 27–38
63. Sirovich L, Kirby M (1987) Low dimensional procedure for the characterization of human faces. J Opt Soc Am 4(3): 519–524
64. Belhumeur P, Hespanha J, Kriegman D (1997) Eigenfaces vs. fisherfaces: Recognition using class specific linear projection. IEEE Trans PAMI 19(7): 711–720

65. Martinez AM, Kak AC (2001) Pca versus ldas. IEEE Trans PAMI 23(2): 228–233
66. Vapnik VN (1995) The nature of statistical learning theory. Springer, Berlin Heidelberg New York
67. Cristianini N, Shawe-Taylor J (2000) An introduction to support vector machines and other kernel-based learning methods. Cambridge University Press
68. The MathWorks (2000) Using matlab: The language of technical computing. The Mathworks, Inc., Natick, MA
69. van der Heijden F, Duin RPW, de Ridder D, Tax DMJ (2004) Classification, parameter estimation, and state estimation: An engineering approach using matlab. Wiley, Chichester
70. Grunau RVE, Johnston CC, Craig KD (1990) Neonatal facial and cry responses to invasive and non-invasive procedure. Pain 42(3): 295–305
71. Warnock F, Sandrin D (2004) Comprehensive description of newborn distress behavior in response to acute pain (newborn male circumcision). Pain 107(3): 242–255

Medical Education Interfaces Through Virtual Patients Based on Qualitative Simulation

Altion Simo and Marc Cavazza

Summary. Cardiac emergency is one field in medicine widely studied and very often experienced in reality. Furthermore, simulation and training issues on this field require sensitive and expensive techniques. In the following, we describe the development of a virtual human to be used for training applications in the field of cardiac emergencies. The system integrates Artificial Intelligence (AI) techniques for simulating medical conditions (shock states) with a realistic visual simulation of the patient in a 3D environment representing an emergency room (ER). It uses qualitative simulation of the cardiovascular system to generate clinical syndromes and simulate the consequences of the trainee's therapeutic interventions. The use of knowledge-based simulation provides a strong basis to integrate the behavioral aspects with the graphical appearance of a patient in the virtual ER. This also supports the creation of an emotional atmosphere. We describe how a subset of cardiac physiology can be modeled using the qualitative process theory and discuss knowledge representation issues. We then present results obtained by the proposed system and the benefits that can be derived from the use of a virtual patient in terms of training. Finally, we explore the problem of integrating multiple pathophysiological models for various aetiologies of shock states. This approach was demonstrated using medicine students who gained good experience which helped them in understanding and handling better these types of emergencies.

1 Introduction

Virtual humans are an important component of intelligent user interfaces. They can serve as intelligent assistants or instructors [1] or be part of complex simulations, where they play an important role for realistically accessing certain situations. In medical critical training applications, they also introduce a sense of emotional involvement. Virtual humans would constitute natural interfaces to knowledge-based systems, as virtual patients displaying the symptoms associated with a given pathology. Yet, not that much research has been dedicated to the integration of knowledge-based systems into 3D virtual patients. While there exist is a substantial amount of research aimed at

A. Simo and M. Cavazza: *Medical Education Interfaces Through Virtual Patients Based on Qualitative Simulation*, Studies in Computational Intelligence (SCI) **48**, 255–290 (2007)
www.springerlink.com

developing virtual patients for surgery, so far very little work has been dedicated to the use of virtual patients in clinical medicine. The main work on 3D virtual patients outside virtual surgery has been that of Badler et al. [2,3] who have described the use of an autonomous virtual human to simulate battlefield casualties in military simulations, however in the field of trauma rather than clinical medicine.

One major limitation of knowledge-based systems in medical education is that they focus on medical knowledge as an object, without putting it in a realistic diagnostic context. A related difficulty, which derives from the "dialog" model used in many systems, is to decide which amount of information should be introduced to the trainee at each step, and how to give a more active role to the trainee. These problems could be addressed by providing a realistic visualization of the clinical situation using a virtual patient in a virtual hospital context. Virtual patients in clinical medicine can be conceived of as visual interfaces to knowledge-based systems, simulating clinical situations from first principles. They offer the potential to embody the medical knowledge in a realistic context, supporting many forms of training and simulation.

The use of a 3D environment not only provides a realistic setting for the training process, but from a diagnostic perspective, creates a situation in which the user has to actively search for visual cues (e.g., clinical signs). In a similar fashion, if the environment contains medical equipment for diagnosis and treatment, the trainee can take initiative in a realistic setting, instead of simply responding to a prompt in the course of a system dialog. To further increase the reality, different visual elements can be used in making an effort of photorealistic representation.

This virtual patient for a specific area of medicine, like cardiac emergencies, uses qualitative simulation for modeling shock states in a virtual patient. Our interest in developing a virtual patient for clinical medicine is not only to provide a realistic tutoring environment, but as well to create an "ideal" interface to medical knowledge-based systems [4] that would be able to visualize clinical situations. The objective of the visualization of clinical situations through a virtual patient is thus to elicit an appropriate diagnostic and therapeutic process in the trainee.

In addition, since this system is targeted at training medical students in emergency decision-making, this is a rationale to try to convey emotional aspects as well, in this highly specific context (i.e., cardiac emergencies).

When showing how qualitative simulation can serve as a central principle for integration of the various aspects of the interface, we strongly emphasize the AI technique used to simulate the patient condition, i.e., qualitative simulation.

The structure of this research is organized as follows. First we try to position our research among other similar work in this area. After a brief reminder of the relations between qualitative simulation and "deep knowledge" and an overview of our system architecture, we describe the qualitative simulation method we have used to model shock states and discuss knowledge representation issues. We then present an extended example from the system, including the visualization of symptoms on the virtual patient. We conclude by discussing the integration of multisystem models around this qualitative model, in order to achieve more complex simulations. Evaluation considerations follow the conclusions drawn at the end.

2 Relation to Previous Work and Motivation

As already stated, virtual humans have been extensively described in Virtual Reality surgery [5] but little work has been dedicated to them in other areas of medicine, in particular clinical medicine, which requires physiological rather than just anatomical modeling.

Most research in virtual patients has actually been carried in this context, largely due to the importance of proper training in the subject and the added value for training of dramatic visual simulations [6, 7].

The above-mentioned Badler et al. work [2, 8, 9] have described the use of an autonomous virtual human to simulate battlefield casualties in military simulations. Their virtual human displays symptoms corresponding to the injuries suffered (Fig. 1) on the battlefield, while the trainee medic controlled by the user would attempt emergency treatment. However, there exist several important differences with our application.

We use physiological models as an "internal" model of the patient itself. This contrasts with the modeling of pathologies themselves through Parallel Transition Networks (PaTNets), which is more in line with causal networks in medicine, and provides a model of the pathology, not an internal model of the patient. For instance a PaTNet for a tension pneumotharax directly associates causes to symptoms and stores variable's evolution for treatment [8]. Using a physiological model provides a stronger integration at various levels of the system and better prospects for knowledge representation. In addition, the same principles are used to represent both normal and pathological cardiac function.

Further, visual appearance can be mapped to the internal model. Treatment can operate on the original model, rather than having a dedicated PaTNet or representation. Of course this is facilitated in our application by the fact that in clinical medicine (especially in cardiology) pathophysiological models relating to the normal function are easier to derive.

Finally, we adopted a first person rather than third-person viewpoint. This creates a stronger user involvement and emphasizes emotional aspects. It follows a setting more similar to [10] than to [9].

As a first step of ours in this direction, the applied research field encompasses a developed and matured environment in both qualitative physiology

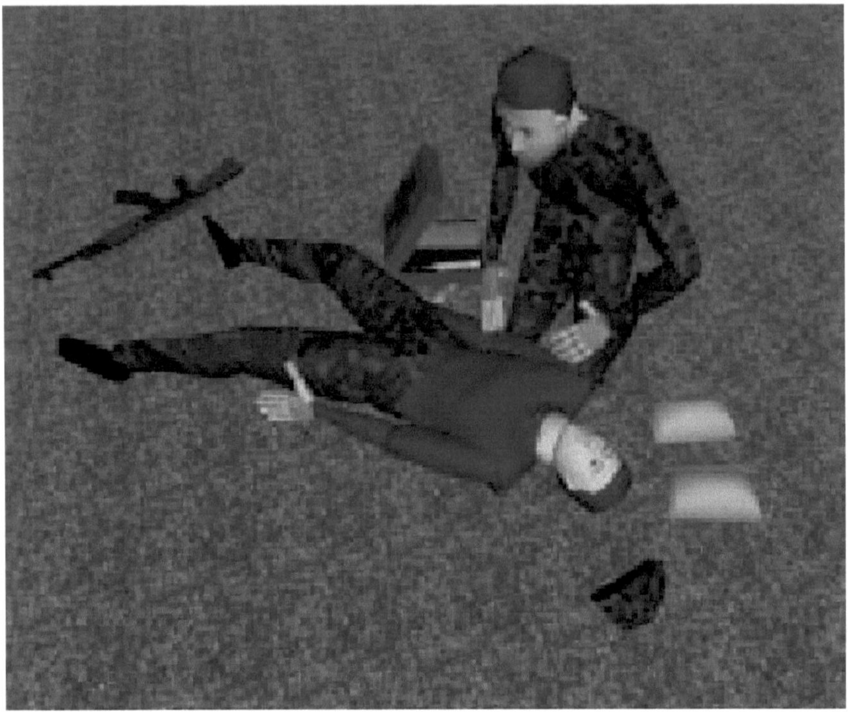

Fig. 1. Virtual human used by Badler et. al. in training applications

for different physiological and pathophysiological knowledge of the human body, and Virtual Reality elements fulfilling the role of visualization in Clinical Medicine. Our developed tools fully integrate deep medical knowledge in an enriched, interactive VR Environment aimed at clinical medicine emergencies, thus providing a novel approach to knowledge representation methods and training tools.

Virtual Reality has been and is being used successfully in several fields of the Medical Sciences. Serious Gaming is one of these successful cases that nowadays are effectively meeting the expectations in this field.

However, our approach is particularly relevant as an effective training tool in medical education. The aim of this research was not only to investigate the use of VR in this field, but also to develop the above interactive tools that can fully support the difficult and time-consuming process of medical education.

As most of the research involving VR in the medical field is done in the visualization of surgical and anatomical medicine, we have chosen the application of VR in an alternative field, that of training for the purposes of clinical medicine, and specifically, in the area of cardiac emergencies. We were aiming not only to have a good visualization of the patient's "internal" state but also to develop a tool which uses VR techniques to support the interactivity and the necessary emotional atmosphere related to the nature of the clinical medicine.

Following the previously conducted research, an experimental investigation was conducted to identify the use of the VR techniques for medical training purposes when treating the emergency problems in the field of clinical medicine. After limitations and current problems were identified, a novel framework was proposed based on Virtual Patients driven by qualitative simulations techniques, thus supporting a new generation of training tools based on pathophysiological reasoning and physiological models.

The rationale behind this new approach is that the integration of qualitative cardiovascular modeling into a virtual environment (VE) will support interactive emergency problem solving. Given the fact that the Artificial Intelligence (AI) layer can produce solutions that match in time the user's interactions, the integration of the AI techniques with real-time 3D VEs can support perfectly the building of training tools. The virtual emergency room (ER) is directly interfaced to the qualitative simulator, but this is far from a trivial solution as in the real medical context such practice might turn into an intractable problem.

Therefore, in order to reach a higher level of integration between the two components (AI and VE) we have found a balanced match with the nature of the trainee interaction model inside a medical related VR environment. Our new approach on this issue is described in details later on. As this solution is based in a real-time 3D graphic environment using an event-based approach, the user can generate and receive in real-time reconfigurations of the situations in a highly sensitive environment like the ER. More specifically in this event based approach, user interaction converted in real time interactions, corresponds to a well-defined scenario taking place in the cardiovascular qualitative simulator, which on the other hand reconfigures and shapes the occurring events in the VE.

The example of the cardiac shock scenario (shown later in the following sections) demonstrates the system behavior. In this context, after initiating the cardiac conditions by manipulating one of the state variables in the cardiovascular qualitative model, an emergency situation develops which asks to be solved (diagnosed and treated) by the trainee in the ER room. The implementation on this approach is described using a proposed example after fully explaining the mechanism beyond it and the finding of a solution (medical treatment) for this case (cardiac shock).

3 System Overview and Architecture

The system presents itself as a 3D environment featuring the virtual patient in an ER. Figure 2 gives an overview of the interface from the user's perspective (first person rendered view of the game). The user can thus see the virtual patient, whose appearance varies according to its clinical condition, as

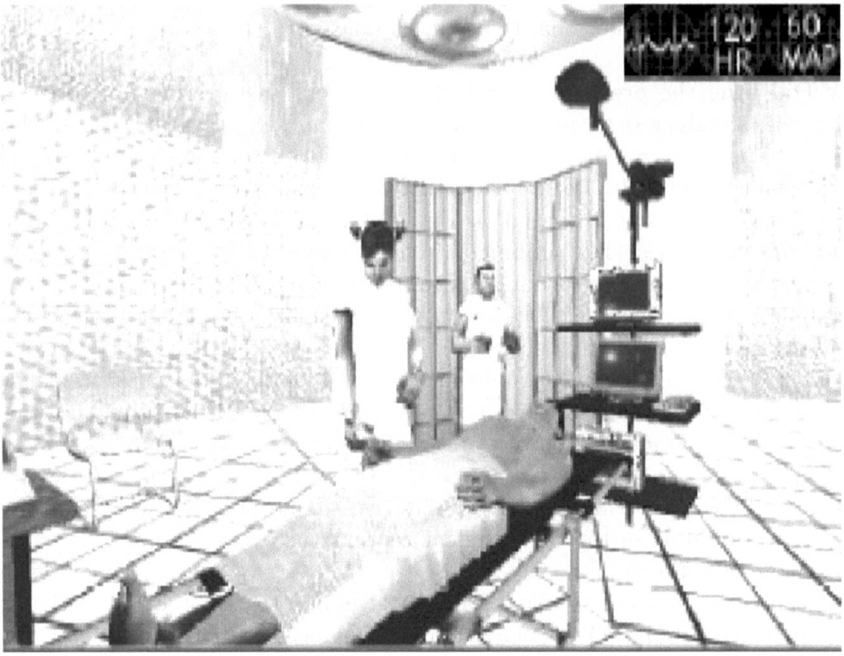

Fig. 2. System overview (user's viewpoint)

well as monitor vital parameters such as heart rate (HR) and mean arterial pressure (MAP). Other parameters are only accessible through specific complementary examination (for instance, pulmonary capillary pressure (PCap), via catheterization) and the trainee demand.

In spite of the virtual patient, the environment is populated with other autonomous agents representing ER nurses. These serve as interface agents, executing user's requests for diagnosis and treatment. The trainees' instructions are transmitted to the nurse using an optional speech recognition (in Japanese), based on a simple command language describing the potential actions and their parameters.

In the first instance, the system generates a clinical condition for the virtual patient. For instance, a cardiogenic shock will be simulated by altering variables such as inotropism (cardiac contractility, by primitively decreasing it), and to some extent other associated variables, such as those dealing with cardiac relaxation. From the initial alteration, the system propagates the consequences of the alteration by simulating various cycles of cardiac processes until a steady-state is reached. The simulation of the patient generates values for all physiological parameters and, as a consequence, provides the trainee with the relevant set of clinical symptoms.

In the virtual ER room (interfaced through the game engine), the trainee can carry out complementary examinations that will assist diagnosis. Finally, she/he will choose a treatment to be administered to the patient; the same

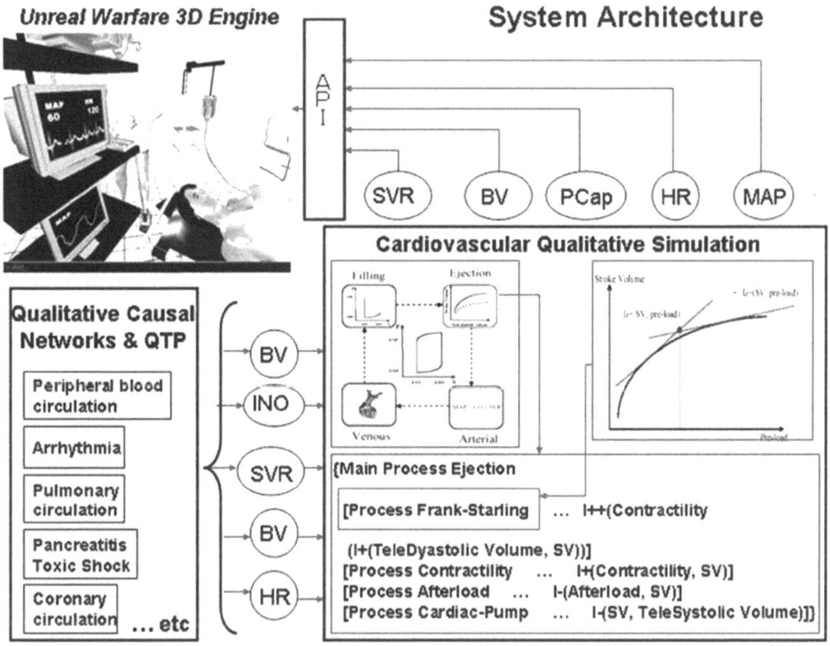

Fig. 3. A detailed view of the architecture for the core system in controlling the graphical and simulation modules

mechanisms will then simulate the impact of treatment and result in a new clinical appearance for the patient.

Figure 3 gives a detailed view on the system signal flows (and parameters that are often used) between the simulation module written in Lisp and the graphical module based on the game engine. It is also important to distinguish between parameters that were chosen for visualization, and other ones which are not visualized directly but nevertheless are important for the simulation. The most important parameters are systemic vascular resistance (SVR), blood volume, HR, MAP, PCap , while the physiological processes can vary from the description of the peripheral blood circulation to the coronary circulation. Also at that time pathological conditions like Arrhythmia, can be modeled. Causality can be interleaved with QTP and they can be finalized in a qualitative simulation package which treats most of the conditional states.

The graphical interface is developed using a state-of-the-art 3D game engine, Unreal Tournament^{TM} with the incorporated advanced Warfare engine, as a development environment [11].

The engine supports high quality graphics, as well as the animation of virtual characters, used for the patient and the nurses. Additionally, it includes an excellent development environment that supports the authoring of animations for virtual humans behavior, as well as various mechanisms (dynamic link libraries and socket-based inter-process communication) for integrating external software, such as the cardiac simulation module and the sound recognition package. Our software architecture is based on UDP socket communication between the 3D graphics engine and the qualitative simulation module, which has been developed in Allegro Common Lisp™. The UDP message format outputs selected physiological parameters to the graphic environment: those that are visible through the monitors and those that impact on the patient's appearance and behavior. These parameters are for instance MAP, HR, SVR, and PCap. In most of the cases, local processing in the form of scripted procedures is required to properly map a value into the graphical environment, e.g., a skin texture. So in conclusion, the set of parameters obtained is interpreted and displayed as clinical signs (e.g., pallor, enlarged jugular veins, etc.), as data on the monitoring devices (HR, MAP), or as results from complementary explorations (e.g., central venous line, Swan Ganz catheter).

All these visual elements can be updated throughout the simulation to reflect deterioration or an improvement of the patient's situation, after a treatment is introduced. The visual appearance of the patient, based on dynamic textures, can reflect a relevant range of shock situations (pallor, "warm shock," cyanosis, etc.). Figure 4 gives a brief description of the system interface and the way the user interacts with it. An actual screenshot of the system in

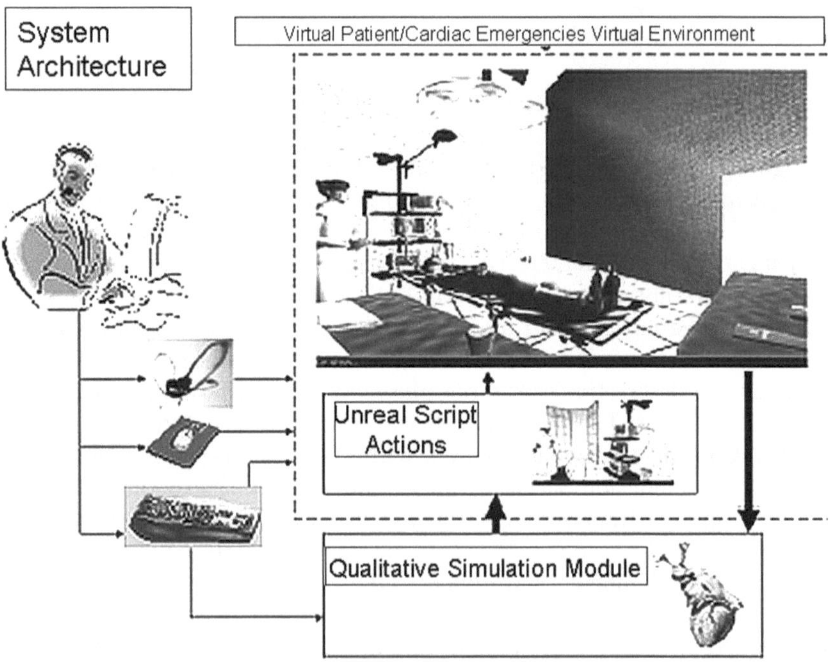

Fig. 4. System interface with respect to the user and its components

action is given toward the end in Sect. 8 where an evaluation discussion is taking place.

4 Qualitative Simulation of the Cardiovascular System

Qualitative simulation aims at modeling the behavior of the cardiovascular system both in normal and pathological circumstances. Cardiac dysfunctions are simulated using the same model with different initial conditions.

Qualitative simulation has been essentially developed for physical systems and mechanical devices [12] and is best known through work in qualitative physics. The main idea consists in reasoning on physical phenomena by abstracting physical descriptions. A pathophysiological model is a model explaining the dynamics of a disease on the basis of the normal behavior of an organ (e.g., heart, liver, etc.) or a physiological system (e.g., endocrine system, haematopoietic system, etc.) affected by that disease. It explicitly represents the dysfunction of the normal system behavior and is a common way to explain the causes and consequences of diseases in medical textbooks and literature [13].

Yet, the same techniques have been used to model physiological systems: for instance, the qualitative simulation (QSIM) approach [14] has been applied to the cardiovascular system by Kuipers as early as 1985 [15]. Pathophysiological models have been extensively used in medical knowledge-based systems as "deep knowledge," i.e., representations from which clinical situations could be generated from first principles rather than having to be encoded explicitly as rules [16]. These models can also be used to simulate the behavior of a physiological system [17–20].

To simulate a pathological process, a primitive variable is altered (e.g., cardiac contractility), and these changes are propagated through the whole system to provide an accurate and realistic description of its state under pathological conditions. The variables used in this context are "orders of magnitude" variables also referred to as qualitative variables (e.g., very low, low, normal, high, and very high). This is also in agreement with the presentation of pathophysiology in most textbooks, which is based on such variables, represented as "+" or "?."

Qualitative process theory (QPT) relies on processes representing the main transformations, encapsulating qualitative variables linked through influence equations. We have defined some 20+ processes corresponding to various physiological mechanisms, such as the determinants of ventricular filling (e.g., ventricular venous return, relaxation, and passive elastance) or ventricular ejection (effects of inotropism, preload, afterload, etc.) as well as various compensatory mechanisms (e.g., baroreceptors). These processes are encapsulated into four macroprocesses: ventricular filling, ventricular ejection, arterial system behavior, venous system behavior. In the course of the simulation, these four macroprocesses are activated in turn, in a way that reflects the cardiac

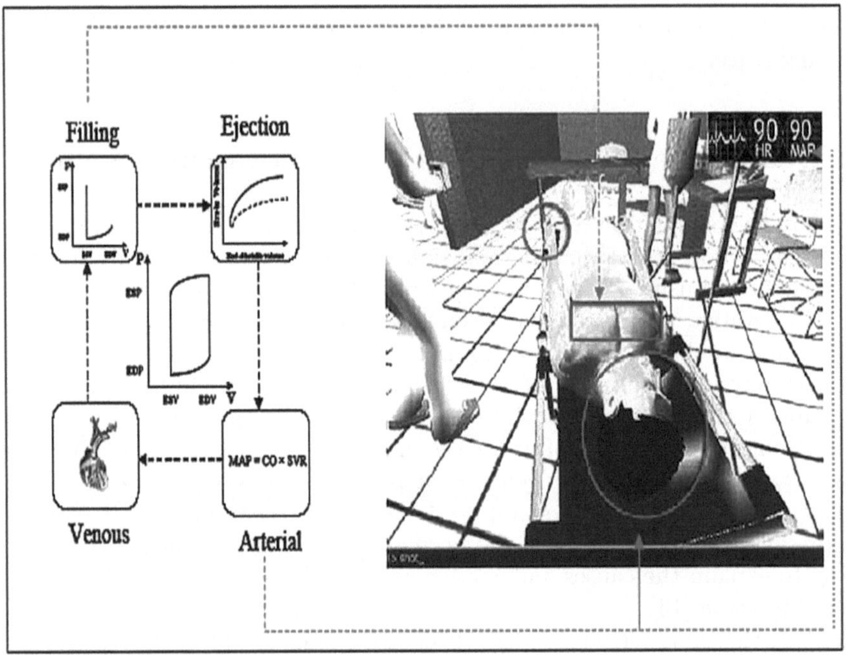

Fig. 5. The four cardiac macroprocesses, P–V curve and VP mapping considerations

cycle (the famous "P–V" curve of a closed process which represents the cardiac contraction cycle, shown in Fig. 5).

The variables we defined are directly adapted from actual qualitative variables used in the description of cardiocirculatory pathophysiology. Hence they can take any of nine values, from "↓↓↓↓" to "↑↑↑↑." Influence equations formalize the relations between variables in terms of their variation. For instance an influence equation such as I+(inotropism, SV) indicates that stroke volume (SV) increases with inotropism, while I–(afterload, SV) indicates that it decreases when afterload increases. Influence equations are generally assumed to be linear considering that they apply to a small set of qualitative values. However, we had to adapt the traditional notion of influence equation to the context of physiological laws, where influences are more complex.

The rationale for the use of qualitative approach in physiology is that numerical simulations of the cardiovascular systems are faced with many limitations: It is sometimes difficult to observe convergence of the set of equations that govern the system, manifesting a difficulty to integrate a large set of experimental equations obtained on subsystems. More importantly, numerical models often behave as black boxes, which make them difficult to interface with other software modules.

Another source of development of qualitative models in physiology was the search for deep knowledge representations for medical knowledge-based systems [21, 22]. These were developed to generate clinical situations from first principles, simplifying the development and maintenance of medical knowledge-based systems.

Our first approach in our research is cardiac emergencies, namely shock states, for which pathophysiological descriptions are readily available [23]. The pathophysiological simulation is based on QPT [14] adapted to the specificity of physiological processes. It is centered on the notion of process, which corresponds to an elementary physiological mechanism (e.g., ventricular filling).

Processes are associated qualitative variables (e.g., end diastolic volume (EDV)) related to each other via influence equations which determine causal links between variables and are used to propagate the consequences of a change in variables' values on other variables in the same process. In this way, the primitive alteration of some qualitative variables (that defines the underlying pathology) is propagated through the whole system.

Cardiology, especially blood pressure regulation, was one main area of application for qualitative modeling: Long [24] developed a causal network, and Kuipers adopted his QSIM approach to cardiac dynamics [15]. In his application, he used equations for cardiac output (CO) and blood pressure such as (1):

$$\text{Cardiac Output} = \text{Heart Rate} \times \text{Stroke Volume} \tag{1}$$

to create a constraint network, through which variable changes are propagated until a completely new state is generated. In his approach, the influence of parameters not part of equations was represented using the M+ operator (for monotonic function, for instance to represent the influence of inotropism on SV). However, physiological equations, unlike physical laws, do not map directly into the observed phenomena, hence they do not represent accurately the behavior of the cardiovascular system (let alone the causal implications). In particular, it is difficult to relate the time course of variable updating to the actual dynamics of the cardiovascular system. Like with causal networks, the dynamics of constraint propagation might not always reflect the actual system dynamics.

Widman [21] proposed another qualitative model of the circulatory system, using a more sophisticated description that emphasized structure/function relationships. In his model, the function of each component of the cardiovascular system is explicitly identified and causal relations link the various functions. For instance, cardiac ventricles are associated in this model to filling and ejection functions in the cardiac contraction cycle.

Since we are using a virtual human as an integrated interface to the simulation system, the latter should underlie a natural mapping between internal processes and the physical appearance of the virtual patient (Fig. 5), as we state at [25].

4.1 Qualitative Processes in the Circulatory System Physiology

As previously mentioned, Forbus has introduced QPT [14], which is centered on the identification of physical processes, within which the causal influence between variables is encapsulated. This approach is much closer to the description of physical phenomena themselves.

QPT has been successful to model complex mechanical devices. It has a real potential for modeling physiological systems as well. Due to the complexity of sub-systems, it is most difficult to derive a consistent set of confluence equations for such systems, which makes other qualitative approaches difficult to use. Besides, it is also necessary to capture a certain ordering of some physiological processes, such as the one that corresponds to the cardiac cycle.

Because physiological knowledge tends to be expressed through processes encapsulating physiological laws [13], the use of a process-based representation facilitates knowledge elicitation as well. The same model accounts for normal and pathological conditions: the latter corresponding to steady-states reached after alterations to normal values of physiological parameters.

The medical knowledge underlying the simulation of circulatory shock states is naturally formalized as physiopathological schemata in intensive care textbooks. The knowledge has been encoded from textbooks [23] descriptions under the supervision of specialized physicians who also participated in the testing of the first prototype (validation though simulation of the main shock states and their treatment). The development of this prototype has also been done in co-operation with consultants from the University of Gifu, School of Medicine.

For instance, Starling's law describes the relation between ventricular ejection and "preload" (the level of ventricular filling prior to contraction), this relation depending on cardiac contractility (inotropism) as well. Causal networks relating the three determinants of cardiac function (contractility, preload, afterload) fail to capture the interrelations between the various determinants [19]. On the other hand, complex inter-relations can be captured in a process-based representation.

The qualitative influence relations are derived from the shape of the curve of Starling's law, and they are used to propagate variable changes as part of the qualitative simulation cycle (which is actually similar to a Pressure–Volume curve in thermodynamics).

The qualitative translation gives two levels of influence depending on the segment of the curve. This can be represented by maintaining two separate influence equations for each segment of the Starling curve, the influence equation to be used being determined by a threshold value of the preload. The threshold value itself depending on inotropism, this representation integrates all influences.

The four corresponding macroprocesses (Figs. 5 and 8) around which the simulation is built comprise the ventricular filling, ventricular ejection, arterial system behavior, and venous system behavior. These processes naturally model the circulatory system, thus introducing an element of structure/function relationship. During a simulation, the four processes are activated in turn, thus reproducing the cardiac cycle. Various cycles of simulation are performed until all qualitative variables reach a steady value. Each macroprocess encapsulates lower-level processes corresponding to elementary physiological phenomena, described by physiological laws (there are some 25 or more processes) [4].

For instance, Frank–Starling's law (Figs. 6 and 7) describes the relation between ventricular ejection and "preload" (the level of ventricular filling prior to contraction), this relation depending on cardiac contractility (inotropism) as well.

The failure of the causal networks to relate the three well-known determinants of cardiac function (contractility, preload, afterload) with respect to different inter-relations between the various corresponding determinants is overcome through some modifications.

One modification consists in including coefficients for the influence relation, which can be modified dynamically to take into account that influence relations can change under different circumstances. For instance the influence of afterload on SV is more important when inotropism is low.

The coefficient used in the influence equation I–(afterload, SV) will dynamically reflect that. A single physiological law may be represented by more than one influence equation. The qualitative translation gives two levels of influence depending on the segment of the curve for the Frank–Starling's law (Fig. 7). This can be represented by maintaining two separate influence equations for each segment of the Frank–Starling curve, the influence equation to be used being determined by a threshold value of the preload. I1+(preload, SV) and I2+(preload, SV), which have different influence coefficients.

[Process *Frank-Starling*

I+(Ino, EDV_{lim})

if EDV > EDV_{lim}

$\alpha = \alpha 1$ else $\alpha = \alpha 2$

I+(α, (EDV, δ-SV))]

Fig. 6. Frank–Starling law mathematics, related to the graph in Fig. 7

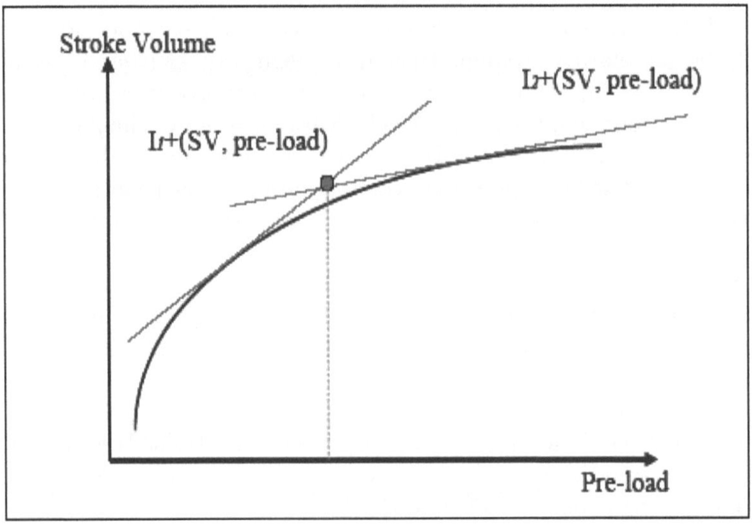

Fig. 7. The Frank–Starling law presented graphically, and the corresponding approaching lines for each curve

The transition point between these two influence equations, i.e., the pre-load value for which the increase of SV is less significant is dynamically computed at each cycle as a function of the inotropic state (the computation is itself a qualitative influence).

As a result, if we consider the determinants of cardiac ejection (whose output is represented by SV), two out of the three influence equations I+(preload, SV), I+(inotropism, SV), I−(afterload, SV) actually use extensions to the original theory to take into account the complex relations between determinants, a phenomenon that is difficult to capture with, for example, standard causal networks.

Overall, our model includes 25 primitive parameters, which account for the main physiological variables: SV, end systolic pressure (ESP) and volume, end diastolic pressure (EDP) and volume, PCap, SVR, inotropism, etc. Each process operates on average on 3 parameters and contains several influence equations. A few more parameters account for system properties that have not been modeled at a finer level of granularity, such as "left atrium function," or "ventricular geometry" (the latter being part of computation of the afterload).

In addition, there are internal variables to the system, through which it is possible to integrate the effects of several influences throughout the cardiac cycles (for instance, the variation in SV).

Temporal aspects are also easier to represent in a process-based approach than with confluence or constraint equations. They are "implicitly" part of the cycle through which the processes are invoked, though this does not address the problem of timescales.

For instance, if we consider the example of a blood loss situation, the first process affected is venous return, which impacts on ventricular filling, then ejection, and finally the arterial system, causing a fall in MAP and triggering short-term mechanisms for maintaining arterial pressure (baroreceptors).

One thing worth mentioning is that the four main processes accounted for the above functionality in circulatory dynamics, venous return, ventricular filling, ventricular contraction, and arterial system behavior (Fig. 5), represent in groups vital cardiac function and the behavior of the arterial and venous system, unlike Widman's model [21].

At each sublevel, we have identified key physiological processes and described relations between qualitative variables involved in these processes, through influence equations inspired from QPT. It is important that we work on orders of magnitude of parameter variation rather than with their absolute value because each of these processes involves a sequence of subprocesses. For instance, ventricular contraction involves subprocesses for ejection, Starling's law, and the effects of afterload.

Influences can be embedded in the description of processes. For instance, the effect of cardiac frequency on ventricular filling (ventricular filling decreases when cardiac frequency is high) can be embedded in one of its subprocesses. Following is some pseudocode for a qualitative process and then one of the methods calculating variations. We can see here clearly how encapsulation happens in this case. Since this simulation part was implemented in Lisp Allegro programming language, it is easier to understand for those who are familiar with this language

```
{Main Process Ejection

[Process Frank-Starling
(...)
I++(Contractility (I+(TeleDyastolic Volume, SV))]

[Process Contractility
(...)
I+(Contractility, SV) ]

[Process Afterload
(...)
I−(Afterload, SV)]

[Process Cardiac-Pump
(...)
I−(SV, TeleSystolic Volume)] }
```

```
(defun Starling ()
"Method enforcing Starling's law "
(let* ((d-EDV (physio_var-variation VTD))
       (EDV (physio_var-value VTD))
       (old-EDV (– EDV d-EDV))
       (p (calcul_p)))
       (unless (= d–EDV 0)
       (cond ((and (>= EDV p) (>= old-EDV p)) nil)
       ((and (<= EDV p) (<= old-EDV p))
(let ((delta (– EDV old-EDV))) (set-DVS delta)))
       ((and (<= EDV p) (>= old-EDV p))
(let ((delta (– EDV p)))
       (set-DVS delta)))
       ((and (>= EDV p) (<= old-EDV p))
(let ((delta (– p old-EDV)))
       (set-DVS delta)))))))
```

Processes can also represent compensatory mechanisms (such as baroreceptors), which are triggered under specific circumstances and play a role in the short-term regulation of arterial pressure.

The described subprocesses, include regulatory mechanisms [26]. A typical process involves between 3 and 7 physiological parameters, taking into account that in some cases both the parameter value and its variation can be required. In addition, embedded procedures are computing key values such as CO and MAP using simple equations (Fig. 8). However, unlike in [15], these equations are not used as actual representations.

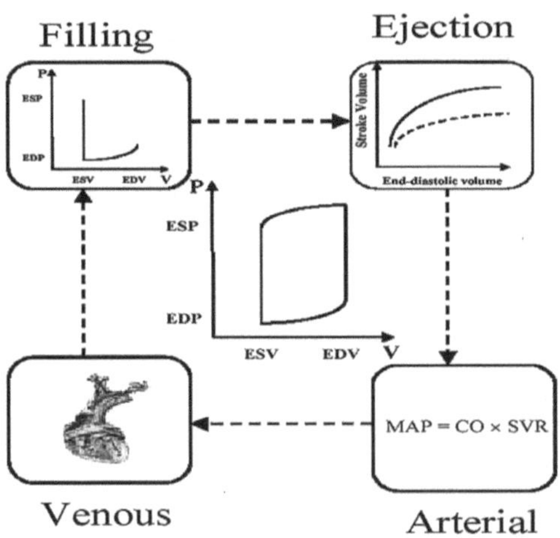

Fig. 8. The cycle of macroprocesses and their relations (the P–V curve)

Figure 8, with its four processes, embodies the closed cyclic P–V curve, which is marked by the values of end systolic volume (ESV), EDV, ESP, EDP.

The arterial process can simply be represented when calculating the MAP as a product of CO, and SVR.

The venous process refers to venous return, while filling as a process is defined again from ESV, EDV, ESP, EDP with the respective P–V curve.

The last process, Ejection, referring to ejection fraction, is the fraction of the EDV ejected at each heart beat and is calculated as the product of SV and the inverse of EDV. It varies according to different factors.

Temporal aspects are also easier to represent in a process-based approach than in one using confluence or constraint equations. For instance, if we consider the example of a blood loss, the first process affected is venous return, which impacts on ventricular filling, then ejection and finally the arterial system, causing a fall in MAP and triggering short-term mechanisms for maintaining arterial pressure (baroreceptors).

The processes are activated as a cycle in the program. Each process is attached to a set of methods corresponding to the influence part of traditional QPT. The postconditions of some processes behave as the preconditions of the next process: in other words, some processes create parameter variations that act as an input for subsequent processes. For instance, cardiac contraction sets the value of the SV, which is a determinant of arterial pressure in the arterial system process, and so on. Hence the updating of variables and propagation of influences follows the structural and temporal cycle of the cardiocirculatory system.

As the virtual patient is developed for educational and training purposes, simulating the effects of therapeutics should be an important part of it. In the context of cardiac shock, a variety of medical treatments is made available: beta-agonists (such as dobutamine), alpha-agonists (norepinephrine or high-dose dopamine), arterial vasodilators, venous vasodilators, mixed vasodilators, adrenaline, fluid infusion, and others.

The effects of the correct therapeutic, beta-agonist are also shown in Fig. 9.

Each drug targets one or more primitive parameters of the simulation accounting for its effects and side effects. For instance, beta-agonists increase inotropism, but also HR. In addition, these effects are dose-dependent and several doses are available: low, moderate, high. This is useful for combined treatments (e.g., Beta-agonists + vasodilators) and also for exploratory treatment (e.g., careful volume expansion).

Some target effects are shown on Table 1. The effects of medical treatment are simulated by modifying the corresponding target variables on the pathophysiological model obtained from the first simulation and running the qualitative simulation again until a new steady-state is obtained, which corresponds to the effects of the therapy in that context. Multiple therapies (e.g., beta-agonists with vasodilators) can be selected. The effects of therapeutics

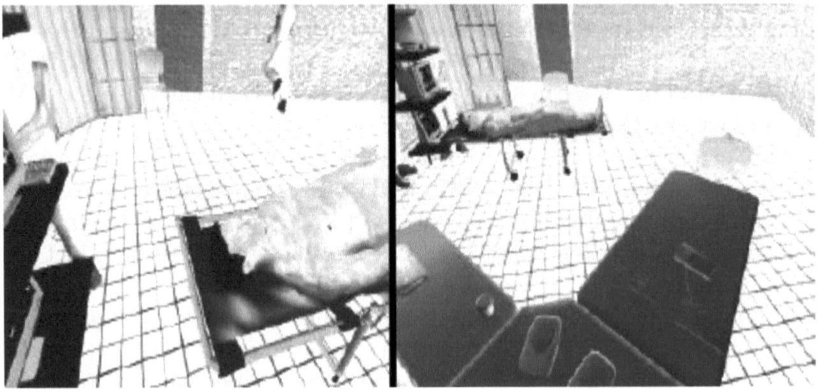

Fig. 9. Changes in the graphical interface before and after application of therapeutics (from *left* to *right*) seen through different viewpoints of the user

Table 1. Target parameters of some common treatments

treatment	target parameter
IV Fluids	blood volume
B−agonist inotropism	HR (heart rate)
vasolidator	SVR (↓)
norepinephrine	SVR (↑)

are simulated in a similar fashion in the graphics (Fig. 9). From the steady-state obtained by simulating cardiogenic shock above, the system is run again after taking into account the modifications introduced by the therapeutic course selected.

They restore inotropism, ejection, and a MAP closer to normal but still low. HR remains high in the acute context and due to the side effect of the drug itself. End-diastolic pressure and PCap decrease. Arterial vasodilators, used alone, improve ejection by decreasing the afterload. The effect of a variation of afterload is greater on a failing heart (when the right treatment is not introduced).

This increases CO but because SVR are decreased, it fails to restore MAP. Finally, isolated fluid expansion initially increases ventricular venous return, but due to a low SV, only contributes to a dangerous elevation of filling pressures and PCap, while CO remains low. This triggers various clinical signs in the patient, such as changes in respiratory rate (onset of pulmonary edema) and under certain circumstances, distension of the jugular veins (Fig. 10). Also in some cases, because this is likely to trigger pulmonary oedema, the breathing animations will be modified to follow a pattern of faster, superficial breathing, reflecting the dyspnoea accompanying pulmonary oedema.

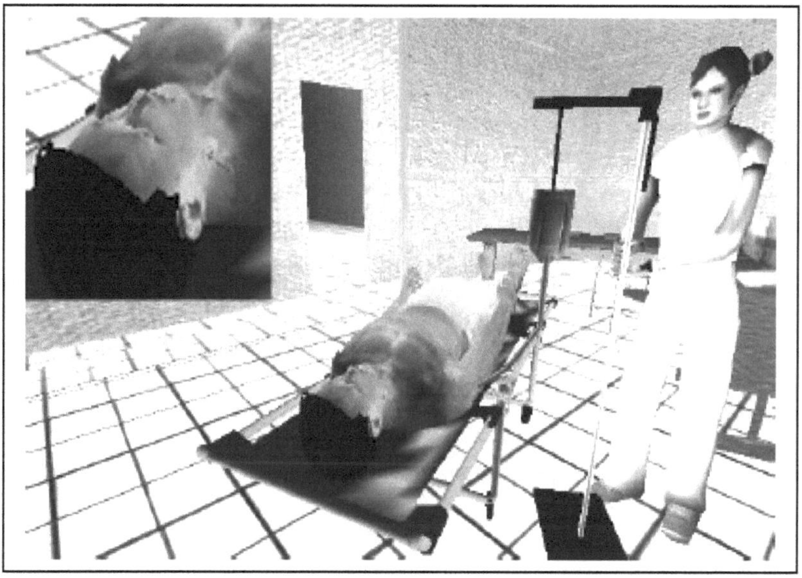

Fig. 10. A visible extended jugular vein situation in a close up of the patient's neck

5 Graphics and Animations: The Interface

The graphic presentation of the interface aims at recreating a realistic environment, which is displayed in a first-person view to the user for maximum involvement.

The system supports different forms of user interaction. The user is allowed to navigate in the virtual environment to observe the patient from various angles (this might be required to observe breathing patterns for instance). It also forces the trainee to actively observe symptoms without having to exaggerate these.

The interface constantly displays vital parameters (HR and MAP) through the usual monitoring devices. Additional investigations can be carried out by instructing nurses: for instance, the user can ask for a reading of PCap, or enquire about patient's diuresis (another parameter whose value qualifies the shock state). The same mechanism applies for selecting a drug therapy. All instructions to the nurses can be issued via an interface menu or, more realistically, by using a speech recognition system.

5.1 Mapping Simulation Parameters into Animations

As the qualitative simulation system corresponds to the virtual patient's physiology, this facilitates a natural mapping between the simulation's results and the patient's appearance. This mapping also applied to the effect of therapeutic drugs, which can be translated directly in terms of the physiological parameters targeted by these drugs (for instance, inotropism or SVR.

The system uses Unreal's dynamic textures to create a realistic appearance: these textures have been edited from real photographs obtained from medical teaching material. For instance, when a shock state appears, the texture will be shifted to pale, sweaty skin for the face. The face texture is under control of MAP mainly, while limb textures are selected using the MAP and SVR parameters.

It is also possible to trigger animations (or modify the "idle animations" of the virtual human) as a function of the overall gravity of the patient's condition (for instance, using the actual level of MAP to qualify the seriousness of the shock state). For associated symptoms, such as dyspnea associated with pulmonary edema, a specific animation can be triggered whenever PCap goes beyond a given threshold, showing the modified breathing pattern. Figure 11 shows various patients' appearances: right-hand side, normal appearance, left-hand side, extremities cyanosis.

The main idea behind virtual patients is that their appearance and behavior should be determined by the pathophysiological models simulating the course of disease. The trainee will have to actively observe the patient to observe clinical signs, which can be used for diagnosis as well as assessing the gravity of the situation. Visually accessible signs can be decomposed into functional signs and inspection signs [3].

Functional signs are related to the patients' behavior and can be simulated using appropriate animations (e.g., for shortness of breath). Patient behavior comprises functional signs such as the level of consciousness and spontaneous movements, pain, and breathing patterns, etc (Fig. 12). Mapping the results of

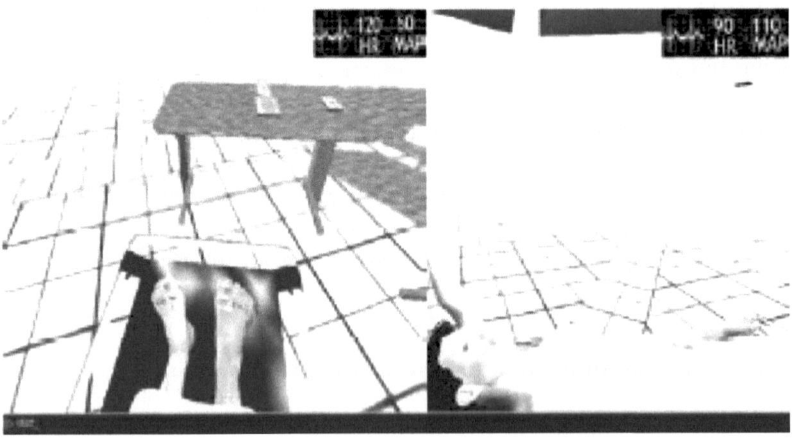

Fig. 11. Patient's appearance in pathological (extremities cyanosis) and normal state (*right*)

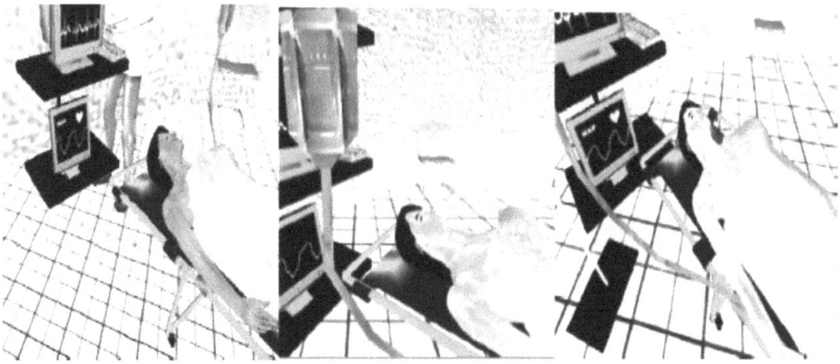

Fig. 12. Functional and inspection signs mapped onto the virtual Patient

the cardiac simulation to these signs involves simple inference from parameter values to the patient reaction.

For instance, as CO decreases so does cerebral perfusion: low CO values can thus be mapped to patient consciousness in the form of changing animations.

Very high ventricular filling pressures result in elevated PCap, which can trigger cardiac edema, manifesting itself in the patient through altered breathing animation patterns.

Inspection signs are symptoms directly visible on the patients, such as sweat, edema, cyanosis, pallor, rashes, etc (Fig. 12). These can be simulated using various forms of dynamic textures (supported by the Unreal^{TM} visualization engine) on the basis of the patient's state as obtained by the pathophysiological simulation. Skin tones depend on peripheral perfusion. Hence, vasodilation (decreased SVR) is accompanied by redness, while vasoconstriction results in intense pallor. The value of the SVR parameter is thus mapped to dynamic textures shifting between various skin appearances (Fig. 12). Additional skin tones are implemented using commercial image processing packages in order to help the diagnosis of certain shock syndromes when they occur (rashes, purpura).

In addition, in the case of Emergency Medicine and Critical Care, *monitoring devices* shown in the above figure visualize in real-time vital physiological parameters, such as HR and MAP. The simulation will give direct access to these parameters by mapping the simulation's variables to preset range values for HR and MAP. Other elements of visualization include EKG curves and blood pressure curves.

Functional signs are thus essentially related to patient animations, such as:

- Head nodding in expression of pain or discomfort
- Hands moving in expression of discomfort
- Antalgic positions (e.g., abdominal pain)
- Spontaneous movements and changes in position
- Breathing rhythm and amplitude

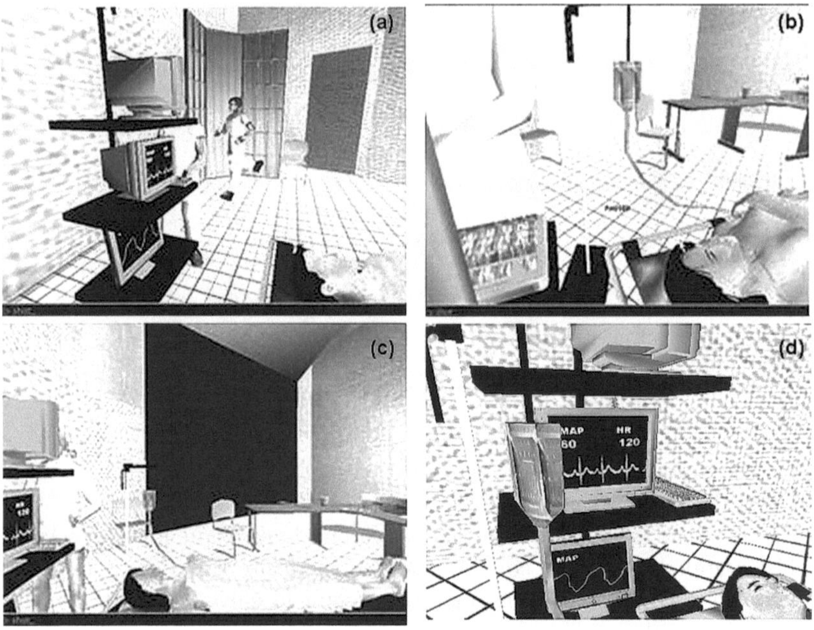

Fig. 13. Clinical signs as part of the overall atmosphere, needed to be discovered by the trainee **(a)** pallor, **(b)** a skin rash situation, **(c)** warm shock, **(d)** normal state

Perhaps the most significant aspect of visualization, as far as diagnosis is concerned, is that of physical signs. The physical signs of shock are well described, and even though many of them are not specific they are important in this context to assess the overall gravity. Several examples of clinical signs are represented on Fig. 13 with the patient in the ER room.

5.2 Emotional Aspects of the Interface

A realistic simulation should render the atmosphere and tension created by the critical nature of the situation. There are several factors that contribute to emotional communication in such a situated context.

The first one is the overall visual realism of the environment as we already have emphasized [27], including its complexity, appearance, lightning, multiple actions and disturbances, background sounds and noises. This recreates the original atmosphere and, unlike some traditional training systems, sometimes requires active exploration of the environment from the trainee to acquire information (for instance, a monitor may not be visible from a given perspective, or a nurse would stand in front of it).

The character's appearance is the second element and the most direct manifestation of the gravity of the situation. In addition to the clinical signs of gravity (e.g., cyanosis or dyspnea, described above), we have implemented behavioral scripts governing spontaneous movements and reactivity (indicating e.g., loss of consciousness, pain, etc.). The latter elements are loosely connected with diagnosis, but play an important role in creating emotional tension and the sense of a grave situation.

The third one is constituted by the additional characters, in this case the nurses. They can be used to give nonverbal feedback on the situation and on the user's decisions, or lack of decisions. This can take place as nonverbal behavior, but is mostly reflected through situated behavior, i.e., the manner in which the nurses will react to the user or carry out their activities. This is implemented by using parameterized models of such activities, tuned in real-time to the gravity of the overall situation. This also follows recent work showing how virtual characters' attitudes could convey emotional content [28].

5.3 Visualization Requirements for the Virtual Patient

Producing a believable virtual patient as presented above requires that relevant symptomatology be reproduced by the system. Various levels of symptoms are commonly distinguished in clinical practice: functional signs, inspection signs, and clinical signs. We already discussed the functional signs as patients' behavior and inspection signs as symptoms. The trainee will have to actively visually observe the patient to distinguish such signs, which can be used for diagnosis as well as assessing the gravity of the situation. Clinical signs are accessible through physical examination only, such as auscultation, palpation of the liver, etc. They would have to be implemented mainly as animations producing an audible or visible result (as there is no haptic feedback): trainee's attention might as well be focused on information provided by monitoring devices or nurses' actions.

In the case of Emergency Medicine and Critical Care, monitoring devices visualize in real-time vital physiological parameters, such as HR and MAP. Physiological parameters that can be classified in three categories:

- Those accessible to clinical measurement. The simulation will give direct access to these parameters by mapping the simulation's variables to preset range values for HR and MAP. Other elements of visualization include EKG curves and pressure curves.
- Those accessible to specific exploration, such as CO or SVR. Such diagnostic procedures (e.g., Swan Ganz catheterization) have to be specifically requested by the trainee and as a result a corresponding animation can be played finally producing the relevant values on a monitor.
- Internal parameters obtained from research in physiology (in laboratory conditions on animal models) but not accessible in routine clinical practice (e.g., ventricular relaxation). The latter cannot be visualized during simulations but can take part in an explanatory process (which rather constitutes a virtual "postmortem" as we already mentioned, but very important in the context of training applications).

6 Integrated Example

Our main goal was that the results provided by the system in terms of the main physiological parameters (MAP, HR, CO, SV, EDV, EDP, etc.) are consistent with the traditional description of these syndromes in the literature, though they are all generated through a complex cycle of simulation.

The actual prototype of the system, integrating all the above features, has been fully implemented. In this section, we describe into more detail a running example from the system, which shows the level of integration achieved between the graphics and the qualitative simulation.

The short-term adaptation to an increase in afterload, to the increase of intrathoracic pressure due to artificial ventilation, acute tachycardia, atrial fibrillation, etc can be observed. These have provided additional validation for the model and can be used to generate more training cases, alone or in combination with acute heart failure.

6.1 Initial Conditions and Simulation

This example is a simulation of cardiogenic shock. This condition can be simulated by primitively decreasing the value of the inotropism parameter, which represents cardiac contractility (and hence cardiac function). The primitive decrease in inotropism starts a cascade of events that is accurately reflected in the simulation of the various physiological processes. Namely, the decrease in inotropism alters SV, and in turn CO and MAP.

Compensatory mechanisms, such as baroreceptors, are triggered, but fail to compensate for the fall in blood pressure. By primitively decreasing the value of the inotropism parameter, we affect the intensity of cardiac contraction. The first process activated is the ejection process (as the site of the inotropism parameter). The main output variable for this process is the SV. The primitive decrease in inotropism causes a decrease in SV of the same order of magnitude. As a consequence, the ESV increases (ESV is updated by a process computing the "mechanical" aspects of the ventricle). The next active process consists in the arterial system, where values of CO and MAP, are computed using the classical equations. In addition, the baroreceptor process reacts to a fall of MAP, triggering an immediate increase in HR, SVR, and venous tone (VT). After the arterial system, the venous system macroprocess is triggered, which contains several processes computing venous return.

The most important influence here is that increased VT (in response to the activation of baroreceptors) increases ventricular venous return. The last process of the cycle is ventricular filling. This one is simplified in our model, which is mostly a left ventricle model, where the role of the right ventricle is part of a coarser model (not modeling specifically right ventricle contraction and pulmonary circulation). Here, ventricular filling is moderately increased by increased venous return due to increased VT: I+(VT, preload). More importantly, this process integrates the variations in ventricular volume.

The (previous) increase in ESV added to the slight increase in venous return causes the EDV to increase.

This example is an important illustration of the integration of effects throughout the cardiac cycle, which enables the integration of multiple dependencies as well as taking into account some dynamic aspects. The second cycle of simulation activates again the ejection process under the new conditions that result from short-term adaptive mechanisms, in particular the variation in preload. However, the increase in preload fails in improving the SV significantly as the influence I+(preload, SV) depends on the levels of inotropism, which is primitively decreased. Hence the qualitative value of SV remains low. Then the arterial system process is triggered again, and the calculations take into account the updated HR and SVR values (as modified by the compensatory mechanisms). The increase in SVR fails to restore MAP for severe alterations of inotropism, just like the increase in HR fails to restore CO.

The system reaches a new equilibrium with a significant drop in MAP and high cardiac frequency. The set of physiological parameters can be mapped onto the patient representation and the monitoring devices: the patient is pale and sweating (low perfusion, vasoconstriction, and sympathic response), his consciousness is modified and the monitoring devices show a low MAP and high HR.

However the full set of physiological parameters is not always visible to the trainee, to reflect the difference between the physiological parameters that have a clinical translation, and those which can be measured by extra investigations (such as PCap or CO) and those inaccessible to examination, and that is part of a pathophysiological 'a posteriori' explanation.

The system finally maps those physiological parameters that have a clinical translation to the virtual patient's appearance. Again, for example, peripheral vasoconstriction will result in pallor and cold extremities, etc., while a prolonged or severe shock state could also result in cyanosis. Depending on the severity of global cardiac dysfunction and the corresponding central venous pressure, jugular veins might become enlarged in the patient.

This state can be difficult to distinguish from other causes of shock on observation alone, which is precisely the purpose of such a training system. Figure 14 shows the specific patient appearance for cardiogenic shock in the current 3D interface and after the right treatment. This is further discussed in Sect. 6.2.

6.2 Choice of Therapeutics and Further Simulation

Once the simulation has reached a steady-state, one of the nurses will prompt the trainee to order a treatment. The system is actually developed as a realistic simulation, in which the user has to directly treat the patient and observe the consequences (Fig. 14), rather than a traditional instructional system in which she/he would first be asked for a diagnosis. The user has a choice between eight major (medical) therapeutics, some of which can be given in association.

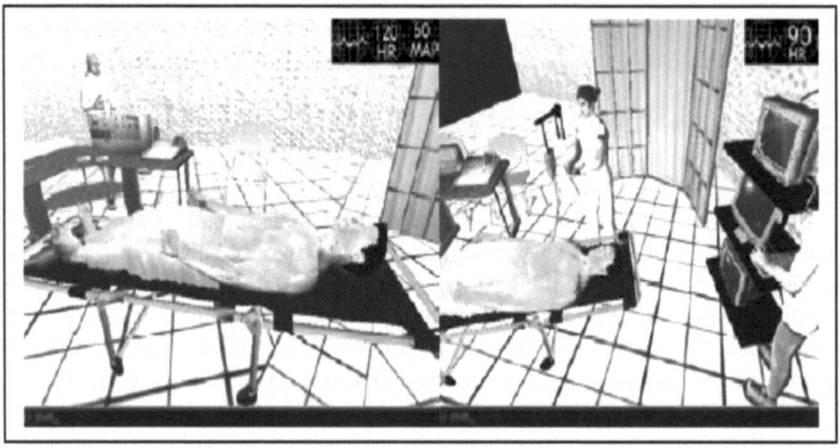

Fig. 14. From left to right: Cardiogenic shock and its final treated situation

A dosage can also be associated to the therapeutic course chosen; for instance, fluid expansion can be conservative or more aggressive, or beta agonists (such as dobutamine) can be given in various dosages.

As we have seen, the effects of therapeutic drugs are simulated by altering the physiological parameters that are targets for the drugs actions: for instance, beta-agonists will increase inotropism (with a side effect of increasing HR as well) and fluid expansion directly increases blood volume. This mechanism is similar to the one for generating the clinical syndrome, and is realistic from a physiological standpoint.

In the above cardiac shock example (Fig. 14), we have selected two courses of action depending on whether the user chooses a correct or a wrong treatment.

Faced with primitive cardiac failure (whatever its aetiology) the appropriate pharmacological treatment at the acute phase consists in administering beta-agonists, which restore inotropism. The qualitative simulation module, starting from the current status (and corresponding values of physiological parameters) simulates another set of cardiac cycles with an increased value for inotropism. This will restore the cardiac contraction process, raising CO, and restoring MAP (a variable for the arterial system process) to a still low, but less life-threatening value. As part of its side effects, the drug maintains an increased HR. In turn, patient appearance is also modified to reflect the improvement.

If failure of the cardiac pump is the main cause of shock, increasing blood volume by fluid expansion will not restore arterial pressure; even worse, it would cause a fluid overload leading to a life-threatening pulmonary edema. When the PCap raises below a certain threshold this tends to cause pulmonary edema (i.e., lungs alveoli are filled with water, preventing normal pulmonary function). In the absence of an accurate modeling of the respiratory system, the patient's breathing pattern is directly altered when PCap raises above a threshold, and corresponding animations are triggered. Needless to say, breathing rhythm is a powerful indicator in the creation of an emotional tension, though this has not been much explored in nonverbal behavior.

The choice of wrong therapeutics course together with possible aggravation of the patient status will also induce adverse behavior from the nurse. The red, yellow, and blue circulated parts in the graphics show the zones where the trainee can look for signs on the VP, in spite of all the above discussed issues.

So in Fig. 15, according to the ordered numbers of the shots, a full scenario of the simulation is given (detection of the shock status and its treatment until

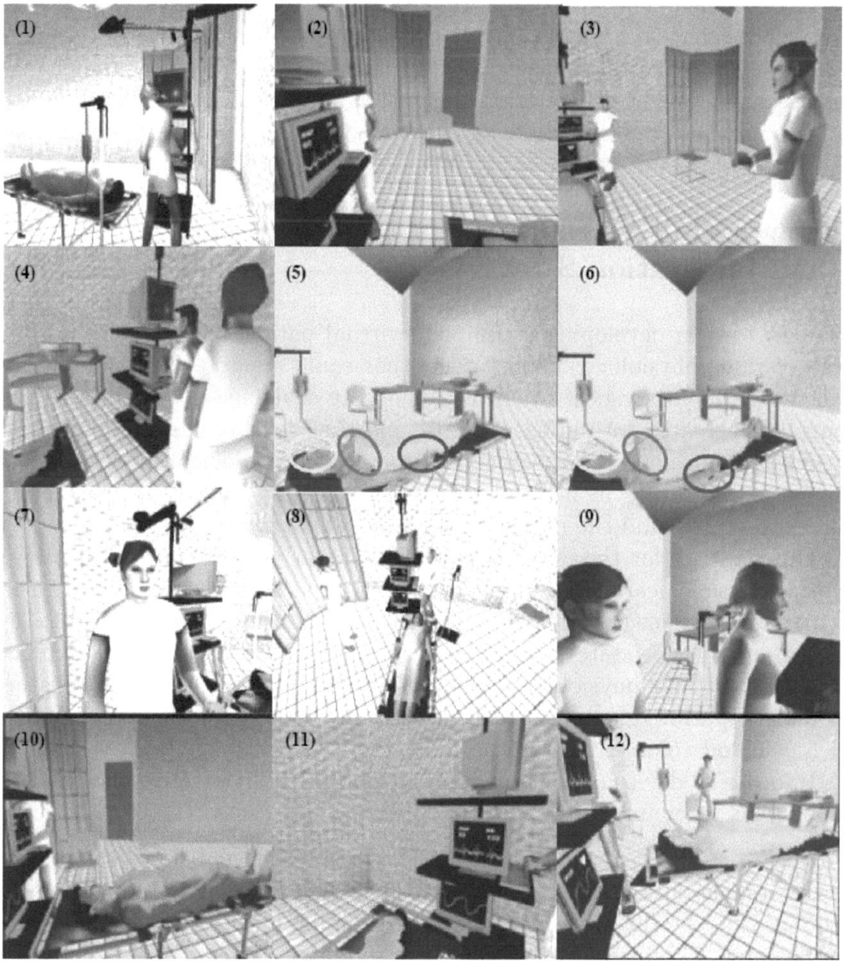

Fig. 15. A series of captured shots from different moments during the simulated scenario

the patient comes to a stable state). After entering the virtual environment (1) presented by the game level, the trainee tries to assess the situation. By reading the monitors (2) the trainee tries to better understand the case he is dealing with. Also by approaching nurses (3, 4) he/she tries to gain some more information if necessary. Then by observing the virtual patient (5, 6) different signs can confirm the hypothesis and clarify the situation. Extra information is introduced by facing and asking the nurses, which according to the case, have their bits and pieces of information to be presented (7–9).

The trainee can assess in spite of the detailed information/situation as well as the overall look of the room and before making his decision of treatment (10). Then once a decision is made and a treatment is administered the trainee can see the progress of its treatment (given the fact that it was the right treatment). The situation of the virtual patient can be accessed (11, 12) through the signs and the reading on the monitors. This constitutes the end of a successful simulation. In the case of an unsuccessful treatment the changes that take place show the deterioration of the patient and if no proper actions are taken in the course of time, an eventual death of the patient will happen.

7 Toward full Virtual Patients: Development and Integration Strategy

The key idea in developing a complete virtual patient is to be able to integrate various physiological subsystems that could support the modeling of a wide range of pathological situations. The main challenge is that these subsystems differ greatly both in their nature and their level of description. From a knowledge representation perspective, classical physiological models appearing in the literature in medical textbooks [23] differ widely in their use of concepts, states, and the nature of the causal links that relate them.

Our strategy for the development of a virtual patient consists in using a central physiological model around which to experiment with the integration of more subsystems (Fig. 16). This central model, originally developed for the simulation of shock states, describes circulatory physiology, with an emphasis on left ventricular physiology and short-term regulation of arterial pressure. Model integration takes place at the level of key variables in the central model, such as blood volume, inotropism, SVR, etc.

In order to devise a principled integration method, we have classified the subsystems to be integrated into the following categories:

Connected pathophysiological models. These represent global evolution of the cardiovascular system in certain pathologies in addition to the simulation produced by the qualitative model. One example is the peripheral model of shock states. This model is essentially a pathophysiological model whose nodes correspond to states and links between states represent a causal as well as temporal relation. The rationale for using a model here directly representing

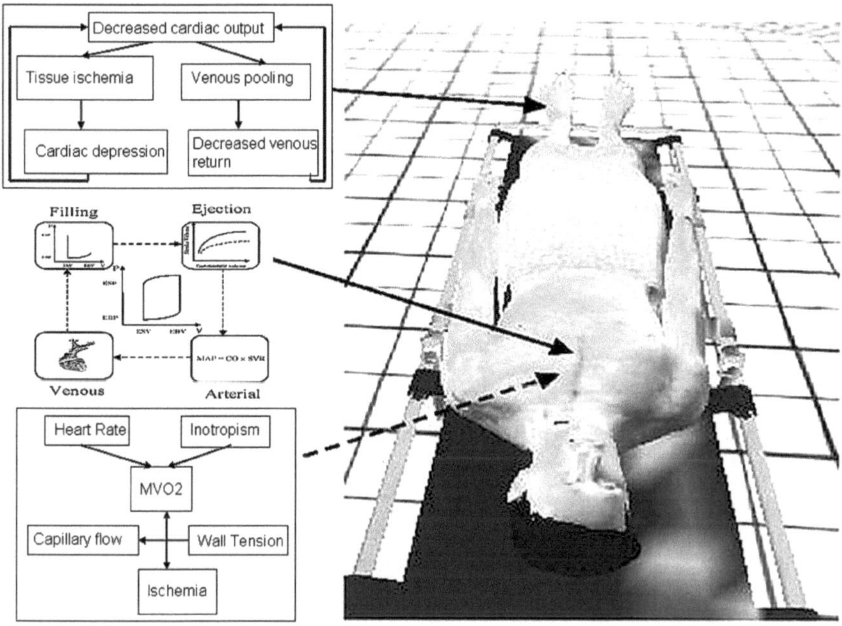

Fig. 16. Integration of different subsystems into the virtual patient model

pathological states, rather than deriving these from first principles, is that it enables work to be at a higher level of description (without having to model microcirculation and tissues metabolism).

External pathophysiological models. These describe the evolution of a disease in an organ system which is not part of the circulatory system but can affect it under pathological circumstances. One example consists in modeling events associated with acute pancreatitis, and its associated shock state (which is interfaced at the level of blood volume and inotropism).

Connected subsystems. This is for instance the case of the coronary circulation, which can be modeled through a causal network involving concepts such as oxygen consumption, cardiac wall tension, etc. It can be interfaced to the cardiac system at the level of inotropism, HR, etc. Other examples include Starling's law of filtration (determining the occurrence of edemas, etc.).

Additional organ systems. These represent all remaining physiological systems in their interconnection with the circulatory system. Examples are the respiratory system (very simply introduced at this stage) and the renal system in its long-term control of arterial pressure (this mainly related to an after treatment of the shock states). They can be interconnected at various levels with both the core models and the other subsystems as described above. Escaffre [29] used de Kleer's [30] confluence theory to implement a qualitative simulation of the *long-term* regulation of blood pressure, hence more centered on the renal system.

Figure 16, gives an in-depth view of the above integration scheme. The top influences block shows the effects, mainly observed at the extremities of the Virtual Patient. The decreased CO has influences on both ways, which through feedback loops are returning the effect in decreasing the CO more. The first way involved goes through tissue ischemia processes and further into cardiac depression, while the other way engages venous pooling which results in a decreased venous return. These two factors influence the decrease of the CO in a regressive process until the shock state is reached. This manifests itself on cold and discolored (not normal lively pink color) extremities, like feet and/or hands.

The second block on the left in Fig. 16. shows the pump function of the heart which we have discussed earlier. Then there is the lowest block in the left side of the figure, which is related to the heart functions as well (thought invisible to the trainee). HR and inotropism have influences over oxygen consumption (MVO2). The connection that exists between the oxygen consumption and Ischemia is inter-related. To this relation is added also the one-way influence of the wall tension (the building wall of the capillars) to the capillary flow. These additional relations in the existing model definitely bring the accuracy of the simulation in a higher level.

These additional models are seamlessly integrated around the cardiovascular model without the need to change the graphical interface. Of course, in order for the trainee to be aware of these other subsystems, additional parameters in the input/output menu are introduced (for some of them it is not necessary, that we define them as interactive parameters, i.e., the trainee cannot change or affect their values, while they can be visible, if appropriate). This definitely completes the scene of a realistic application and furthermore, brings an interesting interface for educational purposes.

8 Conclusions and Discussions

We have described the development of a virtual patient for clinical medicine, which could constitute an ideal interface for many knowledge-based systems in medicine. The need to generate clinical situations from first principles, which justify the development of physiological models, also provides more realistic physiological models that naturally interface with the appearance and behavior of virtual humans. In this context, the development of a virtual patient can be seen as an integration of a visual model and a physiological model, which is also a realistic model of the "internal behavior" of the patient.

As a result in this simulator (Fig. 17), a higher level of integration can be achieved with this approach than in systems in which the virtual human is mainly an interface to traditional knowledge-based systems. Future development includes expanding this system for other stages of cardiac disease treatment (or physiological systems involved) and a better integration of the

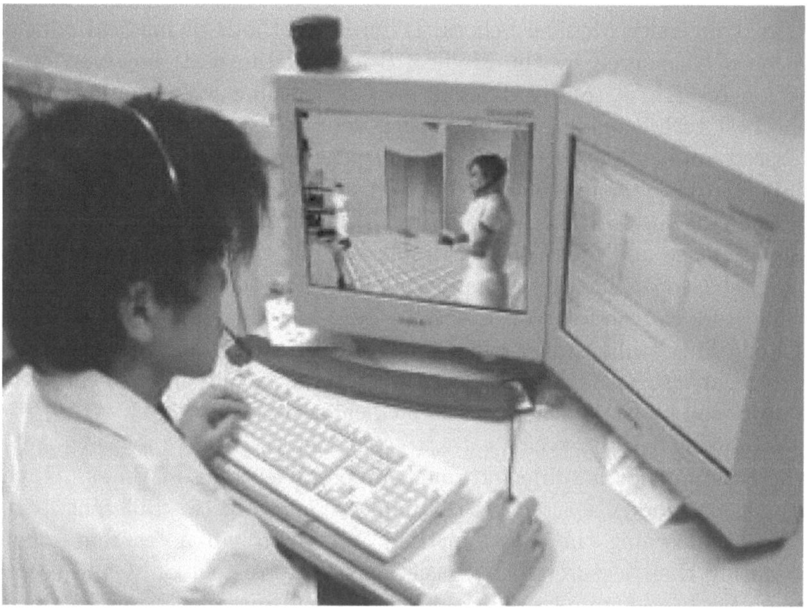

Fig. 17. Actual use of the simulator from medical students

networking possibilities that are offered on this framework in order for this to become a fully collaborative environment.

Our development strategy consists in integrating more physiological subsystems around a core model of the cardiovascular system, which has been implemented and evaluated for the correctness of its simulation results (comparing these with standard literature descriptions of the main shock syndromes). However, the difficulties in adding more subsystems vary greatly according to their nature. Local subsystems (e.g., coronary circulation) are easily integrated into the central model, while complex systems working on a different timescale (e.g., long-term regulation of arterial pressure through the renal system) require modifications to the simulation process, enabling it to integrate various timescales. Our long-term goal is to be able to carry out simulations with multiple integrated and complex subsystems, e.g., circulatory, respiratory, and renal systems, on a more sophisticated scale.

When it was introduced to the medical students of Gifu University, the application drew a lot of attention, this related to the fact that very few students were familiar with the ER room (for various reasons). The lack of experience in this kind of environment promoted their interest in seeing how things take place inside the ER room.

We conducted a formal qualitative evaluation with students who already had knowledge of the cardiovascular system and knew the cardiac physiology involved. From the output of this questionnaire different conclusions were drawn and this served as very good feedback for the respective teachers at Gifu University Medical School. Different methods of medical education have been considered by the Medical School in the past; however, our application brought a totally different way of learning while employing some of the best technologies available, which definitely were superior. In using a VR-based application for educational purposes there are different challenges mainly related to the use of the VR systems. However we will not discuss these issues here as most of the participants in this trial were able to successfully pass this phase and focus on the simulation. Getting them naturalized to a 3D game-based application probably might be the scope of another research.

The student reaction to this system introduction was measured and documented. This evaluation was more qualitative rather than quantitative for the sole purpose of having first a rough estimation on the efficiency, which was approved by the teachers of the medical school.

We considered the recall rates (on certain essential knowledge related to the training) for a subject through different learning methods. The conventional method of learning is textbooks. There are two different learning methods concerning the latest method. First through notes that students take during their lectures, this consisting mainly of text only, and secondly through books, where a combination of text and pictures are used (this also included visiting the ER room, when it is not in use).

These two conventional methods were compared with the proposed VR training simulator in order to we compare the efficiency of knowledge absorbed on the medical students side.

In Fig. 18. the horizontal axis shows the experimental method applied, while the results are grouped in three groups, with the vertical axes being the recall rate (%).The groups "Assimilated using text," "Assimilated using text and figures," and "Assimilated through VR application" are displayed from left to right (differently labeled in the picture). Also there are three recall rates ordered from left to right as "Soon after," "3 days later," and "6 days later". For the participants the training tool was obviously more effective in the general recall tests. We have shown the result for one subject random in Fig. 18 and then an averaged result for all the participating subjects (some 8 students) in Fig. 19. It might happen that the results differ in a wide range; nevertheless they confirm our hypothesis in the efficiency of the proposed system.

We also thought to run the recall rate test for specific details during the emergency situations in a cardiac emergency. Since the application allows modifications in order to emphasize certain situational details, the performance of this method when compared with the recall rates of different detail of other methods can be evaluated as well.

On the other hand, we can also represent the forgetting rates for the introduced concepts of the specific context in the medical knowledge field. By this criterion, also it is concluded that the method was offering a harder-to-forget methodology and knowledge when compared to others. Therefore more effectiveness during studying was offered.

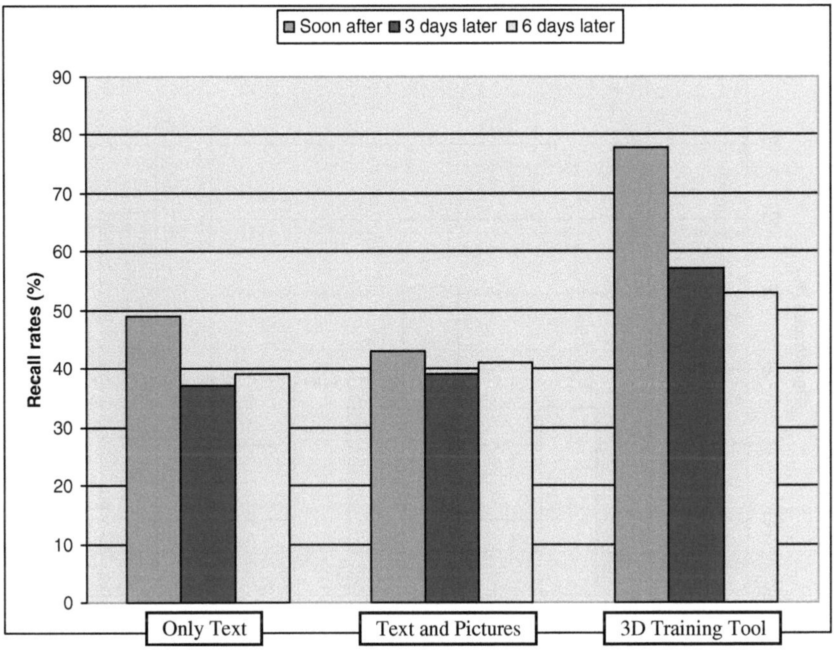

Fig. 18. The results for a random subject

As inferred from Fig. 19 a sophisticated methodology needs to be used in order that the long-term memory on the trained students is more solid. In the short-term it is obvious that the proposed training tool is very effective when compared to other methods.

Following these experimental outputs, it was clear that the proposed system can improve the recall rate of learning and recalling of concepts/procedures when compared to the conventional learning methods, not only on the day the subject was introduced to the knowledge but also in the longer term. Of course this process has room for improvement, not only in the learning strategies, but also in the details employed for this purpose.

It turned out that to have a successful experience for our system's users, different practical issues (related to educational ethics) should be considered and this served as good feedback on our side.

We demonstrated that the proposed approach supports the interactive, first-person training in the medical field (diagnostics and treatment) using VR techniques. The result of this research may have the potential for major developments for shaping the education of medical students. For example, it could be used as a commercial training tool for the graduating students of medical school. It could not only be used for the training simulation of medical students, residents, and health providers, but also it could serve as a start for simulation of advanced distributive learning, while being used as a test bed for further research and validation purposes.

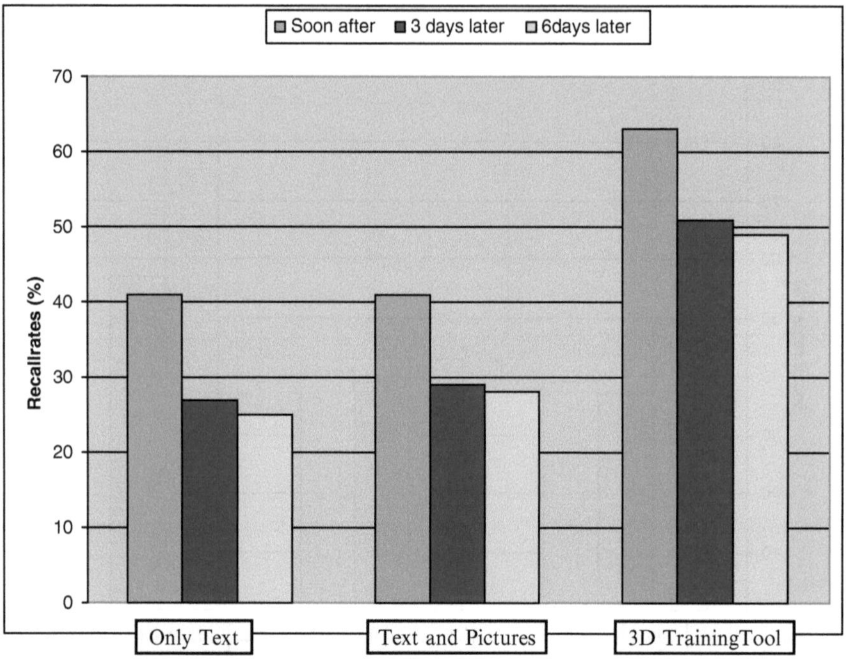

Fig. 19. The result for the average of all the subjects

Acknowledgments

We want to thank the personnel at the Gifu University Hospital (Emergency and First Surgery Section and Lecturers of the Medical School) for their advice on the representation of the ER room and the design of spoken commands. Also we want to thank the people at the Virtual Systems Laboratory near Gifu University, for facilitating the building of the 3D graphic environment.

References

1. Rickel, J., and Johnson, W.L., Animated Agents for Procedural Training in Virtual Reality: Perception, Cognition, and Motor Control. Applied Artificial Intelligence 13:343–382, 1999
2. Badler, N., Webber, B., Clarke, J., Chi, D., Hollick, M., Foster, N., Kokkevis, E., Ogunyemi, O., Metaxas, D., Kaye, J., and Bindiganavale, R. MediSim: Simulated Medical Corpsmen and Casualties for Medical Forces Planning and Training, *National Forum on Military Telemedicine*, IEEE, 1996, pp. 21–28
3. Sticklen, J., and Chandrasekaran, B., Integrating Classification-based Compiled Level Reasoning with Function-based Deep Level Reasoning, Applied artificial Intelligence 3(2–3):275–304, 1989

4. Chi, D., Kokkevis, E., Ogunyemi, O., Bindiganavale, R., Hollick, M., Clarke, J., Webber, B., and Badler, N. Simulated casualties and medics for emergency training, In K.S. Morgan, H.M. Hoffman, D. Stredney, and S.J. Weghorst (Eds.), Medicine Meets Virtual Reality. IOS, Amsterdam, 1997, pp. 486–494
5. Wolfgang Mueller-Wittig, Virtual Surgery, Tutorial 5, VSMM International Conference 25–27 September, 2002, Korea, http://www.vsmm.org/2002/program/tutorial5.htm
6. Halvorsrud, R., Hagen, S., Fagernes, S., Mjelstad, S., and Romundstad, L. Trauma Team Training in a Distributed Virtual Emergency Room. *Medicine Meets Virtual Reality 2003*, Newport Beach, CA, USA
7. Ponder, M., Herbelin, B., Molet, T., Schertenlieb, S., Ulicny, B., Papagiannakis, G., Magnenat-Thalmann, N., and Thalmann, D., Immersive VR Decision Training: Telling Interactive Stories Featuring Advanced Virtual Human Simulation Technologies, *Ninth Eurographics Workshop on Virtual Environments* (EGVE 2003)
8. Chi, D., Clarke, J., Webber, B., and Badler, N. Casualty Modeling for Real-Time Medical Training. Presence 5(4):359–366, 1996
9. Bindiganavale, R., Schuler, W., Allbeck, J., Badler, N., Joshi, A., and Palmer, M., Dynamically Altering Agent Behaviors Using Natural Language Instructions, in Proceedings of Autonomous Agents 2000, (Barcelona, Spain, June 2000), pp. 293–300
10. Swartout, W., Hill, R., Gratch, J., Johnson, W.L., Kyriakakis, C., LaBore, C., Lindheim, R., Marsella, S., Miraglia, D., Moore, B., Morie, J., Rickel, J., Thiebaux, M., Tuch, L., Whitney, R., and Douglas, J., 2001. Toward the Holodeck: Integrating Graphics, Sound, Character and Story, in Proceedings of the Autonomous Agents 2001 Conference, (Montreal, July 2001)
11. Lewis, M., and Jacobson, J., Communications of the ACM, 45, 1, January 2002. Special issue on Games Engines in Scientific Research
12. Weld, D.S., and de Kleer, J., Readings in Qualitative Reasoning about Physical Systems, Morgan Kaufmann, 1990
13. Baan, J. Arntzenius, A.C., and Yellin E.L. (Eds.) *Cardiac Dynamics*. Martinus Nijhoff, The Hague, 1980
14. Forbus, K.D. Qualitative Process Theory. Artificial Intelligence 24(1–3):85–168, 1984
15. Kuipers, B. Qualitative Simulation in Medical Physiology: A Progress Report. Technical Report, MIT/LCS/TM-280, 1985
16. Kuipers, B. Commonsense Reasoning about Causality: Deriving Behaviour from Structure. Artificial Intelligence, 24(1–3):168–204, 1984
17. Bratko, I. Mozetic, I., and Lavrac., N. KARDIO: a Study in Deep and Qualitative Knowledge for Expert Systems. MIT, Cambridge, MA, 1989
18. Bylander T., Smith J.W., and Svirbley J.R., Qualitative Representation of Behaviour in the Medical Domain. Computers and Biomedical Research 21: 367–380, 1988
19. Cavazza, M. Simulation Qualitative en Physiologie Cardiaque, in Proceedings of AFCET/RFIA'91 (Lyon, France, 1991), (in French)
20. Julen, N., Siregar, P., Sinteff, J.-P., and Le Beux, P., A Qualitative Model for Computer-Assisted Instruction in Cardiology, in Proceedings of AMIA 98, pp. 443–447

21. Widman, L.E. Expert System Reasoning About Dynamic Systems by Semi-Quantitative Simulation. Computer Methods and Programs in Biomedicine 29:95–113
22. Coiera, E.W. Monitoring Diseases with Empirical and Model Generated Histories. Artificial Intelligence in Medicine 2:135–147, 1990
23. Guyton, A.C., and Hall, J.E., *Textbook of Medical Physiology*, WB Saunders, 2000
24. Long W.J., Naimi, S., Criscitiello, M.G., Pauker, S.G., Kurzrok, S., and Szolovits, P. Reasoning about Therapy from a Physiological Model, in Proceedings of MEDINFO'86 (Washington DC)
25. Cavazza, M., and Simo, A.A Virtual Patient Based on Qualitative Simulation. ACM Intelligent User Interfaces 2002, Miami, USA
26. Honig, C.R. *Modern Cardiovascular Physiology.* Boston: Little Brown, 1988
27. Simo, A., and Cavazza, M. Visualising Pathophysiological Simulation with a Virtual Patient. *Seventh International Conference on Information Visualization* (IV 2003), London, IEEE Computer Press, pp. 549–554
28. Gratch, J., and Marsella, S., Tears and Fears: Modeling Emotions and Emotional Behaviors in Synthetic Agents, in Proceedings of the 5th International Conference on Autonomous Agents, (Montreal, Canada, June 2001)
29. Escaffre, D. Qualitative Reasoning on Physiological Systems: The Example of the Blood Pressure Regulation. In I. DeLotto and M. Stefanelli (Eds.), Artificial Intelligence in Medicine, Elsevier, New York
30. De Kleer, J."An Assumption-Based TMS," Artificial Intelligence 28(2):127–162, 1986

MIX
Papier aus verantwortungsvollen Quellen
Paper from responsible sources
FSC® C105338

If you have any concerns about our products,
you can contact us on
ProductSafety@springernature.com

In case Publisher is established outside the EU,
the EU authorized representative is:
Springer Nature Customer Service Center GmbH
Europaplatz 3, 69115 Heidelberg, Germany

Printed by Libri Plureos GmbH
in Hamburg, Germany